Injury & Trauma Sourcebook

Learning Disabilit...

Leukemia Sourceb...

Liver Disorders S...

Medical Tests Sou...

Men's Health Con...

Mental Health Dis...

Mental Retardation...

Movement Disorders Sourcebook, 2nd Edition

Multiple Sclerosis Sourcebook

Muscular Dystrophy Sourcebook

Obesity Sourcebook

Osteoporosis Sourcebook

Pain Sourcebook, 3rd Edition

Pediatric Cancer Sourcebook

Physical & Mental Issues in Aging Sourcebook

Podiatry Sourcebook, 2nd Edition

Pregnancy & Birth Sourcebook, 3rd Edition

Prostate & Urological Disorders Sourcebook

Prostate Cancer Sourcebook

Rehabilitation Sourcebook

Respiratory Disorders Sourcebook, 2nd Edition

Sexually Transmitted Diseases Sourcebook, 5th Edition

Sleep Disorders Sourcebook, 3rd Edition

Smoking Concerns Sourcebook

Sports Injuries Sourcebook, 4th Edition

Stress-Related Disorders Sourcebook, 3rd Edition

Stroke Sourcebook, 2nd Edition

Surgery Sourcebook, 2nd Edition

Thyroid Disorders Sourcebook

Transplantation Sourcebook

Traveler's Health Sourcebook

Urinary Tract & Kidney Diseases & Disorders Sourcebook, 2nd Edition

Vegetarian Sourcebook

Women's Health Concerns Sourcebook, 3rd Edition

Workplace Health & Safety Sourcebook

Worldwide Health Sourcebook

... Series

...mation for Teens

...mation for Teens

... Teens,

... Teens

Asthma Information for Teens, 2nd Edition

Body Information for Teens

Cancer Information for Teens, 2nd Edition

Complementary & Alternative Medicine Information for Teens

Diabetes Information for Teens, 2nd Edition

Diet Information for Teens, 3rd Edition

Drug Information for Teens, 3rd Edition

Eating Disorders Information for Teens, 2nd Edition

Fitness Information for Teens, 3rd Edition

Learning Disabilities Information for Teens

Mental Health Information for Teens, 3rd Edition

Pregnancy Information for Teens, 2nd Edition

Sexual Health Information for Teens, 3rd Edition

Skin Health Information for Teens, 2nd Edition

Sleep Information for Teens

Sports Injuries Information for Teens, 3rd Edition

Stress Information for Teens

Suicide Information for Teens, 2nd Edition

Tobacco Information for Teens, 2nd Edition

Domestic Violence
SOURCEBOOK

Fourth Edition

Health Reference Series

Fourth Edition

Domestic Violence

SOURCEBOOK

Basic Consumer Information about Intimate Partner Abuse, Stalking, Sexual Harassment, and Human Trafficking, Including Facts about Risk Factors, Warning Signs, and Forms of Physical, Sexual, Mental, Emotional, and Financial Abuse in Women, Men, Adolescents, Recent Immigrants, Elders, and Other Specific Populations

Along with Facts about Victims and Abusers, Strategies for Preventing and Intervening in Abusive Situations, Guidelines for Managing Emergencies and Making Safety Plans, Interventions through Workplaces and Faith Communities, Tips Regarding Legal Protections, a Glossary of Related Terms, and a Directory of Resources for Further Information

Edited by
Sandra J. Judd

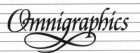

155 W. Congress, Suite 200, Detroit, MI 48226

Bibliographic Note
Because this page cannot legibly accommodate all the copyright notices, the Bibliographic
Note portion of the Preface constitutes an extension of the copyright notice.

Edited by Sandra J. Judd

Health Reference Series
Karen Bellenir, *Managing Editor*
David A. Cooke, MD, FACP, *Medical Consultant*
Elizabeth Collins, *Research and Permissions Coordinator*
Cherry Edwards, *Permissions Assistant*
EdIndex, Services for Publishers, *Indexers*

* * *

Omnigraphics, Inc.
Matthew P. Barbour, *Senior Vice President*
Kevin M. Hayes, *Operations Manager*

* * *

Peter E. Ruffner, *Publisher*
Copyright © 2013 Omnigraphics, Inc.
ISBN 978-0-7808-1261-1
E-ISBN 978-0-7808-1262-8

Library of Congress Cataloging-in-Publication Data

Domestic violence sourcebook : basic consumer information about intimate partner
abuse, stalking, sexual harassment, and human trafficking, including facts about risk
factors, warning signs, and forms of physical, sexual, mental, emotional, and financial
abuse in women, men, adolescents, recent immigrants, elders, and other specific
populations; along with facts about victims and abusers, strategies for preventing
and intervening in abusive situations, guidelines for managing emergencies and
making safety plans, interventions through workplaces and faith communities, tips
regarding legal protections, a glossary of related terms, and a directory of resources
for further information / edited by Sandra J. Judd. -- 4th ed.
    p. cm. -- (Health reference series)
  Includes bibliographical references and index.
  Summary: "Provides basic consumer health information about violence, stalking,
harassment, and other forms of abuse, and discusses the physical, mental, and social
effects of violence against intimate partners, children, teens, the elderly, immigrants,
and other populations; gives strategies for prevention and intervention. Includes
index, glossary of related terms and directory of resources"--Provided by publisher.
  ISBN 978-0-7808-1261-1 (hardcover : alk. paper) 1. Family violence--United States.
2. Victims of family violence--Services for--United States. 3. Sexual abuse victims--
Services for--United States. I. Judd, Sandra J.
  HV6626.2.D685 2012
  362.82'920973--dc23
                                                                    2012030143

Table of Contents

Visit www.healthreferenceseries.com to view *A Contents Guide to the Health Reference Series*, a listing of more than 16,000 topics and the volumes in which they are covered.

Part II: Intimate Partner Abuse

Part III: Abuse in Specific Populations

Part IV: Preventing and Intervening in Domestic Violence

Part V: Emergency Management, Moving Out, and Moving On

Part VI: Additional Help and Information

Preface

About This Book

The scope of domestic violence in our society is staggering. Its victims include men and women and people of every age, race, ethnicity, religion, sexual orientation, and economic level. According to the National Coalition Against Domestic Violence, an estimated 1.3 million women each year (and one in every four women during her lifetime) will experience domestic violence. One in twelve women and one in forty-five men have been stalked, and one in six women has experienced an attempted or completed rape. Many of those caught in the cycle of domestic violence feel isolated and powerless and do not know the avenues of help available to them.

Domestic Violence Sourcebook, Fourth Edition offers information to victims of domestic violence and to those who care about them. It defines domestic abuse, describes the risk factors for abuse, and offers tips for recognizing abuse. It describes the different types of abuse, including rape, physical violence, emotional and verbal abuse, stalking, and human trafficking. Information about abuse in specific populations—including the gay, lesbian, bisexual, and transgender communities, immigrant communities, teen and elder populations, and within the military—is also included. In addition, the book discusses tips for building healthy relationships and intervening in abusive situations, and it offers detailed guidelines for managing emergency situations, protecting oneself before, during, and after a separation from an abuser, navigating the legal system, and preventing workplace violence. The book concludes with a glossary of related terms and directories of resources for additional help and information.

How to Use This Book

This book is divided into parts and chapters. Parts focus on broad areas of interest. Chapters are devoted to single topics within a part.

Part I: Facts about Domestic Violence, Stalking, and Sexual Harassment provides basic information about what domestic violence is, which characteristics and situations place victims at risk, and how victims, abusers, and those wanting to help can identify abuse. It also explains what stalking and sexual harassment are and what victims can do to increase their safety and end the abuse.

Part II: Intimate Partner Abuse describes the different types of intimate partner abuse and their physical, emotional, and socioeconomic effects. It also describes the effect domestic violence has on children exposed to it and discusses the co-occurrence of child abuse and intimate partner abuse.

Part III: Abuse in Specific Populations provides information about child abuse, teen dating violence, abuse of men, elder abuse, and abuse in the lesbian, gay, bisexual, and transgender population. It also describes the special issues involved when the abuse occurs within the military, when the abuser is a police officer, or when the abuse occurs within the immigrant community. The part concludes with a discussion of human trafficking and the types of assistance available to its victims.

Part IV: Preventing and Intervening in Domestic Violence explains how to recognize and build healthy relationships. It also discusses how parents, caretakers, friends, co-workers, healthcare providers, and others can intervene in cases of abuse, and it describes measures employers can take to prevent violence in the workplace.

Part V: Emergency Management, Moving Out, and Moving On discusses why victims stay with their abusers and details what victims will need to know if they decide to leave. It explains the steps involved in calling the police, preserving and collecting evidence, and documenting abuse. It describes the sources of help available to victims of domestic abuse and offers suggestions for safety planning, safeguarding children, and protecting pets. It also provides detailed information about internet safety and identity protection and describes how to navigate the legal system.

Part VI: Additional Help and Information includes a glossary of terms related to domestic violence and directories of resources offering additional help and support, including domestic violence hotlines, child abuse reporting numbers, and programs offering shelter for pets of domestic violence victims.

Bibliographic Note

This volume contains documents and excerpts from publications issued by the following U.S. and other government agencies: Agency for Healthcare Research and Quality; Centers for Disease Control and Prevention (CDC); Federal Bureau of Investigation (FBI); National Center for Posttraumatic Stress Disorder; National Health Information Center; Office on Women's Health; Social Security Administration; U.S. Computer Emergency Readiness Team; U.S. Department of Health and Human Services; U.S. Department of Homeland Security; U.S. Department of Justice; and the Veterans Administration.

In addition, this volume contains copyrighted documents from the following organizations and individuals: A.D.A.M., Inc.; Advocates for Human Rights; Alabama Coalition Against Domestic Violence; American Bar Association; American Humane Association; American Society for the Prevention of Cruelty to Animals; Animal Legal and Historical Center; Aurora Center for Advocacy and Education; A Call to Men; Centre for Research and Education on Violence against Women and Children; Child Witness to Violence Project; Children's Hospital of Pittsburgh; Colorado Bar Association Family Violence Program; Corporate Alliance to End Partner Violence; Cyberbullying Research Center; Gary Direnfeld; Domestic Abuse Helpline for Men and Women; Domestic Abuse Intervention Programs; Endocrine Today; Evelyn Jacobs Ortner Center on Family Violence; FaithTrust Institute; Futures without Violence; HealthDay/Scout News LLC; Helpguide; Houston Area Women's Center; Humane Society of the United States; Indiana Coalition Against Sexual Assault; Johns Hopkins Center for Gun Policy and Research; Kansas State University Counseling Services; T. K. Logan; LoveisRespect.org; Mecklenburg County (NC) Women's Commission; Men Can Stop Rape; Michigan State University Safe Place; National Coalition Against Domestic Violence; National Coalition for the Homeless; National Committee for the Prevention of Elder Abuse; National Crime Prevention Council; National Network to End Domestic Violence—WomensLaw. org; Nemours Foundation; New York State Office for the Prevention of Domestic Violence; Ohio State University Research Communications;

Prairie View A & M University Department of Public Safety; PsychCentral; Rape, Abuse & Incest National Network; Safe Havens Interfaith Partnership Against Domestic Violence; A Safe Passage; San Diego County District Attorney; Santa Clara County Office of Women's Policy; Start Strong; United Nations Development Fund for Women; University of Michigan Health System; University of Nevada Cooperative Extension; Utah State University Affirmative Action/Equal Opportunity; Vermont Office of the Attorney General; Washington State Coalition Against Domestic Violence; West Virginia Foundation for Rape Information and Services; Diane Wetendorf; Wisconsin Office of Justice Assistance; Women's Aid Federation of England; Women's Justice Center; and Workplaces Respond to Domestic and Sexual Violence.

Full citation information is provided on the first page of each chapter or section. Every effort has been made to secure all necessary rights to reprint the copyrighted material. If any omissions have been made, please contact Omnigraphics to make corrections for future editions.

Acknowledgements

Thanks go to the many organizations, agencies, and individuals who have contributed materials for this *Sourcebook* and to medical consultant Dr. David Cooke and prepress services provider WhimsyInk. Special thanks go to managing editor Karen Bellenir and permissions coordinator Liz Collins for their help and support.

About the Health Reference Series

The *Health Reference Series* is designed to provide basic medical information for patients, families, caregivers, and the general public. Each volume takes a particular topic and provides comprehensive coverage. This is especially important for people who may be dealing with a newly diagnosed disease or a chronic disorder in themselves or in a family member. People looking for preventive guidance, information about disease warning signs, medical statistics, and risk factors for health problems will also find answers to their questions in the *Health Reference Series*. The *Series*, however, is not intended to serve as a tool for diagnosing illness, in prescribing treatments, or as a substitute for the physician/patient relationship. All people concerned about medical symptoms or the possibility of disease are encouraged to seek professional care from an appropriate healthcare provider.

A Note about Spelling and Style

Health Reference Series editors use *Stedman's Medical Dictionary* as an authority for questions related to the spelling of medical terms and the *Chicago Manual of Style* for questions related to grammatical structures, punctuation, and other editorial concerns. Consistent adherence is not always possible, however, because the individual volumes within the *Series* include many documents from a wide variety of different producers and copyright holders, and the editor's primary goal is to present material from each source as accurately as is possible following the terms specified by each document's producer. This sometimes means that information in different chapters or sections may follow other guidelines and alternate spelling authorities. For example, occasionally a copyright holder may require that eponymous terms be shown in possessive forms (Crohn's disease *vs.* Crohn disease) or that British spelling norms be retained (leukaemia *vs.* leukemia).

Locating Information within the Health Reference Series

The *Health Reference Series* contains a wealth of information about a wide variety of medical topics. Ensuring easy access to all the fact sheets, research reports, in-depth discussions, and other material contained within the individual books of the series remains one of our highest priorities. As the *Series* continues to grow in size and scope, however, locating the precise information needed by a reader may become more challenging.

A Contents Guide to the Health Reference Series was developed to direct readers to the specific volumes that address their concerns. It presents an extensive list of diseases, treatments, and other topics of general interest compiled from the Tables of Contents and major index headings. To access *A Contents Guide to the Health Reference Series*, visit www.healthreferenceseries.com.

Medical Consultant

Medical consultation services are provided to the *Health Reference Series* editors by David A. Cooke, MD, FACP. Dr. Cooke is a graduate of Brandeis University, and he received his M.D. degree from the University of Michigan. He completed residency training at the University of Wisconsin Hospital and Clinics. He is board-certified in Internal Medicine. Dr. Cooke currently works as part of the University of Michigan Health System and practices in Ann Arbor, MI. In his free time, he enjoys writing, science fiction, and spending time with his family.

Our Advisory Board

We would like to thank the following board members for providing guidance to the development of this series:

Health Reference Series Update Policy

The inaugural book in the *Health Reference Series* was the first edition of *Cancer Sourcebook* published in 1989. Since then, the *Series* has been enthusiastically received by librarians and in the medical community. In order to maintain the standard of providing high-quality health information for the layperson the editorial staff at Omnigraphics felt it was necessary to implement a policy of updating volumes when warranted.

Medical researchers have been making tremendous strides, and it is the purpose of the *Health Reference Series* to stay current with the most recent advances. Each decision to update a volume is made on an individual basis. Some of the considerations include how much new information is available and the feedback we receive from people who use the books. If there is a topic you would like to see added to the update list, or an area of medical concern you feel has not been adequately addressed, please write to:

Editor
Health Reference Series
Omnigraphics, Inc.
155 W. Congress, Suite 200
Detroit, MI 48226
E-mail: editorial@omnigraphics.com

Part One

Facts about Domestic Violence, Stalking, and Sexual Harassment

Chapter 1

What Is Domestic Violence?

Chapter Contents

Section 1.1

Domestic Violence: Basic Facts

Excerpted from "Understanding Intimate Partner Violence,"
Centers for Disease Control and Prevention, 2011.

Intimate partner violence (IPV) occurs between two people in a close relationship. The term "intimate partner" includes current and former spouses and dating partners. IPV exists along a continuum from a single episode of violence to ongoing battering.

IPV includes four types of behavior:

- Physical violence is when a person hurts or tries to hurt a partner by hitting, kicking, or other type of physical force.

- Sexual violence is forcing a partner to take part in a sex act when the partner does not consent.

- Threats of physical or sexual violence include the use of words, gestures, weapons, or other means to communicate the intent to cause harm.

- Emotional abuse is threatening a partner or his or her possessions or loved ones, or harming a partner's sense of self-worth. Examples are stalking, name-calling, intimidation, or not letting a partner see friends and family.

Often, IPV starts with emotional abuse. This behavior can progress to physical or sexual assault. Several types of IPV may occur together.

Why is IPV a public health problem?

IPV is a serious problem in the United States:

- Nearly three in ten women and one in ten men in the United States have experienced rape, physical violence, and/or stalking by a partner with IPV-related impact.[1]

- IPV resulted in 2,340 deaths in 2007. Of these deaths, 70 percent were females and 30 percent were males.[2]

4

- The medical care, mental health services, and lost productivity (e.g., time away from work) cost of IPV was an estimated $5.8 billion in 1995. Updated to 2003 dollars, that's more than $8.3 billion.[3,4]

These numbers underestimate the problem. Many victims do not report IPV to police, friends, or family.[1] Victims may think others will not believe them or that the police cannot help.[1]

How does IPV affect health?

IPV can affect health in many ways. The longer the violence goes on, the more serious the effects.

Many victims suffer physical injuries. Some are minor, like cuts, scratches, bruises, and welts. Others are more serious and can cause death or disabilities. These include broken bones, internal bleeding, and head trauma.

Not all injuries are physical. IPV can also cause emotional harm. Victims may have trauma symptoms. This includes flashbacks, panic attacks, and trouble sleeping. Victims often have low self-esteem. They may have a hard time trusting others and being in relationships. The anger and stress that victims feel may lead to eating disorders and depression. Some victims even think about or commit suicide.

IPV is linked to harmful health behaviors as well. Victims may try to cope with their trauma in unhealthy ways. This includes smoking, drinking, taking drugs, or having risky sex.

Who is at risk for IPV?

Several factors can increase the risk that someone will hurt his or her partner. However, having these risk factors does not always mean that IPV will occur.

Risk factors for perpetration (hurting a partner) include:

- Being violent or aggressive in the past

- Seeing or being a victim of violence as a child

- Using drugs or alcohol, especially drinking heavily

- Not having a job, or other life events that cause stress

How can we prevent IPV?

The goal is to stop IPV before it begins. There is a lot to learn about how to prevent IPV. We do know that strategies that promote healthy behaviors in relationships are important. Programs that teach young people skills for dating can prevent violence. These programs can stop violence in dating relationships before it occurs.

We know less about how to prevent IPV in adults. However, some programs that teach healthy relationship skills seem to help stop violence before it ever starts.

References

1. Black MC, Basile KC, Breiding MJ, Smith SG, Walters ML, Merrick MT, Chen J, Stevens MR. The National Intimate Partner and Sexual Violence Survey (NISVS): 2010 Summary Report. Atlanta, GA: National Center for Injury Prevention and Control, Centers for Disease Control and Prevention; 2011.

2. Department of Justice, Bureau of Justice Statistics. Intimate partner violence. [cited 2011 Jan 07]. Available from URL: http://bjs.ojp.usdoj.gov/index.cfm?ty=tp&tid=971#summary.

3. Centers for Disease Control and Prevention (CDC). Costs of intimate partner violence against women in the United States. Atlanta (GA): CDC, National Center for Injury Prevention and Control; 2003. [cited 2006 May 22]. Available from: URL: www.cdc.gov/ncipc/pub-res/ipv_cost/ipv.htm.

4. Max W, Rice DP, Finkelstein E, Bardwell RA, Leadbetter S. The economic toll of intimate partner violence against women in the United States. *Violence and Victims* 2004; 19(3):259–72.

Section 1.2

Myths and Truths about Domestic Violence

"Myths and Truths," reprinted with permission from Mecklenburg County Community Support Services Women's Commission, © 2012. For additional information, visit http://CSS.CharMeck.org and click on Women's Commission.

Myth 1: Battering is rare. Battering is extremely common. One-third to one-half of all women in the United States will be assaulted by their intimate partner at some time in their life.

Myth 2: Domestic violence occurs only in low income, poorly educated families. This behavior crosses all socioeconomic, racial, and religious lines. Doctors, ministers, psychologists, police officers, judges, and other professionals have battered their wives.

Myth 3: Women are just as violent as men. There are rare cases where a woman batters a man, and battering occurs in homosexual relationships also, but in the greatest majority (around 95 percent) of cases it is a man battering a woman.

Myth 4: All members of the family must change for the violence to stop. Only the perpetrator has the ability to stop the violence. Battering is a behavioral choice. Many women who are battered make numerous attempts to change their behavior in the hope that this will end the abuse. This does not work.

Myth 5: Domestic violence is usually a one-time event, an isolated incident. Battering is a pattern. Once violence begins in a relationship it almost always escalates both in frequency and severity.

Myth 6: Battered women choose to stay in the violent relationship. Many battered women leave their abusers permanently, and despite many obstacles, succeed in building a life free of violence. Almost all battered women leave at least once. The perpetrator dramatically escalates his violence and coercive tactics when she leaves (or tries to):

- Fifty to 75 percent of all homeless women and children are fleeing domestic violence.

- A woman is at a 75 percent greater risk of being killed or injured when attempting to leave.

- Every month, more than fifty thousand women in the United States seek a restraining/protective order.

- There are three times more animal shelters than safe houses for victims in this country.

Myth 7: Men who batter are often good fathers and should have joint custody. Of the men who batter their female partner, 70 percent sexually or physically abuse their children. More than three million children every year witness domestic violence, and this causes as much psychological damage as though they were assaulted themselves.

Section 1.3

The Cycle of Abuse

"The Common Pattern of Domestic Violence," by Toby D. Goldsmith, M.D., and Maria Vera, Ph.D. © 2010 Psych Central (www.psychcentral .com). All rights reserved. Reprinted with permission.

In 1979, psychologist Lenore Walker found that many violent relationships follow a common pattern or cycle. The entire cycle may happen in one day or it may take weeks or months. It is different for every relationship and not all relationships follow the cycle—many report a constant stage of siege with little relief.

This cycle has three parts:

- **Tension-building phase:** Tension builds over common domestic issues like money, children, or jobs. Verbal abuse begins. The victim tries to control the situation by pleasing the abuser, giving in or avoiding the abuse. None of these will stop the violence. Eventually, the tension reaches a boiling point and physical abuse begins.

- **Acute battering episode:** When the tension peaks, the physical violence begins. It is usually triggered by the presence of an external event or by the abuser's emotional state—but not by the victim's behavior. This means the start of the battering episode is unpredictable and beyond the victim's control. However, some experts believe that in some cases victims may unconsciously provoke the abuse so they can release the tension and move on to the honeymoon phase.

- **The honeymoon phase:** First, the abuser is ashamed of his behavior. He expresses remorse, tries to minimize the abuse, and might even blame it on the partner. He may then exhibit loving, kind behavior followed by apologies, generosity, and helpfulness. He will genuinely attempt to convince the partner that the abuse will not happen again. This loving and contrite behavior strengthens the bond between the partners and will probably convince the victim, once again, that leaving the relationship is not necessary.

This cycle continues over and over, and may help explain why victims stay in abusive relationships. The abuse may be terrible, but the promises and generosity of the honeymoon phase give the victim the false belief that everything will be all right.

Section 1.4

Progression of Abuse

"Dating and Domestic Violence," reprinted with
permission from the Prairie View A & M University website,
http://www.pavmu.edu, © 2012. All rights reserved.

Dating or domestic violence is not a disagreement; it represents a violation of trust. Violence against women is the leading cause of injury to women between the ages of fifteen and forty-four. It encompasses a wide range of acts committed by one partner against another in a relationship. These acts can include breaking objects, hurting pets, yelling, driving to endanger, isolating family members from others, and controlling resources like money, vehicles, credit, and time. This can occur in a variety of relationships: co-habitual, dating, married, separated, divorced, heterosexual, or gay/lesbian. Control is the goal of domestic violence—the abuser develops a cycle of violence, which grows in severity and frequency. It is a learned pattern of behavior whose effects, without intervention, become more destructive over time and can become lethal. The progression of violence is:

- **Pre-battering violence:** Verbal abuse, hitting objects, throwing objects, and making threats.

- **Beginning levels:** Slapping, pinching, kicking, pulling of hair.

- **Severe levels:** Choking, beating with objects (sticks, ball bats, etc.), use of weapons, and sexual assault.

One in three women in battering relationships are sexually assaulted. While drinking and drug use do not cause battering, these elements can create a violent situation. When chemical dependency is involved, both the injuries and lethality of abuse may increase.

Chapter 2

Prevalence of Domestic Abuse

Trends in Family Violence

The rate of family violence fell between 1993 and 2002 from an estimated 5.4 victims to 2.1 victims per 1,000 U.S. residents age twelve or older. Throughout the period family violence accounted for about one in ten violent victimizations.

Reported and Unreported Family Violence

Family violence accounted for 11 percent of all reported and unreported violence between 1998 and 2002. Of these roughly 3.5 million violent crimes committed against family members, 49 percent were crimes against spouses, 11 percent were sons or daughters victimized by a parent, and 41 percent were crimes against other family members.

The most frequent type of family violence offense was simple assault. Murder was less than half of 1 percent of all family violence between 1998 and 2002.

About three-fourths of all family violence occurred in or near the victim's residence.

Forty percent of family violence victims were injured during the incident. Of the 3.5 million victims of family violence between 1998 and 2002, less than 1 percent died as a result of the incident.

Excerpted from "Family Violence Statistics," U.S. Department of Justice, June 2005 (these are the most recent statistics available at this time).

The majority (73 percent) of family violence victims were female. Females were 84 percent of spouse abuse victims and 86 percent of victims of abuse at the hands of a boyfriend or girlfriend.

While about three-fourths of the victims of family violence were female, about three-fourths of the persons who committed family violence were male.

Most family violence victims were white (74 percent), and the majority were between ages twenty-five and fifty-four (65.7 percent). Most family violence offenders were white (79 percent), and most were age thirty or older (62 percent).

Fatal Family Violence

About 22 percent of murders in 2002 were family murders. Nearly 9 percent were murders of a spouse, 6 percent were murders of sons or daughters by a parent, and 7 percent were murders by other family members.

Females were 58 percent of family murder victims. Of all the murders of females in 2002, family members were responsible for 43 percent.

Children under age thirteen were 23 percent of murder victims killed by a family member, and just over 3 percent of nonfamily murder victims.

The average age among sons or daughters killed by a parent was seven years, and four out of five victims killed by a parent were under age thirteen.

Eight in ten murderers who killed a family member were male. Males were 83 percent of spouse murderers and 75 percent of murderers who killed a boyfriend or girlfriend.

In 2002 family murders were less likely than nonfamily murders to involve a firearm (50 percent versus 68 percent). Parents were the least likely family murderers to use a firearm (28 percent), compared to spouses (63 percent) or other family members (51 percent).

Among incidents of parents killing their children, 19 percent involved one parent killing multiple victims.

Family Violence Reported to Police

Approximately 60 percent of family violence victimizations were reported to police between 1998 and 2002. The reporting rate among female victims was not significantly greater than the reporting rate among male victims.

The most common reason victims of family violence cited for not reporting the crime to police was that the incident was a "private/personal matter" (34 percent). Another 12 percent of nonreporting family violence victims did not report the crime in order to "protect the offender."

Among the 2.1 million incidents of family violence reported to police between 1998 and 2002, 36 percent resulted in an arrest.

Family Violence Recorded by Police

Family violence accounted for 33 percent of all violent crimes recorded by police in eighteen states and the District of Columbia in 2000. Of these more than 207,000 family violence crimes, about half (53 percent, or 110,000) were crimes between spouses.

Among crimes recorded by police, 2 percent of family violence involved a firearm, compared to 6 percent of nonfamily violence. A weapon was used in 16 percent of family and 21 percent of nonfamily violence.

About 6 percent of all violent crime recorded by police in 2000 involved more than one offender victimizing a lone victim. The exception was stranger crime, in which 14 percent of incidents involved multiple offenders victimizing a lone victim.

About 49 percent of family violence crimes recorded by police resulted in an arrest. Males comprised 77 percent of suspected family violence offenders arrested in 2000.

State Prosecution of Family Assault

Of the approximately 1,500 defendants charged with felony assault during May 2000 in the state courts of eleven large counties, about a third were charged with family violence.

Among felony assault defendants charged with family violence in state courts, 84 percent had at least one prior arrest for either a felony or a misdemeanor (not necessarily for family violence), and 73 percent had been previously convicted of some type of felony or misdemeanor (not necessarily family violence).

Nearly half of felony assault defendants charged with family violence were released pending case disposition.

Among the 1,500 felony assault cases, the probability of the case leading to conviction (felony or misdemeanor) was greater for family assault defendants (71 percent) than nonfamily assault defendants (61 percent).

State courts sentenced 83 percent of persons convicted of assault (both family and nonfamily) to either prison or jail. Among felony assault defendants convicted in state courts, 68 percent of incarceration sentences for family assault were to jail, 62 percent of incarceration sentences for nonfamily assault were to prison, and 45 percent of persons sent to prison for family assault received a sentence of more than two years, compared to 77 percent of nonfamily assault offenders sent to prison.

Family Violence Offenders in Prison

Of the nearly five hundred thousand men and women in state prisons for a violent crime in 1997, 15 percent were there for a violent crime against a family member.

Nearly half of all the family violence offenders in state prisons were serving a sentence for a sex offense against a family member. More than three-quarters of parents convicted of a violent crime against their son or daughter were in prison for a sex offense.

Of the crimes for which family violence offenders were in prison:

- most were against a female (78 percent);

- more than half were against a child under age eighteen;

- more than a third were against a child under age thirteen.

About 90 percent of offenders in state prisons for family violence had injured their victim:

- Fifty percent of family violence victims were raped or sexually assaulted.

- Twenty-eight percent of the victims of family violence were killed.

- Fifty percent of offenders in state prisons for spousal abuse had killed their victims.

- Of state prison inmates imprisoned for a crime against their son or daughter, 79 percent had raped or sexually assaulted the child, and another 10 percent had killed the child.

Among family violence offenders in state prisons in 1997:

- most were male (93 percent);

- six out of ten were white, while about a quarter were black;

- about 80 percent were between ages twenty-five and fifty-four.

Among offenders whose incarceration in state prisons was for family violence, 23 percent had used a weapon to commit their crime. The comparable percentage among state prisoners incarcerated for nonfamily violence was higher—46 percent.

Chapter 3

Characteristics of Abusers and Victims

Chapter Contents

Section 3.1

Who Are the Abusers?

"Who Are the Abusers of Domestic Violence?" by Toby D. Goldsmith, M.D., and Maria Vera, Ph.D. © 2010 Psych Central (www.psychcentral. com). All rights reserved. Reprinted with permission.

Abusers don't wear signs that say, "I'm an abuser." They can be doctors, lawyers, judges, nurses, policemen, clergymen, mechanics, janitors, or the unemployed. They could be white, black, Asian, Hispanic, or Native American. They may have had five previous spouses, or may have never been married.

However, research shows that abusers are likely to have some common characteristics. In general, abusers:

- are less educated than the abused partner;

- come from a lower socioeconomic group than the abused partner;

- need great amounts of attention;

- are possessive, jealous, and controlling of their partner;

- fear being abandoned by the partner;

- are emotionally dependent on the partner;

- have low self-esteem;

- have rigid expectations of the relationship;

- have poor impulse control and low frustration tolerance;

- are prone to explosive rage;

- use children to exert power over partner;

- blame their partners for their own abusive behavior;

- lie to keep the victim psychologically off balance;

- manipulate the victim and others to get on their good side;

- have very traditional beliefs about the roles of men and women (if a man is abusing a woman).

Section 3.2

Who Are the Victims?

"Who Are the Victims of Domestic Violence?" by Toby D.
Goldsmith, M.D., © 2012 Psych Central (www.psychcentral.com).
All rights reserved. Reprinted with permission.

Domestic violence can happen in any relationship, regardless of ethnic group, income level, religion, education, or sexual orientation. Abuse may occur between married people, or between unmarried people living together or in a dating relationship. It happens in heterosexual, gay, and lesbian relationships.

However, researchers have found that some people are more likely to become the victims of domestic violence. A likely victim:

- has poor self-image;

- puts up with abusive behavior;

- is economically and emotionally dependent on the abuser;

- is uncertain of his or her own needs;

- has low self-esteem;

- has unrealistic belief that he or she can change the abuser;

- feels powerless to stop violence;

- believes that jealousy is proof of love.

While abuse can happen to anyone, women are by far the most frequent victims and men are the most frequent abusers. The U.S. Department of Justice estimates that 95 percent of the assaults on partners or spouses is committed by men against women.

Again, the victims often have some common characteristics. Women who are victims of domestic violence often:

- abuse alcohol or other substances;

- have been previously abused;

- are pregnant;

- are poor and have limited support;
- have partners who abuse alcohol or other substances;
- have left their abuser;
- have requested a restraining order against the abuser;
- are members of ethnic minority or immigrant groups;
- have traditional beliefs that women should be submissive to men;
- do not speak English.

Chapter 4

Risk Factors for Domestic Violence

Chapter Contents

Section 4.1

Why Do Abusers Abuse?

Domestic violence is a pattern of controlling and coercive conduct that serves to deprive victims of safety and autonomy. Perpetrators believe they are entitled to power and control over their partners and perceive all interactions within relationships through a prism of compliance or disobedience. Perpetrators use abusive tactics to reinforce their rules and maintain absolute control over their victims.

Perpetrators come from all races, religions, socioeconomic classes, areas of the world, educational levels, and occupations.

They often appear charming and attentive to outsiders, and even to their partners, at first. Many perpetrators are very good at disguising their abusive behavior to appear socially acceptable. Once they develop a relationship with a partner, however, they become more and more abusive.

Characteristics

Domestic violence perpetrators:

- seek control of the thoughts, beliefs, and conduct of their partner;
- restrict all of the victim's rights and freedoms;
- punish their partner for breaking their rules or challenging the perpetrator's authority.

Men who batter:

- minimize the seriousness of their violence;
- believe they are entitled to control their partner;
- use anger, alcohol/drug use, and stress as excuses for their abusive behaviors;
- blame the victim for the violence.

A batterer covers up his violence by denying, minimizing, and blaming the victim. He often convinces his partner that the abuse is less serious than it is, or that it is her fault. He may tell her that "if only" she had acted differently, he wouldn't have abused her. Sometimes he will say, "You made me do it."

Victims of abuse do not cause violence. The batterer is responsible for every act of abuse committed.

Domestic violence is a learned behavior. It is learned through:

- observation;

- experience;

- culture;

- family;

- community (peer group, school, etc.).

Abuse is not caused by:

- mental illness: personality disorders, mental illness, and other problems may compound domestic violence, but the abusive behavior must be addressed separately.

- genetics.

- alcohol and drugs: many men blame their violence on the effects of drug and alcohol use. Alcohol abuse is present in about 50 percent of battering relationships. Research shows that alcohol and other drug abuse is commonly a symptom of an abusive personality, not the cause. Men often blame their intoxication for the abuse, or use it as an excuse to use violence. Regardless, it is an excuse, not a cause. Taking away the alcohol does not stop the abuse. Substance abuse must be treated before or in conjunction with domestic violence treatment programs.

- out-of-control behavior.

- anger.

- stress.

- behavior of the victim.

- problems in the relationship.

A batterer abuses because he wants to, and thinks he has a "right" to his behavior. He may think he is superior to his partner and is entitled to use whatever means necessary to control her.

Some ways batterers deny and minimize their violence:

- "I hit the wall, not her head."
- "She bruises easily."
- "She just fell down the steps."
- "Her face got in the way of my fist."

Characteristics of a potential batterer:

- Jealousy
- Controlling behavior
- Quick involvement
- Unrealistic expectations
- Isolation of victim
- Blames others for his problems
- Blames others for his feelings
- Hypersensitivity
- Cruelty to animals or children
- "Playful" use of force during sex
- Verbal abuse
- Rigid sex roles
- Jekyll and Hyde type personality
- History of past battering
- Threats of violence
- Breaking or striking objects
- Any force during an argument
- Objectification of women
- Tight control over finances
- Minimization of the violence
- Manipulation through guilt
- Extreme highs and lows
- Expects her to follow his orders

- Frightening rage
- Use of physical force
- Closed mindedness

Manipulation

Abusers often try to manipulate the "system" by:

- Threatening to call Child Protective Services or the Department of Human Resources and making actual reports that his partner neglects or abuses the children.
- Changing lawyers and delaying court hearings to increase his partner's financial hardship.
- Telling everyone (friends, family, police, etc.) that she is "crazy" and making things up.
- Using the threat of prosecution to get her to return to him.
- Telling police she hit him, too.
- Giving false information about the criminal justice system to confuse his partner or prevent her from acting on her own behalf.
- Using children as leverage to get and control his victim.

Abusers may try to manipulate their partners, especially after a violent episode. He may try to "win" her back in some of these ways:

- Invoking sympathy from her, her family and friends
- Talking about his "difficult childhood"
- Becoming overly charming, reminding her of the good times they've had
- Bringing romantic gifts, flowers, dinner
- Crying, begging for forgiveness
- Promising it will "never happen again"
- Promising to get counseling, to change

Abuse gets worse and more frequent over time.

Section 4.2

Individual, Relational, Community, and Societal Risk Factors

"Intimate Partner Violence: Risk and Protective Factors,"
Centers for Disease Control and Prevention, September 20, 2010.

Risk factors are associated with a greater likelihood of intimate partner violence (IPV) victimization or perpetration. They are contributing factors and may or may not be direct causes. Not everyone who is identified as "at risk" becomes involved in violence.

Some risk factors for IPV victimization and perpetration are the same. In addition, some risk factors for victimization and perpetration are associated with one another; for example, childhood physical or sexual victimization is a risk factor for future IPV perpetration and victimization.

A combination of individual, relational, community, and societal factors contribute to the risk of becoming a victim or perpetrator of IPV. Understanding these multilevel factors can help identify various opportunities for prevention.

Risk Factors for Intimate Partner Violence

Individual Risk Factors

- Low self-esteem

- Low income

- Low academic achievement

- Young age

- Aggressive or delinquent behavior as a youth

- Heavy alcohol and drug use

- Depression

- Anger and hostility

- Antisocial personality traits

24

- Borderline personality traits
- Prior history of being physically abusive
- Having few friends and being isolated from other people
- Unemployment
- Emotional dependence and insecurity
- Belief in strict gender roles (e.g., male dominance and aggression in relationships)
- Desire for power and control in relationships
- Perpetrating psychological aggression
- Being a victim of physical or psychological abuse (consistently one of the strongest predictors of perpetration)
- History of experiencing poor parenting as a child
- History of experiencing physical discipline as a child

Relationship Factors

- Marital conflict: Fights, tension, and other struggles
- Marital instability: divorces or separations
- Dominance and control of the relationship by one partner over the other
- Economic stress
- Unhealthy family relationships and interactions

Community Factors

- Poverty and associated factors (e.g., overcrowding)
- Low social capital: lack of institutions, relationships, and norms that shape a community's social interactions
- Weak community sanctions against IPV (e.g., unwillingness of neighbors to intervene in situations where they witness violence)

Societal Factors

- Traditional gender norms (e.g., women should stay at home, not enter workforce, and be submissive; men support the family and make the decisions)

Section 4.3

Power and Control Model

Introductory text excerpted from "FAQ about the Wheels" and graphic reprinted from "Power and Control Wheel," © 2012 Domestic Abuse Intervention Programs. All rights reserved. Reprinted with permission. For additional information, visit www.theduluthmodel.org.

Battering is one form of domestic or intimate partner violence. It is characterized by the pattern of actions that an individual uses

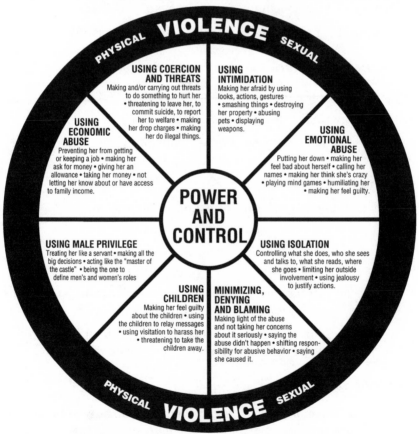

Figure 4.1. *Power and control wheel.*

to intentionally control or dominate his intimate partner. That is why the words "power and control" are in the center of the wheel. A batterer systematically uses threats, intimidation, and coercion to instill fear in his partner. These behaviors are the spokes of the wheel. Physical and sexual violence holds it all together—this violence is the rim of the wheel.

The Power and Control Wheel makes the pattern, intent, and impact of violence visible.

Section 4.4

Theories of Violence

A common understanding of the causes of domestic violence can help communities develop more effective responses to the violence; such an understanding helps avoid conflicting responses that could undermine efforts to protect victims and hold batterers accountable.

When the battered women's movement in the United States began in the early 1970s, the prevailing theory of why men batter was based on psychopathology. According to this theory, men who abused their wives were mentally ill and could be cured through medication or psychiatric treatment. Researchers found, however, that the behavior of perpetrators of domestic violence did not correspond to profiles of individuals who were mentally ill. Batterers attack only their intimate partners. People who suffer from mental illnesses such as schizophrenia do not limit their violence to their intimate partners.

Initial studies also characterized battered women as mentally ill. The results of these first studies, however, were distorted because the studies examined women who were in mental hospitals; their batterers, who were calm and credible in contrast to their wives, were asked about the cause of their partners' condition and thus given an opportunity to minimize and deny their partners' account of the abuse. In reality, however, battered women are not mentally ill, and many of those who were institutionalized were misdiagnosed because of a failure to recognize or understand the physical and psychological effects of domestic violence.[1]

Researchers next theorized that violence was learned. They argued that men battered because they had learned violence in their families as children, and women sought out abusive men because they saw their mothers being abused. This was the "learned behavior" theory of violence. Yet women who witness domestic violence are not any more likely to be battered as adults. (A recent study reported by the Family Violence Prevention Fund does indicate, however, that women who were physically or sexually abused as children may be more likely to be abused as adults.)

Although research does show that boys who witness abuse in the home are seven times more likely to batter, many men who witnessed violence as children vow not to use violence and do not grow up to be batterers. A more consistent explanation for the relationship between witnessing and battering is that witnessing is one of many sources of information; men also receive information from the larger society that it is appropriate to control your wife and to enforce this control through violence. Further, as emphasized in batterers' intervention programs, boys who witnessed domestic violence and grew up to be batterers learned more than just violence; rather, they learned—and thus can unlearn—lessons about the respective roles of men and women that contribute to their abusive behavior as adults.

Closely related to the "learned behavior" theory were the theories that described violence as the result of a loss of control. For example, many believed that men are abusive when they drink because the alcohol causes them to lose control. Others explained men's violence as a result of an inability to control their anger and frustration. These theorists argued that gendered societal expectations prevented men from expressing anger and frustration; these feelings would build up until the man lost control and released his feelings through the use of violence.

This "loss of control" theory is contradicted by batterers' behavior. Batterers' violence is carefully targeted to certain people at certain times and places. For example, batterers "choose not to hit their bosses or police officers, no matter how angry or 'out of control' they are."[2]

Abusers also follow their own "internal rules and regulations about abusive behaviors." They often choose to abuse their partners only in private, or may take steps to ensure that they do not leave visible evidence of the abuse. Batterers also chose their tactics carefully—some destroy property, some rely on threats of abuse, and some threaten children. Through these decisions, "perpetrators are making choices about what they will or will not do to the victim, even when they are claiming they 'lost it' or were 'out of control.' Such decision making indicates that they are actually in control of their abusive behaviors."[3] In fact, a recent study reported by the Family Violence Prevention Fund indicates that many batterers become more controlled and calm as their aggressiveness increases.

Another theory that was advanced was the "learned helplessness" theory. Lenore Walker, a psychologist in the United States, studied the behavior of women who stay in violent relationships. Walker hypothesized that women stay in abusive relationships because constant abuse strips them of the will to leave.

The learned helplessness theory, however, did not account for the fact that there are many social, economic, and cultural reasons a woman might chose to stay in an abusive relationship. Women often have very rational reasons for staying—they may fear retaliation against themselves or their children, or they may not be able to financially support themselves or their children. They may be ostracized by their family and community if they leave.

Further, the learned helplessness theory is inconsistent with the fact that women surviving in abusive relationships attempt to leave many times and routinely act in very conscious ways to try to minimize the abuse directed at them and to protect their children. As Dobash and Dobash explain, "[w]omen are usually persistent and often tenacious in their attempts to seek help, but pursue such help through channels that prove to be most useful and reject those that have been found to be unhelpful or condemning." Battered women do not live their lives in a state of "learned helplessness." On the contrary, they often engage in a process of "staying, leaving and returning." During this process,

> women make active and conscious decisions based on their changing circumstances: they leave for short periods in order to escape the violence and to emphasize their disaffection in the hope that this will stop the violence. In the beginning, they are generally not attempting to end the relationship, but are negotiating to reestablish the relationship on a non-violent basis.[4]

In addition, the learned helplessness theory was based on perceived characteristics ostensibly shared by battered women, such as low self-esteem, a tendency to withdraw, or perceptions of loss of control. Those who espoused the theory, however, rarely took into account the fact that these "characteristics" might be, in fact, the physical and psychological effects of the abuse.

Finally, the static model of "learned helplessness" is contradicted by the fact that the violence, and the woman's reaction to the violence, often changes over time. The first episode of violence is generally minor; victims may be surprised and shocked, and may not anticipate that it will occur again. Rather, as Dobash and Dobash explain, "they believe, as anyone might, in the potential for reform and are still committed to the relationship." Victims may begin to then

> look to their own actions for an explanation. This is not surprising in societies which allocate to wives the responsibility for happy husbands and families; women are expected to ask how their behavior "caused" their husband's violence. Women eventually realize that solutions to the man's violence do not reside in a change of their own behavior. For some this realization comes fairly quickly while others take longer to overcome such culturally constructed notions.[4]

The "learned helplessness" theory was accompanied by a resurgence of the psychopathology; theorists argued that women stayed in abusive relationships because they suffered from a personality disorder that caused them to seek out abusive relationships as a means of self-punishment, or were addicted to abusive relationships. Many also maintained that women were co-alcoholics with their spouses and thus could be "treated" through alcohol addiction programs. These theories were inconsistent with the fact that women had very rational reasons for staying in relationships. In addition, while battered women may be subject to an increased risk of substance abuse, this is a consequence, not a cause, of the abuse.

The "cycle of violence" was the next theory to gain popularity in the United States. This theory was based on the belief that men did not express their frustration and anger because they had been taught not to show their feelings. The man's tension built until he exploded and became violent. The tension was released, and the couple enjoyed a "honeymoon" period, during which the husband was apologetic and remorseful.

This theory, however, was not consistent with women's experiences. Many women never experienced a honeymoon period. Others stated that there was no gradual buildup of tension, but rather unpredictable, almost random, episodes of battering. This theory also did not explain why men directed their explosions of rage only against their intimate partners. Dobash and Dobash explain that

> the conception of a cycle of violence is static rather than dynamic and changing, does not deal with intentionality, and the notion

of the third phase as a "honeymoon" phase belies the experience of women who indicate that even the process of "making-up" or reconstructing the relationship is carried out against the background of a personal history of violence and coercion and in the context of few viable alternatives to the violent relationship.[4]

This theory was often paired with the "family/relationship conflict" model. According to this model, "both the man and the woman contribute to violence in an intimate relationship." This model assumes either that the relationship is characterized by mutual violence, or that "in many cases a wife provokes her husband by 'below-the-belt' arguments prompting a violence response from her husband." The woman's behavior contributes to the buildup of tension in the man, until the man explodes in a violent rage, followed by a honeymoon period.

Theories based on "mutual" violence do not take into account the different ways that men and women use violence in intimate relationships. Further, any theory that describes violence as a response to "provocation" from the other partner is simply another form of victim blaming. Nor does this model account for instances in which a husband explodes over trivial issues or starts beating his wife while she is asleep.[5]

What was missing from all of these theories was a recognition of batterers' intent to gain control over their partners' actions, thoughts, and feelings. The current understanding of abuse, represented by the "Power and Control Wheel," evolved out of many discussions with battered women and batterers through the Domestic Abuse Intervention Project (DAIP) in Duluth. The Power and Control Wheel describes the different tactics an abuser uses to maintain power and control over his partner.

In an abusive relationship, the batterer uses the pattern of tactics described in the Power and Control Wheel to reinforce his use of physical violence. Violent incidents are not isolated instances of a loss of control, or even cyclical expressions of anger and frustration. Rather, each instance is part of a larger pattern of behavior designed to exert and maintain power and control over the victim.

The Power and Control Wheel is based on the assumption that the purpose of the violence is to exert power and control over another. The elements that formed the basis of earlier theories—a boy witnessing abuse as a child, or substance abuse—may be contributing factors, but are not the "cause" of the violence. Rather, the batterer consciously uses these tactics to ensure the submissiveness of his partner. As Schecter and Ganley explain, perpetrators of domestic violence bring into their intimate relationships certain expectations of who is in charge and what the acceptable mechanisms are for enforcing that dominance. Those attitudes and beliefs, rather than the victim's behavior, determine whether or not perpetrators are domestically violent.[6]

The exercise of male violence, through which women's subordinate role and unequal power are enforced and maintained, is, in turn, tolerated and reinforced by political and cultural institutions and economic arrangements.

Over time, however, DAIP began to realize that even this theory—that batterers use violence to gain control and power—did not sufficiently capture the phenomenon of violence. While the Power and Control Wheel (i.e., coercive behaviors that establish power and control) did describe women's experiences, batterers in batterers' intervention programs did not articulate a desire for power and control when they talked about their use of these behaviors. Consequently, DAIP began to conceptualize violence within the larger context of society. Under this theory, violence is

a logical outcome of relationships of dominance and inequality—relationships shaped not simply by the personal choices or desires of some men to [dominate] their wives but by how we, as a society, construct social and economic relationships between men and women and within marriage (or intimate domestic relationships) and families. Our task is to understand how our response to violence creates a climate of intolerance or acceptance to the force used in intimate relationships.[7]

Adapted from Loretta Frederick's Presentation on Theories of Violence at the Domestic Violence Workshop, sponsored by the Bulgarian Centre for Human Rights, the Gender Project for Bulgaria Foundation, and The Advocates for Human Rights, in Plovdiv, Bulgaria, on June 2, 1997.

Notes

1. From Joan Zorza, Batterer Manipulation and Retaliation in the Courts: A Largely Unrecognized Phenomenon Sometimes Encouraged by Court Practices, Violence Against Women 47–48 (Joan Zorza ed., 2002).

2. From Ethel Klein et al., Ending Domestic Violence: Changing Public Perceptions/Halting the Epidemic 6 (1997).

3. From Anne L. Ganley and Susan Schechter, Domestic Violence: A National Curriculum for Family Preservation Practitioners 19 (1995).

4. From R. Emerson Dobash and Russel P. Dobash, Women, Violence and Social Change 222–23, 225, 229–32 (1992).

5. From Michael Paymar, Building a Coordinated Community Response to Domestic Violence: An Overview of the Problem 3–4 (1994).

6. From Schechter and Ganley, Domestic Violence: A National Curriculum for Family Preservation Practitioners 19 (1995).

7. From Ellen L. Pence, Some Thoughts on Philosophy, in Coordination Community Responses to Domestic Violence: Lessons from the Duluth Model 25, 29–30 (Melanie F. Shepard and Ellen L. Pence, eds., 1999).

Section 4.5

Economic Stress and Intimate Partner Violence

"Economic Distress and Intimate Partner Violence,"
U.S. Department of Justice, January 5, 2009.

Financial strain, unemployment, and living in economically disadvantaged neighborhoods can impact rates and severity of intimate partner violence.[1] The National Institute of Justice (NIJ) has funded a number of studies that have shown relationships between the following:

- Financial strain and intimate partner violence

- Employment and intimate partner violence

- Economically disadvantaged neighborhoods and intimate partner violence

Financial Strain and Intimate Partner Violence

Intimate partner violence is more likely to occur when couples are under financial strain.[2] Researchers in one study found a strong relationship between couples worried about financial strain (subjective feelings of financial strain[3]) and the likelihood of intimate partner violence. The violence for couples experiencing low levels of subjective financial strain was 2.7 percent, compared to 9.5 for couples experiencing high levels of subjective financial strain.

Repeat victimization of women is more frequent in couples feeling financial strain. Results of a study showed that women in relationships in which the couples experience low levels of financial strain report less than 2 percent of repeat victimizations or being injured by their male partners, while just over 5 percent of women in relationships in which the couples experience high levels of subjective strain report repeat victimizations or being injured by their male partners.

Financial strain may keep women in abusive relationships. A review of census and survey data revealed that women at greatest risk of intimate partner violence tend to be those in relationships where the couple has few economic resources, experience high subjective stress about finances, experience higher unemployment, and live in proximity to economically disadvantaged neighborhoods. The choice to stay or leave violent relationships may be based on the decision that a partner's economic contribution to the relationship outweighs the risk of violence. It also may compel women to live with men's violent behavior rather than seek help or take other steps to leave the violent relationship.

Employment and Intimate Partner Violence

Unstable employment increases the risk of intimate partner violence. The study showed that for couples where the male was always employed, the rate of intimate partner violence was 4.7 percent. When men experienced one period of unemployment the rate rose to 7.5 percent and when men experienced two or more periods of unemployment the rate of intimate partner violence rose to 12.3 percent.

Women who are victims of intimate partner violence may experience unstable employment. Women who were recently abused (but not those abused only in the past) experienced unstable employment for up to two years.[4]

Intimate partner violence can lead to both mental and physical health problems, which decreases a woman's ability to retain employment. Researchers interviewed 1,311 women in Illinois once a year for three years and found that intimate partner violence contributes to stress-related physical and mental health problems for as long as a year after the abuse has occurred. Specifically, the researchers found:

- Women who had reported abuse by their partner rated their health as poorer and their need for mental health services as greater a year later as compared to nonabused women.

- Women with abusive partners also reported more stress-related concerns and emotional problems.

- Women with abusive partners reported more headaches, ulcers, and back problems than did nonabused women. (Chronic intimate partner violence is associated with poor health).

These health problems decrease women's ability to retain employment even as long as two years after the abuse occurred.

Economically Disadvantaged Neighborhoods and Intimate Partner Violence

Violence against women in intimate relationships occurred more often, was more severe, and was more likely to be repeated in economically disadvantaged neighborhoods. A study showed that the rate of intimate partner violence in economically disadvantaged neighborhoods is 8.7 percent, compared with 4.3 percent in more economically advantaged neighborhoods.

Women in economically disadvantaged neighborhoods were more likely to be victimized repeatedly or injured severely by their partners then women who lived in more advantaged neighborhoods (6 percent versus 2 percent, respectively).

African Americans and whites with the same economic characteristics have similar rates of intimate partner violence. However, African Americans have a higher overall rate of intimate partner violence, due in part to higher levels of economic distress and more frequent residence in economically disadvantaged neighborhoods.

Notes

1. While research shows that these factors individually affect the risk of intimate partner violence, they may interact or combine in ways that are not completely understood. Thus addressing only one of the three factors may not reduce the intimate partner violence.

2. This study looked at data from the National Survey of Families and Households to examine whether employment instability and financial strain were related to the risk for intimate partner violence against women.

3. Subjective financial strain was defined as perceptions of financial inadequacy and was operationalized by combining responses to questions about satisfaction with finances and questions regarding worry about money.

4. This study defined employment instability as the number of periods of unemployment for men between waves of the National Survey of Families and Households.

Section 4.6

Repressed Emotions and Domestic Violence

"Domestic Violence Often Comes from Men Who Repress Emotions, Feel Threatened, Study Finds," December 2002. Reprinted with permission from Ohio State University Research Communications, © 2002. Reviewed by David A. Cooke, M.D., FACP, July 2012.

A new study suggests that the way abusive men try to manage stress in their relationships and other parts of their lives may be associated with their violent outbursts.

Results showed abusive men were likely to view stressful circumstances as personally threatening, while trying to avoid the situation or repress emotional responses.

The findings indicate that abusive men don't show signs of depression or other reactions to the stress they're under. Instead, the feelings of stress build up and are released in bursts of violence, said Kristi Williams, co-author of the study and assistant professor of sociology at Ohio State University.

That's not an excuse for violence, she said, but understanding how abusers respond to stress may help mental health professionals intervene more appropriately.

"Our study suggests that violent behavior is a likely response among people with particular methods of evaluating and coping with stress," Williams said.

Williams conducted the study with Debra Umberson of the University of Texas at Austin and Kristin Anderson of Western Washington University. The study was published in a recent issue of the *Journal of Health and Social Behavior*.

The study included thirty-four men who had a history of domestic violence, most of whom were participating in a rehabilitation program in Texas. They were matched with a sample of thirty nonviolent subjects who were similar in socio-demographic factors.

All of the study participants completed a variety of questionnaires that examined levels of stress in their lives; how they responded to stress, anger, and hostility; and other psychological issues. The researchers also conducted in-depth interviews with the participants and asked them to discuss the sources of strain and satisfaction in their relationships, the worst and most recent arguments with their female partners, and their general attitudes about family relationships.

The results showed that, in general, the violent subjects reported significantly higher levels of stress in their lives than did the nonviolent subjects. Surprisingly, though, the violent men did not differ from others in the level of psychological distress they reported. In other words, the violent men did not show signs of depression, loneliness, or other indications that they were dealing with a lot of stress in their lives.

This was consistent with the finding that violent men were more likely to report that they repressed emotions—for example, saying that, when they are depressed, they try to take their mind off their problems rather than confronting them.

"People who repress emotions and feelings are not necessarily free of distress," she said. "They are simply free of traditional symptoms of psychological distress, such as depression. This may lead to a buildup of frustration that results in an outburst of violence."

In addition, violent men were more likely to view stressful situations as personally threatening, Williams said. These were situations in which the men said they did not feel fully in control of their lives. Violent men were most likely to feel threatened by issues involving their relationship with their partner. The in-depth interviews showed that "violent men are more likely to perceive their partner's behavior as threatening, regardless of the objective qualities of the behavior," Williams said.

Men who showed both tendencies—viewing stressful situations as threatening and repressing emotions—were three-and-a-half times more likely to commit domestic violence than those who didn't share that combination of traits, the study found.

The situation was even worse for men who tended to avoid or withdraw from conflicts with their partners. Men who felt threatened and who avoided conflict were eight times more likely than others to commit domestic violence.

Personal control plays a key factor in domestic violence, according to Williams.

"Issues of control surfaced throughout the in-depth interviews," she said. "Men who engage in domestic violence are more likely to feel they are at the mercy of people or situations in their lives. That's probably one reason why they perceive many events as more threatening to them personally."

Williams said researchers have tended to view violence as either a symptom of a psychiatric problem or a criminal behavior to achieve some goal, such as violence used in a robbery. However, these results suggest violence may also be an expression of distress that some people use in response to a stressful situation. In this case, violence is a way of externalizing feelings of distress that occur as a result of problems in their relationships. These men react with violence, while others may externalize stress in other ways, such as by abusing drugs or alcohol or showing suicidal behaviors, she said. Still others internalize stress by becoming depressed.

"It's not a way of excusing violence, but we hope that more clearly understanding the socio-psychological processes that can lead to domestic violence may help practitioners design more effective interventions that could prevent abuse," she said.

Section 4.7

Domestic Violence Linked to Substance Abuse and Unemployment

"Battering Linked to Substance Abuse and Unemployment," reprinted with permission from the Corporate Alliance to End Partner Violence, © 2012. All rights reserved. For additional information, visit www.caepv.org.

Men who abuse alcohol and drugs tend to batter their wives and girlfriends more often than others, according to two recent studies in the *New England Journal of Medicine*. One study at eight emergency departments around the country looked at 915 injured women, including 256 hurt by husbands or male partners. The women were asked about the habits and lives of the men.

The first study found more than three times the risk of domestic violence when husbands or male partners abuse alcohol or drugs, go in and out of jobs, or break up with the women. They also found that perpetrators of violence against women tend to be former or estranged husbands or ex-boyfriends. The study found that the risk of being injured from a domestic violence incident was:

- 3.6 times higher if the male partner abused alcohol;

- 3.5 times greater if he used illegal drugs;

- 3.1 times higher if he didn't have a steady job.

The researchers also found that women involved with men who were high school dropouts were 2.5 times more likely to be the victims of domestic violence.

The second study analyzed the factors for both domestic violence and other violence against women in a poor west Philadelphia neighborhood. It found that the male partners of the injured women were more than three times more likely to have used cocaine and more than four times more likely to have an arrest record than the male partners of women in the control group. One-third of the women who were attacked tested positive for cocaine. In the Philadelphia study, 53 percent of violent injuries to the women had been perpetrated by persons other than their partners, including neighbors, family members, or other women.

The Pennsylvania study also found that injured women differed from other women in several ways. The researchers noted that "Women who had been injured by a partner tended to be socially isolated, to have low self-esteem, and to have few sources of social or financial support."

Section 4.8

Domestic Violence in the Wake of Disasters

"Disasters and Domestic Violence," United States Department of Veteran Affairs, National Center for PTSD, December 20, 2011.

Two questions require attention when considering the implications of domestic violence for postdisaster recovery.

The first question is whether domestic violence increases in prevalence after disasters. There are only minimal data that are relevant to this question. Mechanic et al.[1] undertook the most comprehensive examination of intimate violence in the aftermath of a disaster after the 1993 Midwestern flood. A representative sample of 205 women who were either married or cohabitating with men and who were highly exposed to this disaster acknowledged considerable levels of domestic violence and abuse. Over the nine-month period after flood onset, 14 percent reported at least one act of physical aggression from their partners, 26 percent reported emotional abuse, 70 percent verbal abuse, and 86 percent partner anger. Whether these rates of physical aggression are greater than normal is not known because studies of domestic violence from previous years and under normal conditions have shown the existence of rates of violence as low as 1 percent and as high as 12 percent.

A few studies have produced evidence that supports the above. Police reports of domestic violence increased by 46 percent following the eruption of the Mt. St. Helens volcano.[2] One year after Hurricane

Hugo, marital stress was more prevalent among individuals who had been severely exposed to the hurricane (e.g., life threat, injury) than among individuals who had been less severely exposed or not exposed at all.[3] Within six months after Hurricane Andrew, 22 percent of adult residents of the stricken area acknowledged having a new conflict with someone in their household.[4] In a study of people directly exposed to the bombing of the Murrah Federal Building in Oklahoma City, 17 percent of noninjured persons and 42 percent of persons whose injuries required hospitalization reported troubled interpersonal relationships.[5]

The second question is whether domestic violence, regardless of the reasons how or why it occurs, influences women's postdisaster recovery. An important finding from Mechanic et al.'s (2001) study was that the presence of domestic violence strongly influenced women's postdisaster mental health. Thirty-nine percent of women who experienced post-flood partner abuse developed post-flood PTSD, compared to 17 percent of women who did not experience post-flood abuse. Fifty-seven percent of women who experienced post-flood partner abuse developed post-flood major depression, compared to 28 percent of nonabused women. Similarly, Norris and Uhl[3] found that as marital stress increased, so too did psychological symptoms such as depression and anxiety. Likewise, Norris et al.[4] found that six and thirty months after Hurricane Andrew, new conflicts and other socially disruptive events were among the strongest predictors of psychological symptoms.

These findings take on additional significance when it is remembered that not only are women generally at greater risk than men for developing postdisaster psychological problems, but women who are married or cohabitating with men may be at even greater risk than single women.[6,7] In contrast, married status is often a protective factor for men.[8,9] It also has been found that the severity of married women's symptoms increases with the severity of their husbands' distress, even after similarities in their exposure have been taken into account.[7]

In summary, although the research regarding the interplay of disaster and domestic violence is not extensive and little of it has been derived from studies of incidents of mass violence, the available evidence does suggest that services related to domestic violence should be integrated into other mental health services for disaster-stricken families. Screening for women's safety may be especially important. Helping men find appropriate ways to manage and direct their anger will benefit them and their wives. It will also help their children, as children are highly sensitive to postdisaster conflict and irritability in the family.[7,10]

Summary of Empirical Findings

- Although there is little conclusive evidence that domestic violence increases after major disasters, research suggests that its postdisaster prevalence may be substantial.

- In the most relevant study, 14 percent of women experienced at least one act of post-flood physical aggression and 26 percent reported post-flood emotional abuse over a nine-month period.

- One study reported a 46 percent increase in police reports of domestic violence after a disaster.

- Other studies show that substantial percentages of disaster victims experience marital stress, new conflicts, and troubled interpersonal relationships.

- There is more conclusive evidence that domestic violence harms women's abilities to recover from disasters.

- In the most relevant study, 39 percent of abused women developed postdisaster post-traumatic stress disorder (PTSD), compared to 17 percent of other women, and 57 percent of abused women developed postdisaster depression, compared to 28 percent of other women.

- Marital stress and conflicts are highly predictive of postdisaster symptoms.

- In light of the fact that, in general, married women are a high-risk group for developing postdisaster psychological problems, it seems advisable to integrate violence-related screenings and services into programs for women, men, and families.

References

1. Mechanic, M., Griffin, M., and Resick, P. (2001). The effects of intimate partner abuse on women's psychological adjustment to a major disaster. Manuscript submitted for publication.

2. Adams, P. R., and Adams, G. R. (1984). Mount Saint Helen's ashfall. *American Psychologist*, 39, 252–60.

3. Norris, F. H., and Uhl, G. A. (1993). Chronic stress as a mediator of acute stress: The case of Hurricane Hugo. *Journal of Applied Social Psychology*, 23, 1263–84.

4. Norris, F. H., Perilla, J. L., Riad, J. K., Kaniasty, K., and Lavizzo, E. A. (1999). Stability and change in stress, resources, and

psychological distress following natural disaster: Findings from Hurricane Andrew. *Anxiety, Stress, and Coping*, 12, 363–96.

5. Shariat, S., Mallonee, S., Kruger, E., Farmer, K., and North, C. (1999). A prospective study of long-term health outcomes among Oklahoma City bombing survivors. *Journal of the Oklahoma State Medical Association*, 92, 178–86.

6. Brooks, N., and McKinlay, W. (1992). Mental health consequences of the Lockerbie disaster. *Journal of Traumatic Stress*, 5, 527–43.

7. Gleser, G. C., Green, B. L., and Winget, C. N. (1981). *Prolonged psychological effects of disaster: A study of Buffalo Creek*. New York: Academic Press.

8. Fullerton, C. S., Ursano, R. J., Tzu-Cheg, K., and Bharitya, V. R. (1999). Disaster-related bereavement: Acute symptoms and subsequent depression. *Aviation, Space, and Environmental Medicine*, 70, 902–9.

9. Ursano, R. J., Fullerton, C. S., Kao, T. C., and Bhartiya, V. R. (1995). Longitudinal assessment of posttraumatic stress disorder and depression after exposure to traumatic death. *Journal of Nervous and Mental Disease*, 183, 36–42.

10. Wasserstein, S. B., and LaGreca, A. (1998). Hurricane Andrew: Parent conflict as a moderator of children's adjustment. *Hispanic Journal of Behavioral Science*, 20, 212–24.

Chapter 5

Detecting Abuse

Chapter Contents

Section 5.1

Comparing Healthy and Abusive Relationships

Excerpted from "Healthy Relationships 101," a brochure published by the Aurora Center for Advocacy and Education (www.umn.edu/aurora), © 2012. Reprinted with permission.

Healthy Relationships . . .

Nonthreatening Behavior

- Talk and act so that both partners feel safe and comfortable doing and saying things

Respect

- Listen to each other nonjudgmentally
- Partners are emotionally affirming and understanding
- Value opinions
- Engage in consensual sexual activity

Trust and Support

- Support each other's goals in life
- Respect each other's right to have own feelings, friends, activities, and opinions

Honesty and Accountability

- Accept responsibility for self
- Acknowledge past use of violence
- Admit when wrong

- Communicate openly and truthfully

Responsible Parenting

- Share parental responsibilities
- Are a positive, nonviolent role model for children

Shared Responsibility

- Mutually agree on a fair distribution of work
- Make family decisions together

Abusive Relationships . . .

Use Intimidation

- Incite fear by using looks, actions, and gestures
- Smash things
- Destroy property
- Abuse pets
- Display weapons

Use Emotional Abuse

- Put partner down
- Call partner names
- Make partner think they're crazy
- Play mind games
- Humiliate partner
- Make partner feel guilty

Use Isolation

- Control what partner does and reads, who partner sees and talks to, and where partner goes
- Limit partner's outside involvements
- Use jealousy to justify actions

Minimize, Deny, and Blame

- Make light of abuse and do not take partner's concerns about it seriously
- Say the abuse didn't happen
- Shift responsibility for abusive behavior
- Say partner caused the abuse

Use Children

- Make partner feel guilty about the children
- Use the children to relay messages
- Use visitation to harass partner
- Threaten to take the children away

Use Privilege and Power

- Treat partner like a servant
- Make all the big decisions
- Act like the "Master of the Castle"
- Is the one to define and enforce gender roles

Use Economic Abuse

- Prevent partner from getting or keeping a job
- Make partner ask for money
- Give partner an allowance
- Take partner's money
- Deny partner knowledge about or access to family income

Adapted from Health Partners, Discover: "Here's What Healthy and Abusive Relationships Look Like," Summer 1996.

Section 5.2

Indicators of Domestic Violence

"Domestic Violence Warning Signs," © Michigan State University Safe Place (http://www.msu.edu/~safe). Reprinted with permission. Reviewed by David A. Cooke, M.D., FACP, July 2012.

There is no way to tell for sure if someone is experiencing domestic violence. Those who are battered, and those who abuse, come in all personality types. Battered women are not always passive with low self-esteem, and batterers are not always violent or hateful to their partner in front of others. Most people experiencing relationship violence do not tell others what goes on at home. So how do you tell?

Here are some signs to look for.

Injuries and excuses: In some cases, bruises and injuries may occur frequently and be in obvious places. When this happens, the intent of the batterer is to keep the victim isolated and trapped at home. When black eyes and other bruising is a result of an assault, the person being battered may be forced to call in sick to work, or face the embarrassment and excuses of how the injuries occurred. In other cases, bruises and other outward injuries never occur. When there are frequent injuries seen by others, the one being battered may talk about being clumsy, or have elaborate stories of how the injuries occurred. The truth about the source of injuries will not usually be told unless the one told could be trusted and/or the one being battered wants help to end the relationship.

Absences from work or school: When severe beatings or other trauma related to violence occurs, the one being battered may take time off from his or her normal schedule. If you see this happening, or the person is frequently late, this could be a sign of something (such as relationship violence) occurring.

Low self-esteem: Some battered women have low self-esteem, while others have a great deal of confidence and esteem in other areas of their life (at work, as a mother, with hobbies, etc.) but not within their relationship. In terms of dealing with the relationship, a sense of

49

powerlessness and low self-esteem may exist. A battered woman may believe that she could not make it on her own without her partner and that she is lucky to have him in her life.

Accusations of having affairs: This is a common tactic used by batterers as an attempt to isolate their partners and as an excuse for a beating. It could include accusations of looking at other men, wanting to be with other men, or having affairs with the man bagging groceries at the local supermarket. Friends of the couple may observe this at times, but what is seen in public is usually only a small fraction of what the battered woman experiences at home.

Personality changes: People may notice that a very outgoing person, for instance, becomes quiet and shy around his or her partner. This happens because the one being battered "walks on eggshells" when in the presence of the one who is abusive to him or her. Accusations (of flirting, talking too loudly, or telling the wrong story to someone) have taught the abused person that it is easier to act a certain way around the batterer than to experience additional accusations in the future.

Fear of conflict: As a result of being battered, some may generalize the experience of powerlessness with other relationships. Conflicts with co-workers, friends, relatives, and neighbors can create a lot of anxiety. For many, it is easier to give in to whatever someone else wants than to challenge it. Asserting one's needs and desires begins to feel like a battle, and not worth the risks of losing.

Not knowing what one wants or how one feels: For adults or children who have experienced violence from a loved one, the ability to identify feelings and wants, and to express them, may not exist. This could result in passive-aggressive behavior. Rather than telling others what you want, you say one thing but then express your anger or frustration in an aggressive manner (such as scratching his favorite car, burning dinner, or not completing a report on time for your boss).

Blaming others for everything: The abuse, which usually includes the batterer blaming others for everything that goes wrong, is usually targeted at a partner or ex-partner. For example, a simple drive somewhere could turn into a violent situation if the batterer blames the partner and/or children for getting them lost. Co-workers and relatives may observe this type of behavior, and it may be directed at others as well.

Self-blame: You may notice someone taking all of the blame for things that go wrong. A co-worker may share a story about something that happened at home and then take all of the blame for whatever occurred. If you notice this happening a lot, it may be a sign that the one taking all of the blame is being battered.

Aggressive or care-taking behavior in children: Children who live in violent homes may take that experience with them to school and to the playground. Often the class bully is a child who sees violence in his home (directed at mom, or at some or all of the children in the home). Children who seem very grownup and are sensitive and attentive to others' needs may see violence at home as well.

Section 5.3

Helping Increase the Ability of Physicians to Identify Abuse Victims

Excerpted from "Family Violence Prevention Program Significantly Improves Ability to Identify and Facilitate Treatment for Patients Affected by Domestic Violence," Agency for Healthcare Research and Quality (AHRQ), March 11, 2011. AHRQ Health Care Innovations Exchange. Service Delivery Innovation Profile: Family Violence Prevention Program Significantly Improves Ability to Identify and Facilitate Treatment for Patients Affected by Domestic Violence (Kaiser Permanente-Northern California). In AHRQ Health Care Innovations Exchange, http://www.innovations.ahrq.gov. Rockville (MD): cited 2012 July 22. Available: http://www.innovations.ahrq.gov.

What They Did

The Family Violence Prevention Program seeks to improve the identification, prevention, and treatment of domestic violence by approaching it as a serious health issue that should be "diagnosed" during a physician office visit (just like other health conditions). The program's coordinated approach includes four components: a supportive environment that encourages identification; routine, physician-led inquiry; referral to onsite mental health resources; and linkages to community resources. Each component is described in more detail below.

Environment that supports identification: Kaiser Permanente Northern California facilities support the disclosure of domestic violence to providers by continually exposing patients to information on the topic. Brochures about domestic violence (in English, Spanish, and Chinese) are placed throughout Kaiser Permanente facilities in areas that are easily accessible to patients, such as physician offices, lounge areas, and restrooms. Other prominently displayed materials include posters (placed in examination rooms) and brochures with local resources. Domestic violence information is available online in text, stories, videos, and podcast.

Routine physician inquiry of at-risk patients: Kaiser Permanente providers in all departments routinely inquire about domestic violence as part of general physical examinations for all women between the ages of eighteen and sixty-five years and for male or female patients of any age who present with "red-flag" conditions, such as a suspicious injury, headaches, gastrointestinal or genitourinary conditions, chronic pain, depression, or substance use. Depending on the physician's comfort level with an individual patient, physicians may ask about domestic violence directly ("Within the last year, has your partner hit, slapped, kicked, or otherwise physically hurt you?"; "Are you afraid of your partner?") or as part of the routine update on medications, allergies, or change in health conditions. Most commonly, however, it is part of a relationship-building interaction ("Who do you live with?" "How are things at home?" "Do you ever feel physically or emotionally threatened or hurt by your partner/spouse?").

- *Physician resources:* Physicians have access to a variety of materials designed to facilitate patient screening, including toolkits to assist with reporting to law enforcement when required, examination room posters that can help facilitate the discussion, pocket reference cards, and online clinician reference information and tools. An intranet site linked to the electronic medical record includes care pathways, referral information to mental health and community resources, and online training for clinicians.

Referral to onsite services: When domestic violence is identified, a physician communicates support for the patient, documents the findings, provides community resource information, and refers the patient to onsite services based on an established protocol. Onsite services provided by mental health clinicians include an evaluation for co-occurring psychiatric conditions (e.g., posttraumatic stress disorder, anxiety, and depression), a danger assessment, and assistance with safety planning.

Community linkages: The onsite mental health clinicians refer patients to community resources as needed, including twenty-four-hour crisis response services, long-term counseling, support groups, legal assistance, emergency and transitional housing, and children's services.

Continuous feedback: Using diagnostic information from automated databases, department- and facility-specific feedback is provided twice a year, which facilitates trending over time and guides local and regional quality improvement efforts.

Did It Work?

Results

The program has led to a sixfold increase in the number of patients identified as being victims of domestic violence, a high percentage of these patients receiving follow up services, and high levels of member satisfaction.

Sixfold increase in patients identified: In 2000, approximately 1,022 patients were diagnosed with domestic violence; by 2008, that figure had increased to more than 4,000. Information provided in February 2011 indicates that by 2010 more than 6,200 patients had been diagnosed. In addition, the site of identification has shifted—most patients are now identified in less acute settings, such as primary care.

High follow-up rates: Since the program began, more than 50 percent of members diagnosed with domestic violence have had a follow-up visit with a Kaiser Permanente mental health clinician within sixty days.

High member satisfaction: An analysis based on twenty-five thousand member satisfaction surveys revealed a strong correlation between recalling the physician asking about home and family relationships (an area probed in one survey question) and being "very satisfied" with the care received. This was demonstrated across age, gender, and ethnic groups.

How They Did It

Planning and Development Process

Kaiser Permanente Northern California used a four-phase implementation process for the program. Key elements of each phase are highlighted below:

- **Phase 1:** Identified physician champions for the project, created an implementation team, and developed a protocol for referral to mental health services for patients identified with domestic violence.

- **Phase 2:** Developed clinician tools for evaluation, documentation, and reporting; provided training and tools to mental health clinicians receiving referrals; developed quality improvement measures; and identified local community domestic violence advocacy organizations.

- **Phase 3:** Provided training and tools to physicians and other clinicians and staff via grand rounds, department meetings, videos, and online training modules; placed appropriate materials in examination rooms, waiting areas, and restrooms and created a mechanism for restocking these materials; and established relationships with local community advocacy organizations and law enforcement.

- **Phase 4:** Developed an outreach and publicity plan (including placing articles in member newsletters); increased collaboration between medical facility and community advocacy agencies; incorporated assessment, documentation, and referral tools into the electronic medical record; developed online domestic violence and workplace training for managers, brochures for employees, and increased awareness of Kaiser Permanente's Employee Assistance Program as a resource for employees; and incorporated domestic violence training into yearly staff trainings and new employee orientation.

Adoption Considerations

Getting Started with This Innovation

Identify an MD champion: An MD champion serves as the voice of the program, highlighting domestic violence as an important health issue that should be addressed by clinicians and develops strategies for full implementation of the program.

Create a multidisciplinary implementation team: The identification, prevention, and treatment of domestic violence require the involvement of practitioners from multiple disciplines; representatives from each of these disciplines should be involved in program development and implementation.

Provide flexibility in screening techniques: Physicians should be given multiple options so they can incorporate domestic violence inquiry into their practices in a way that is comfortable and natural for them.

Design a referral protocol: Physicians will be more likely to ask patients about domestic violence if they have a clear, straightforward protocol to guide next steps after identifying a victim of domestic violence and feel confident that the patient will receive services and resources. The protocol should include referral for patients in crisis and noncrisis situations. Mental health clinicians should receive specific domestic violence training so that they are familiar with domestic violence assessment, safety planning materials, and information about local advocacy organizations.

Develop a supportive environment: A supportive environment will put domestic violence at the forefront of patients' minds, thus encouraging them to discuss domestic violence with a provider and/or directly access resources. Have resources available in print and online.

Partner with domestic violence advocacy services: For facilities or healthcare organizations that do not have onsite mental health or social work services, the patient should be given resource and crisis information and the opportunity to call a local or national domestic violence hotline while in the clinic. Information about available mental health resources should be offered.

Sustaining This Innovation

Identify qualitative and quantitative measures to ensure continuous quality improvement: This will ensure that clinicians and administrators can evaluate the program's impact on an ongoing basis and make adjustments as needed.

Include domestic violence prevention as a health plan, facility, and department goal: Striving to meet a goal keeps domestic violence identification and referral present in the thoughts of providers and administrators.

Use a consistent approach based on systems-model thinking: When disseminating the program, identify facility-based champions and multidisciplinary teams that will use the "systems-model" approach to domestic violence prevention. Provide regional leadership the resources to ensure consistency of services across facilities/departments, incorporation into new services (particularly call center, electronic medical record, and online), and alignment with other health initiatives.

Integrate domestic violence response into existing systems and daily workflow: Incorporate domestic violence into clinical practice processes and tools such as the electronic medical record and advice and call center protocols.

References

1. Tjaden P, Thoennes N. Extent, nature, and consequences of intimate partner violence. Washington, DC: U.S. Department of Justice; 2000.

2. Adult female victims of intimate partner physical domestic violence, in Data Points. Sacramento, CA: California Women's Health Survey, Office of Women's Health, California Department of Health Services; 2001.

3. Thompson RS, Bonomi AE, Anderson M, et al. Intimate partner violence: prevalence, types, and chronicity in adult women. *Am J Prev Med*. 2006; 30(6):447–57.

4. Rivara F, Anderson ML, Fishman P, et al. Healthcare utilization and costs for women with a history of intimate partner violence. *Am J Prev Med*. 2007; 32(2):89–96.

5. Bonomi AE, Thompson RS, Anderson M, et al. Intimate partner violence and women's physical, mental and social functioning. *Am J Prev Med*. 2006; 30(6):458–66.

6. U.S. Centers for Disease Control and Prevention. Understanding intimate partner violence fact sheet 2006. Available at: http://www.cdc.gov/ncipc/dvp/ipv_factsheet.pdf.

7. Felitti VJ, Anda RF, Nordenberg D, et al. Relationship of childhood abuse and household dysfunction to many of the leading causes of death in adults: the adverse childhood experiences (ACE) study. *Am J Prev Med*. 1998; 14(4):245–58.

8. Costs of intimate partner violence against women in the United States. Atlanta, GA: National Center for Injury Prevention and Control, Centers for Disease Control and Prevention; 2003.

9. McCaw B, Kotz K. Family violence prevention program: another way to save a life. *The Permanente Journal*. 2005 Winter; 9(1):65–68.

10. Rodriguez MA, Bauer HM, McLoughlin E, et al. Screening and intervention for intimate partner abuse: practices and attitudes of primary care physicians. *JAMA*. 1999; 282:468–74.

Section 5.4

Self-Test: Am I Being Abused?

Excerpted from "Am I Being Abused," U.S. Department of Health and
Human Services Office on Women's Health, May 18, 2011.

It can be hard to know if you're being abused. You may think that
your husband is allowed to make you have sex. That's not true. Forced
sex is rape, no matter who does it. You may think that cruel or threatening words are not abuse. They are. And sometimes emotional abuse
is a sign that a person will become physically violent.

Following is a list of possible signs of abuse. Some of these are illegal. All of them are wrong. You may be abused if your partner does
any of the following things:

- Monitors what you're doing all the time

- Unfairly accuses you of being unfaithful all the time

- Prevents or discourages you from seeing friends or family

- Prevents or discourages you from going to work or school

- Gets very angry during and after drinking alcohol or using drugs

- Controls how you spend your money

- Controls your use of needed medicines

- Decides things for you that you should be allowed to decide (like
  what to wear or eat)

- Humiliates you in front of others

- Destroys your property or things that you care about

- Threatens to hurt you, the children, or pets

- Hurts you (by hitting, beating, pushing, shoving, punching, slapping, kicking, or biting)

- Uses (or threatens to use) a weapon against you

- Forces you to have sex against your will

- Controls your birth control or insists that you get pregnant

- Blames you for his or her violent outbursts

- Threatens to harm himself or herself when upset with you

- Says things like, "If I can't have you then no one can."

If you think someone is abusing you, get help. Abuse can have serious physical and emotional effects. No one has the right to hurt you.

Section 5.5

Self-Test: Am I an Abuser?

"Am I a Good Boy/Girlfriend?" © 2012 LoveisRespect.org. All rights reserved. Reprinted with permission. Additional information and resources are available at www.loveisrespect.org.

Are you a good boyfriend or girlfriend? Answer yes or no to the following questions to find out. Make sure to write down your responses. At the end, you'll find out how to score your answers.

Do I:

1. forget to thank my partner when they do something nice for me?

2. ignore my partner's calls if I don't feel like talking?

3. get jealous when my partner makes a new friend?

4. have trouble making time to listen to my partner when something is bothering them?

5. discourage my partner from trying something new like joining a club?

6. call, text, or drive by my partner's house a lot?

7. get upset when my partner wants to hang out with their friends or family?

8. make fun of my partner or call them names?

9. criticize my partner for their taste in music or clothing?

10. make fun of my partner's appearance?

11. accuse my partner of flirting or cheating even if I'm not sure that's what happened?

12. take out my frustrations on my partner, like snapping at them or giving them attitude?

13. throw things if I'm mad at my partner or do things like hit walls or drive dangerously?

14. read my partner's texts or go through their personal things, like their wallet or purse?

15. tell my partner they are the reason for my bad mood even if they aren't?

16. try to make my partner feel guilty about things they have no control over?

17. sometimes say things to my partner knowing that they are hurtful?

18. make my partner feel bad about something nice they did for me that I didn't like, even though I know they tried their best?

19. talk down to or embarrass my partner in front of others?

20. have sex with my partner even if I think they don't want to go that far?

Scoring: So Are You a Good Boyfriend/Girlfriend?

Give yourself one point for every "Yes" you answered to questions one through four and five points for all "Yes" answers to numbers five through twenty. Don't give yourself any points for any "No" answers.

Now that you're finished and have your score, the next step is to find out what it means. Simply take your total score and see which of the categories below apply to you.

Score: 0 Points

If you got zero points, congratulations! You make a good boyfriend/ girlfriend! It sounds like you're very mindful of your actions and respectful of your partner's feelings —these are the building blocks of a healthy relationship. Keeping things on a good track takes work, so stay with it! As long as you and your partner continue like this, your relationship should grow in a healthy direction.

Score: 1–2 Points

If you scored one or two points, there may be a couple of things in your relationship that could use a little attention. Nobody is perfect, but it is important to be mindful of your actions and try to avoid hurting your partner. Remember, communication is key to building a healthy relationship!

Score: 3–4 Points

If you scored three or four points, it's possible that some of your actions may hurt your partner and relationship. While the behaviors may not be abusive, they can worsen over time if you don't change. Read about the different types of abuse, so that you can keep your relationship safe and healthy.

Score: 5 Points or More

If you scored five or more points, some of your actions may be abusive. You may not realize it, but these behaviors are damaging. The first step to improving your relationship is becoming aware of your unhealthy actions and admitting they are wrong. It's important to take responsibility for the problem and get help to end it. An unhealthy pattern is hard to change, so chat with a peer advocate for more information on how to get help.

Chapter 6

Stalking

Chapter Contents

Section 6.1

Stalking: What It Is and What You Can Do About It

What Is Stalking?

Any unwanted contact that communicates a threat or places the victim in fear. This communication could involve repeated visual or physical contact; verbal, written, or implied threats; nonconsensual communication; or a combination of these measures.

Effects of Stalking on Victims

Stalking victims often live in constant fear that at any moment their safety and lives may be threatened. Never knowing when the threat may become a violent reality, stalking victims experience higher levels of anxiety, severe depression, social dysfunction, and insomnia, causing significant disruption and alteration of daily life.

Three Broad Categories of Stalking

- **Intimate or former intimate partner stalking:** The stalker and victim may be married or divorced, may live together or have lived together in the past, may be serious or casual sexual partners, or former sexual partners. There may be a history of sexual or domestic violence in the relationship as well.

- **Acquaintance stalking:** The stalker and victim might know each other casually, as in a co-worker or neighbor relationship.

- **Stranger stalking:** The stalker and victim do not know each other. This also includes cases where the victim may be a celebrity.

Know the Facts: Stalking Statistics

- During a twelve-month period an estimated 3.4 million persons age eighteen or older were victims of stalking.

- Females experienced twenty stalking victimizations per one thousand females age eighteen or older.

- The rate of stalking victimizations for males was approximately seven per one thousand males eighteen or older.

- Persons age eighteen to nineteen and twenty to twenty-four experienced the highest rates of stalking victimization.

- One in seven victims reported they moved as a result of the stalking.

- Approximately 60 percent do not report victimization to the police.

(From the United States Department of Justice SVS: Stalking Victimization in the United States Report.)

Stalking and Technology

Computers and Internet

If stalkers have access to a victim's computers, they can track them by looking at the history or websites visited on the computer. Spyware software on computers (sometimes sent through e-mail) can send stalkers a copy of every keystroke made, including passwords, websites visited, and e-mail sent by victims.

Stalkers can also use the internet to contact or post things about the victim on message board or discussion forums. They may also verbally attack or threaten victims in chat rooms. Some stalkers will post threatening or personal information about the victim, including the victim's full name and address. Often stalkers will e-mail the victim, or fill their inbox with spam, and have been known to send viruses or other harmful programs to victims' computers.

Phones

Telephones and cellular phones can be used to threaten or harass. Cell phones also have features that can be used against victims:

- **Caller ID spoofing:** Spoofing is a tool used by stalkers to change the Caller ID on your phone or cellular phone to show any desired number they want.

- **Cell phone global positioning system (GPS):** Stalkers can enable the GPS on your cellular phone to locate where you are at all times.

Hidden Cameras

Stalkers use small hidden cameras to monitor their victims and learn their routines. Stalkers use information they gather to exert power and control their victims. Small wireless high-resolution cameras can be hidden in smoke detectors, children's lamps, behind a pin-sized hole in a wall, and can even be activated remotely.

I'm Being Stalked, What Should I Do?

Notify the police: This is the first thing victims of stalking incidents should do. They should notify the police department where they live and where they work.

Keep a record of your stalker: The victim should maintain a detailed record of each encounter with the stalker. Included in this record of incidents should be dates, times, locations, complete description of the offender, words spoken, actions taken during the incident, actions taken afterward, and names of witnesses.

Seek a protection order: Court-ordered protection orders are intended to keep the stalker away from the victim by making it illegal for the stalker to have contact with the victim. In most jurisdictions, a person who violates this order can be found in contempt of court and jailed or fined. A person who violates a protection order is guilty of a criminal offense, usually a misdemeanor, but sometimes a felony, and is subject to criminal prosecution.

Develop and implement a safety plan: A safety plan is designed to clearly state what to do if you ever need to leave your home and abuser. Creating a safety plan in advance will help you to retain control during your escape. Leaving is very dangerous and it is very important to plan in advance to maintain safety.

What Should I Do in Advance?

- Have important numbers nearby (police, friends, family, shelter, hotlines).

- Ask a neighbor to beware of suspicious activity in your home and to call police for help.

- Plan an escape route and practice it often. Plan an escape route from work as well.

- Keep a "ready bag" packed with all of your important documents (driver's license and registration, birth certificates, social security cards, insurance papers, etc.), extra cash, address book, prescription medications, clothes, cell phone, etc. Keep it hidden, but easy to grab quickly.

- Think about where you could go if you needed to leave in an emergency. Have more than one place in mind.

- Leave extra money, car keys, and copies of important documents with someone you trust.

- Open a savings account or get a credit card in your name.

- Have a "code word" to use with your family and others you trust.

How You Can Help Someone Being Stalked

- Encourage them to seek help.
- Be a good listener.
- Offer your support.
- Ask how you can help.
- Educate yourself about stalking.
- Avoid any confrontations with the stalker. This could be dangerous for you and your friends.

Stalking Myths and Facts

Myth: Only celebrities are stalked.

Fact: 1.4 million people are stalked every year in the United States. We may hear more about celebrity stalking cases in the media, but the vast majority of stalking victims are ordinary citizens.

Myth: If you ignore stalking, it will go away.

Fact: Stalkers seldom "just stop." In fact, behaviors can turn more and more violent as time goes on. Victims should seek help form advocates, law enforcement, and the courts to intervene to stop stalking.

Myth: Stalking is creepy but not dangerous.

Fact: Stalking is creepy and dangerous. Three out of four women who were murdered by an intimate partner had been previously stalked by the killer.

Myth: Stalking is annoying but not illegal.

Fact: Stalking is a crime under the laws of all fifty states, and the federal government.

Myth: You can't be stalked by someone you are still dating.

Fact: If your current partner tracks your every move or follows you around in a way that causes you fear, that is stalking.

Myth: Modern surveillance technology is too expensive and confusing for most stalkers to use.

Fact: Stalkers can buy surveillance software and hardware for cheap and can easily track victims' every move on a computer.

Myth: If you confront the stalker, he'll go away.

Fact: Stalkers can be unreasonable and unpredictable. Confronting or trying to reason with a stalker can be dangerous.

Section 6.2

Security Tips for Stalking Victims

What to Do about Stalkers

State your decision directly and clearly when you do not want to have further contact with a pursuer. Do not state reasons or negotiate. Then stop all contact and communication with that person. Do not respond to escalation or have a person who is not a police officer intervene for you. Do not display fear or concern to the stalker. Carefully evaluate the stalker's communications and actions. Design a plan that minimizes encounters and maximizes safety.

Safety Strategies

- Call the police and file a crime report. When making a subsequent report, tell the officer the number assigned to the original report.

- Ask the officer for an emergency protective order if you are in immediate danger. Restraining orders may serve to incite the perpetrator. Be prepared to seek temporary safety at a shelter or with others if you are in imminent danger.

- Implement preventive measures such as installing dead bolt locks and outside lighting, vary routes taken, stay in public areas, and inform trusted neighbors regarding the situation.

- Assist the police by keeping a log of current and past events. Keep phone message tapes and items sent in the mail.

- As a last resort, change jobs and move to a new location. Consult with the police department about ways to maintain privacy of information that could be used to locate you.

Security Recommendations for Stalking Victims

Residence Security

- Be alert for any suspicious persons.

- Positively identify callers before opening doors. Install a wide-angle viewer in all primary doors.

- Install a porch light at a height that would discourage removal.

- Install dead bolts on all outside doors. If you cannot account for all keys, change door locks. Secure spare keys. Place a dowel in sliding glass doors and all sliding windows.

- Keep garage doors locked at all times. Use an electric garage door opener.

- Install adequate outside lighting.

- Trim shrubbery. Install locks on fence gates.

- Keep fuse box locked. Have battery lanterns in residence.

- Install a loud exterior alarm bell that can be manually activated in more than one location.

- Maintain an unlisted phone number. Alert household members to unusual and wrong number calls. If such activity continues, notify local law enforcement agency.

- Any written or telephone threat should be treated as legitimate and must be checked out. Notify the appropriate law enforcement agency.

- All adult members of the household should be trained if you plan to keep a firearm for protection in its use. It should be stored out of reach of children.

- Household staff should have a security check prior to employment and should be thoroughly briefed on security precautions. Strictly enforce a policy of the staff not discussing family matters or movement with anymore except police.

- Be alert for any unusual packages, boxes, or devices on the premises. Do not disturb such objects.

- Maintain all-purpose fire extinguishers in the residence and in the garage. Install a smoke detector system.

- Tape emergency numbers on all phones.

- When away from the residence for an evening, place lights and radio on a timer. For extended absences, arrange to have deliveries suspended.

- Intruders will attempt to enter unlocked doors or windows without causing a disturbance. Keep doors and windows locked.

- Prepare an evacuation plan. Brief household members on plan procedures. Provide ladders or rope for two-story residences.

- A family dog is one of the least expensive but most effective alarm systems.

- Know the whereabouts of all family members at all times.

- Children should be accompanied to school or bus stops.

- Routes taken and time spent walking should be varied.

- Require identification of all repairmen and salesmen prior to permitting entry into residence.

- Always park in a secured garage if available.

- Inform trusted neighbor regarding situation. Provide neighbor with photo or description of suspect and any possible vehicles.

- Inform trusted neighbors of any anticipated extended vacations, business trips, etc.

- During vacations, etc., have neighbors pick up mail and newspapers.

- If residing in an apartment with on-site manager, provide the manager with a picture of the suspect. If in a secured condominium, provide information to the doorman or valet.

Office Security

- Central reception should handle visitors and packages.

- Office staff should be alert for suspicious people, parcels, and packages that do not belong in the area.

- Establish key and lock control. If keys possessed by terminated employees are not retrieved, change the locks.

- Park in secured area if at all possible.

- Have your name removed from any reserved parking area.

- If there is an on-site security director, make him/her aware of the situation. Provide him/her with suspect information.

- Have secretary or co-worker screen calls if necessary.

- Have a secretary or security personnel screen all incoming mail (personal) or fan letters.

- Be alert to anyone possibly following you from work.

- Do not accept any package unless you personally ordered an item.

Personal Security

- Remove home address on personal checks and business cards.

- Place real property in a trust, and list utilities under the name of the trust.

- Utilize a private mailbox service to receive all personal mail.

- File for confidential voter status or register to vote utilizing mailbox address.

- Destroy discarded mail.

- Phone lines can be installed in a location other than the person's residence and call-forwarded to the residence.

- Place residence rental agreements in another person's name.

- The person's name should not appear on service or delivery orders to the residence.

- Do not obtain a mailbox with the United States Post Office.

- Mailbox address now becomes the person's official address on all records and in all rolodexes. It may be necessary or more convenient to list the mailbox as "Suite 123" or "Apartment #123" rather than "Box 123."

- File a change of address card with the post office giving the mailbox address as the person's new address. Send postcards to friends, businesses, etc., giving the mailbox address and requesting that they remove the old address from their files and rolodexes.

- All current creditors should be given a change of address card to the mailbox address. (Some credit reporting agencies will remove past addresses from credit histories if a request is made. We recommend this be done.)

- File a change of address with the Department of Motor Vehicles (DMV) to reflect the person's new mailbox address. Get a new driver's license with the new address on it.

Vehicle Security

- Park vehicles in well-lit areas. Do not patronize parking lots where car doors must be left unlocked and keys surrendered; otherwise surrender only the ignition key. Allow items to be placed in or removed from the trunk only in your presence.

- When parked in the residence garage, turn the garage light on and lock the vehicle and garage door.

- Equip the gas tank with a locking gas cap. The hood-locking device must be controlled from inside the vehicle.

- Visually check the front and rear passenger compartments before entering the vehicle.

- Select a reliable service station for vehicle service.

- Keep doors locked while vehicle is in use.

- Be alert for vehicles that appear to be following you.

- When traveling by vehicle, plan ahead. Know the locations of police stations, fire departments, and busy shopping centers.

- Use a different schedule and route of travel each day. If followed, drive to a police station, fire department, or busy shopping center. Sound the horn to attract attention.

Section 6.3

Documenting and Reporting Stalking

Excerpted from "Tracking the Stalker: What You Need to Know about Documenting the Stalker's Actions," created by T. K. Logan, Ph.D., University of Kentucky. Copyright 2012 T. K. Logan. All rights reserved. Reprinted with permission. To view this document online, along with additional information, visit http://outrageus.org.

Are You Being Stalked?

Is someone repeatedly following or watching you, showing up unexpectedly, or communicating with you in ways that seem obsessive or make you concerned or afraid for your safety?

Stalking is a pattern of behavior that usually is very frightening, unpredictable, and dangerous. The stalker might be someone you have had a relationship with or someone you don't know or have barely met. Stalking can begin at any time including while you are in a relationship with a partner, or even after a no contact order has been issued. Stalking is a crime in most states, although the legal definitions vary from state to state.

Why Should I Keep a Log of the Stalker's Actions?

Document the intentional nature of the stalker's actions: Logging or tracking the stalker's actions will increase your credibility if and when you seek help from others. Not only will it help you remember specific dates, times, and details but it will show others that you are not talking about a few minor instances that could be dismissed as "accidental." Tracking all of the things the stalker does shows others that what the stalker is doing is intentional, not accidental.

Collect evidence: Even though you may not want to involve the police or the court system at this point, having this information can be crucial if you ever do decide to pursue help through the court. The log, if you collect all of the information you need, may show a course of conduct, document your fears, and provide police with corroborating evidence or guide police to what evidence needs to be collected.

Help others understand: Detailing the full scale of the tactics the stalker is using against you and the harms or losses you have suffered because of the stalker can increase others' awareness of how harmful this is to you and your family. This is key to getting others to take the stalking seriously.

Increase your safety: Stalking logs can show patterns and areas of risk and provide information that can help you target your safety. Keeping a log of the stalker's behaviors can also help others identify ways in which they may be able to increase your safety and intervene with the stalker.

What Should I Include in the Log?

Incident description: Date, time, and specific description and location of the incident. Include everything, even if it seems small or insignificant and even if you are not sure it was the stalker. It is unlikely that all of the things that are happening to you during the course of stalking are coincidental.

Corroborating evidence: All evidence should be preserved, including time, date, and location of each incident, and full name(s) and phone number(s) of any witness(es). When possible, take pictures or videos. All evidence should be dated. If the police are involved, they should collect and preserve evidence, including photographs. Keep all notes, e-mails, text messages, gifts, and pictures.

Whether or not the police are involved, be sure to write as much detail as possible about where and when the incident occurred, even if you do not have any other evidence. It is possible that police can get evidence through surveillance videos from stores or other businesses, or by tracing phone numbers.

All receipts for repairs from damages should be kept along with pictures or other evidence of damage. Also keep in mind that your cell phone and computer may be "crime scenes" containing important evidence.

Police or court system notification and response or other agency notification and responses: You may or may not decide to involve the police, the court system, or other offices (e.g., probation and parole, victim services), but if you called the police or other agencies (e.g., probation officer, prosecutor, victim services), be sure to write down who you talked to, the date and time of your contact, badge number or other employee identification, and the outcome of that interaction (e.g., report taken, no action taken). Also, any accommodations at your place of work or other places you frequent should be noted. If possible, have security document any work disturbance and accommodations.

Why this "contact/incident" made you feel concerned for your safety or upset: It is important to document the specific fear or emotional distress the incident caused you. This is primarily focusing on your immediate reaction to the contact or incident. Also, be certain to explain the context of the incident, including past threats or behaviors that make this particular incident seem so frightening or harmful to you. Remember that police and others do not know the stalker as well as you do and you may need to help them understand what happened and what it meant to you. The log is a good place to help explain how certain actions convey threats of harm.

Impact: Be sure to document how the incident impacted your life (e.g., any ways it changed your life, work, or routines, any financial costs to you). This may be short-term or longer-term impact from contact or incident.

I Don't Want to Write Everything Down; I Just Want It to Go Away!

Many victims of stalking just want to move on with their lives. Writing about everything the stalker is doing can be uncomfortable, hard, and time consuming. Unfortunately, ignoring or reasoning with the stalker often does not deter the stalker. Stalkers often persist in making life miserable for their target. This is why it is so critical to take active control of your safety and to document everything that the stalker does.

One key to making this work for you is to find some way to document or track the stalker's actions in a manner that is comfortable for you. It may mean keeping a small notebook in your purse to pull out anytime you need it. Or you can document the events on a formal documentation log, or in a password-protected file on your computer or phone. Choose the easiest, safest, and most comfortable way to record what is happening so that you document the stalking as consistently as possible (including the elements that were mentioned above for each incident). It is important to see the whole picture and pattern of stalking behaviors. Also be sure to keep backup copies (either electronically or in paper form) in case something happens to your original.

Find someone who can support you during this process. Having a close and trusted friend or family member or an advocate who can support you during this process is critical. He or she may be able to help you maintain the log and to provide the emotional support that you need.

Is It Safe for Me to Write All This Down and Keep It?

Safety must be kept as your primary concern at all times. You will want to keep your log in a safe place, with a trusted friend or family member, or you may want to keep it electronically and password protected.

It is also important to stick to the facts when documenting incidents. Try to keep emotion and other details out of the log except where necessary to document the impact stalking has had on you and your family. Keep in mind the information in the log could potentially be used as evidence by police or the courts and if this happens, information in the log may be seen by the court and other people involved in the case.

Section 6.4

Stalking Legislation

"Federal Stalking Laws," © 2011 West Virginia Foundation
for Rape Information and Services (www.fris.org). All rights reserved.
Reprinted with permission.

What Are the United States Statutes for Stalking?

In addition to state statutes, stalking victims should be aware of federal legislation that makes it a crime to cross a state line in order to stalk another person, a spouse or partner.

Note: The laws cited below were current as of April 2011.

18 U.S.C. 2261A Interstate Stalking (1996; 2000; 2006)

Whoever:

1. travels in interstate or foreign commerce or within the special maritime and territorial jurisdiction of the United States, or enters or leaves Indian country, with the intent to kill, injure, harass, or place under surveillance with intent to kill, injure, harass, or intimidate another person, and in the course of, or as a result of, such travel places that person in reasonable fear

of the death of, or serious bodily injury to, or causes substantial emotional distress to that person, a member of the immediate family (as defined in section 115 [18 USCS § 115]) of that person, or the spouse or intimate partner of that person; or

2. with the intent:

    A. to kill, injure, harass, or place under surveillance with intent to kill, injure, harass, or intimidate, or cause substantial emotional distress to a person in another state or tribal jurisdiction or within the special maritime and territorial jurisdiction of the United States; or

    B. to place a person in another state or tribal jurisdiction, or within the special maritime and territorial jurisdiction of the United States, in reasonable fear of the death of, or serious bodily injury to: (i) that person; (ii) a member of the immediate family (as defined in section 115 [18 USCS § 115]) of that person; or (iii) a spouse or intimate partner of that person; [and] uses the mail, any interactive computer service, or any facility of interstate or foreign commerce to engage in a course of conduct that causes substantial emotional distress to that person or places that person in reasonable fear of the death of, or serious bodily injury to, any of the persons described in clauses (i) through (iii) of subparagraph (B); shall be punished as provided in section 2261(b) of this title [18 USCS § 2261(b)].

18 U.S.C. 2261 Interstate Domestic Violence (1994; 2000; 2006)

a. Offenses:

    1. Travel or conduct of offender. A person who travels in interstate or foreign commerce or enters or leaves Indian country or within the special maritime and territorial jurisdiction of the United States with the intent to kill, injure, harass, or intimidate a spouse, intimate partner, or dating partner, and who, in the course of or as a result of such travel, commits or attempts to commit a crime of violence against that spouse, intimate partner, or dating partner, shall be punished as provided in subsection (b).

    2. Causing travel of victim. A person who causes a spouse, intimate partner, or dating partner to travel in interstate or foreign commerce or to enter or leave Indian country by

force, coercion, duress, or fraud, and who, in the course of, as a result of, or to facilitate such conduct or travel, commits or attempts to commit a crime of violence against that spouse, intimate partner, or dating partner, shall be punished as provided in subsection (b).

b. Penalties: A person who violates this section or section 2261A [18 USCS § 2261A] shall be fined under this title, imprisoned:

1. for life or any term of years, if death of the victim results;

2. for not more than twenty years if permanent disfigurement or life-threatening bodily injury to the victim results;

3. for not more than ten years, if serious bodily injury to the victim results or if the offender uses a dangerous weapon during the offense;

4. as provided for the applicable conduct under chapter 109A [18 USCS §§ 2241 et seq.] if the offense would constitute an offense under chapter 109A [18 USCS §§ 2241 et seq.] (without regard to whether the offense was committed in the special maritime and territorial jurisdiction of the United States or in a federal prison); and

5. for not more than five years, in any other case, or both fined and imprisoned.

6. Whoever commits the crime of stalking in violation of a temporary or permanent civil or criminal injunction, restraining order, no-contact order, or other order described in section 2266 of title 18, United States Code, shall be punished by imprisonment for not less than one year.

18 U.S.C.2262 Interstate Violation of a Protective Order

a. Offenses:

1. Travel or conduct of offender. A person who travels in interstate or foreign commerce, or enters or leaves Indian country or within the special maritime and territorial jurisdiction of the United States, with the intent to engage in conduct that violates the portion of a protection order that prohibits or provides protection against violence, threats, or harassment against, contact or communication with, or physical proximity to, another person, or

that would violate such a portion of a protection order in the jurisdiction in which the order was issued, and subsequently engages in such conduct, shall be punished as provided in subsection (b).

2. Causing travel of victim. A person who causes another person to travel in interstate or foreign commerce or to enter or leave Indian country by force, coercion, duress, or fraud, and in the course of, as a result of, or to facilitate such conduct or travel engages in conduct that violates the portion of a protection order that prohibits or provides protection against violence, threats, or harassment against, contact or communication with, or physical proximity to, another person, or that would violate such a portion of a protection order in the jurisdiction in which the order was issued, shall be punished as provided in subsection (b).

b. Penalties: A person who violates this section shall be fined under this title, imprisoned:

1. for life or any term of years, if death of the victim results;

2. for not more than twenty years if permanent disfigurement or life-threatening bodily injury to the victim results;

3. for not more than ten years, if serious bodily injury to the victim results or if the offender uses a dangerous weapon during the offense;

4. as provided for the applicable conduct under chapter 109A [18 USCS §§ 2241 et seq.] if the offense would constitute an offense under chapter 109A (without regard to whether the offense was committed in the special maritime and territorial jurisdiction of the United States or in a federal prison); and

5. for not more than five years, in any other case, or both fined and imprisoned.

18 U.S.C. 875(c) Interstate Communications

c. Whoever transmits in interstate or foreign commerce any communication containing any threat to kidnap any person or any threat to injure the person of another, shall be fined under this title or imprisoned not more than five years, or both.

47 U.S.C. 223(a) Obscene or Harassing Telephone Calls in the District of Columbia or in Interstate or Foreign Communications

This statute makes it a federal crime, punishable by up to two years in prison, to use a telephone or other telecommunications device to annoy, abuse, harass, or threaten another person at another number.

a. Prohibited acts generally: Whoever:

1. in interstate or foreign communications:

    A. by means of a telecommunications device knowingly (i) makes, creates, or solicits, and (ii) initiates the transmission of, any comment, request, suggestion, proposal, image, or other communication which is obscene or child pornography, with intent to annoy, abuse, threaten, or harass another person;

    B. by means of a telecommunications device knowingly (i) makes, creates, or solicits, and (ii) initiates the transmission of, any comment, request, suggestion, proposal, image, or other communication which is obscene or child pornography, knowing that the recipient of the communication is under eighteen years of age, regardless of whether the maker of such communication placed the call or initiated the communication;

    C. makes a telephone call or utilizes a telecommunications device, whether or not conversation or communication ensues, without disclosing his identity and with intent to annoy, abuse, threaten, or harass any person at the called number or who receives the communications;

    D. makes or causes the telephone of another repeatedly or continuously to ring, with intent to harass any person at the called number; or

    E. makes repeated telephone calls or repeatedly initiates communication with a telecommunications device, during which conversation or communication ensues, solely to harass any person at the called number or who receives the communication; or

2. knowingly permits any telecommunications facility under his control to be used for any activity prohibited by paragraph (1) with the intent that it be used for such activity, shall be fined under title 18 or imprisoned not more than two years, or both.

Section 6.5

Stalking Statistics

Excerpted from "Stalking Victimization in the United States,"
U.S. Department of Justice, January 2009.

During a twelve-month period an estimated fourteen in every one thousand persons age eighteen or older were victims of stalking.

An estimated 5.9 million U.S. residents age eighteen or older experienced behaviors consistent with either stalking or harassment in the twelve months preceding the SVS interview.[1] Of the 5.9 million victims, more than half experienced behavior that met the definition of stalking. Approximately fourteen per one thousand persons age eighteen or older experienced the repetitive behaviors associated with stalking in addition to feeling fear or experiencing behaviors that would cause a reasonable person to feel fear. Harassment victims, who experienced a course of conduct consistent with stalking but who did not report feeling fear, experienced these behaviors at a rate of ten victimizations per one thousand persons age eighteen or older.

About half (46 percent) of all stalking victims experienced at least one unwanted contact per week. Many victims of stalking reported being stalked over a period of months or years, and 11 percent of victims said they had been stalked for five years or more. The fears and emotional distress that stalking engenders are many and varied. About one in five victims feared bodily harm to themselves, and one in six feared for the safety of a child or other family member. About one in ten stalking victims feared being killed by the stalker. About four in ten stalkers threatened the victim or the victim's family, friends, co-workers, or family pet.

The most common type of stalking behavior victims experienced was unwanted phone calls and messages.

With the exception of receiving unwanted letters, e-mails, or other correspondence, stalking victims were more likely than harassment victims to experience all forms of unwanted behaviors. In particular, victims of stalking experienced higher levels of three unwanted behaviors most commonly associated with stalking. These included an offender following or spying on the victim, showing up at places without a legitimate reason, or waiting outside (or inside) places for the victim. Stalking victims were about three times more likely to report experiencing these three behaviors than individuals who were harassed. For example, 34 percent of stalking victims reported that the offender followed or spied on them, compared with 11 percent of harassment victims who reported experiencing this behavior. Thirty-one percent of stalking victims reported that the offenders showed up in places where they had no legitimate purpose being; approximately 10 percent of harassment victims reported this type of unwanted behavior. Also, 29 percent of stalking victims stated that the offender waited in places for them, while 8 percent of harassment victims reported this type of behavior.

Risk of victimization varies more for stalking than for harassment.

Females were at higher risk of stalking victimization than males. During the study period, females experienced twenty stalking victimizations per one thousand females age eighteen or older. The rate of stalking victimization for males was approximately seven per one thousand males age eighteen or older. Males and females were equally likely to experience harassment.

Age: As with victimization risk more generally, risk of being stalked diminished with age. Persons age eighteen to nineteen and twenty to twenty-four experienced the highest rates of stalking victimization. About thirty per one thousand persons age eighteen to nineteen and twenty-eight per one thousand persons age twenty to twenty-four were stalked during 2006.

Race and Hispanic origin of victim: Asians and Pacific Islanders (seven per one thousand persons age eighteen and older) were less likely to experience stalking than whites (fourteen per one thousand), blacks (twelve per one thousand), and persons of two or more races (thirty-two per one thousand). Despite apparent racial differences, no other consistent patterns of risk for stalking victimization emerged. Non-Hispanics were more likely than Hispanics to experience stalking. During the study period, non-Hispanics experienced about fourteen stalking victimizations per one thousand individuals age eighteen and older. The rate for Hispanics during this period was eleven stalking victimizations per one thousand persons age eighteen or older.

Marital status: The rate of stalking victimization for individuals who were divorced or separated was thirty-four per one thousand individuals age eighteen or older—a higher rate of victimization than for persons of other marital status. Individuals who had never been married (seventeen per one thousand individuals) were at a lower risk of stalking victimization than divorced or separated persons, but were at a higher risk of stalking victimization than persons who were married (nine per one thousand) or widowed (eight per one thousand).

Income: As with crime more generally, a pattern of decreasing risk for stalking victimization existed for persons residing in households with higher incomes. Individuals in households with an annual income under $7,500 and $7,500 to $14,999 were equally likely to be stalked but more likely to be victimized than were persons in households with an annual income at or above $25,000.

Victims were more likely to be stalked by an offender of the same age and race.

Offender age: Individuals were more likely to be stalked by offenders of similar age. Nearly half of victims age twenty-one to twenty-nine were stalked by offenders perceived to also be in their twenties, and 38 percent of victims age thirty to thirty-nine perceived the offender to also be in their thirties.

Race: Similar to other types of victimization, stalking is primarily intraracial in nature. Most (83 percent) white stalking victims perceived the offender to be white, compared to 66 percent of black stalking victims who perceived the offender to be black. This pattern of intraracial victimization changes for persons of other races. Despite apparent differences, persons of other races were equally likely to be stalked by an offender who was black, white, or of another race.[2]

Offender gender: Males were as likely to report being stalked by a male as a female offender. Forty-three percent of male stalking victims stated that the offender was female, while 41 percent of male victims stated that the offender was another male. Female victims of stalking were significantly more likely to be stalked by a male (67 percent) rather than a female (24 percent) offender.

Stalking is unlike most crimes because a course of conduct designed to create fear in another person does not necessarily require that the victim come into contact with the offender. For example, a victim may receive repeated threatening correspondence without knowing the source of the communication. Sixteen percent of male stalking victims and approximately 10 percent of female stalking victims were not able to identify the gender of the offender.

Number of offenders: About six in ten stalking victims stated that the perpetrator was a single offender. A much lower percentage of victims reported being stalked by two (18 percent) or three (13 percent) offenders.

Relationship: About a tenth of all victims were stalked by a stranger, and nearly three in four of all victims knew their offender in some capacity. Stalking victims most often identified the stalker as a former intimate (21.5 percent) or a friend, roommate, or neighbor (16.4 percent).

Employment status of the offender: Forty-two percent of stalking victims stated that the offender was employed during the time stalking occurred. Victims were equally likely to report that the offender was unemployed or that the victim was unable to ascertain the employment status of the offender.

Problems with the law: Thirty-six percent of stalking victims stated that the offender had some previous interaction with law enforcement. A similar percentage of victims (38 percent) were unable to identify whether the offender had problems with the law prior to the stalking victimization.

One in ten victims reported that the stalking started five years or more before the survey.

Over half of all victims reported that the stalking or harassment began "less than a year ago." Harassment victims had characteristically experienced the harassing behavior for a shorter period leading up to the interview (six months or less). Stalking victims were most likely to be stalked once or twice a week or with no set pattern. Nearly a quarter of all victims reported that they were stalked almost every day (16.9 percent) or at least once a day (6 percent).

Victim perception of why stalking began: The most common reasons victims perceived for the stalking were retaliation, anger, spite (37 percent), or desire to control the victim (33 percent). About one in six victims believed the stalking started to keep him or her in the relationship with the offender, and one in ten reported the stalking began while living with the offender. About a tenth of victims did not know why the stalking began.

Cyberstalking and electronic monitoring: More than one in four stalking victims reported some form of cyberstalking was used, such as e-mail (83 percent) or instant messaging (35 percent). Electronic monitoring was used to stalk one in thirteen victims. Video or digital cameras were equally likely as listening devices or bugs to be used to electronically monitor victims (46 percent and 42 percent). Global positioning system (GPS) technology comprised about a tenth of the electronic monitoring of stalking victims.

One in seven victims reported they moved as a result of the stalking.

The most common types of actions victims took to stop the stalking from continuing were to change usual activities outside of work or school, stay with family, or install caller ID or call blocking. The least frequent actions taken were to alter one's appearance or get pepper spray, a gun, or some other kind of weapon. Forty percent of stalking victims did not change their usual activities outside of work or school, take protective actions, or change their personal information.

Help from others: Seven in ten victims of stalking sought help to protect themselves or to stop the stalking. Victims were most likely to enlist the help of family or friends, followed by asking people not to release information about them (43 percent versus 33 percent). About 7 percent of victims contacted victim services, a shelter, or a helpline.

Reasons stalking stopped: At the time of the interview, three in five of the victims reported the stalking had stopped, while about two in five reported it was ongoing. The most common victim perceptions for why the unwanted contacts stopped were that the police warned the stalker (15.6 percent), the victim talked to the stalker (13.3 percent), or a friend or relative intervened (12.2 percent). About a tenth of victims attributed the cessation of the unwanted behavior to obtaining a restraining, protection, or stay away order.

Emotional impact: For stalking victims, the most common fear cited was not knowing what would happen next. Nine percent of stalking victims reported their worst fear was death. Twenty-nine percent of stalking victims feared the behavior would never stop. More than half of the stalking victims feared bodily harm to themselves, their child, or another family member.

More than seven in ten of all victims felt angry or annoyed at the beginning of the unwanted contacts or as they progressed. Stalking victims were about twice as likely as harassment victims to feel anxious or concerned at the beginning of the unwanted contacts (52.7 percent versus 25.4 percent). As the unwanted contacts progressed, about 15 percent of stalking victims felt depressed or sick, and 1 percent reported feeling suicidal.

Workplace impact: Of the 79 percent of stalking victims who had a job during the twelve months preceding the interview, about one in eight lost time from work because of fear for their safety or to pursue activities such as obtaining a restraining order or testifying in court. Seven percent of victims lost time from work for activities such as changing a phone number, moving, or fixing or replacing damaged property. For one in seven of these victims, a day or less was lost from work. More than half of victims lost five or more days from work. About 130,000 victims reported that they had been fired from or asked to leave their jobs because of the stalking.

Financial impact of stalking on victim: About three in ten of stalking victims accrued out-of-pocket costs for things such as attorney fees, damage to property, child care costs, moving expenses, or changing phone numbers. About a tenth of victims spent less than $250, while 13 percent spent $1,000 or more. About 296,000 stalking victims lost pay from work. Over half of the victims lost less than $1,000 of pay, and 8 percent of victims lost $5,000 in pay or more.

Stalkers commit various types of crimes against their victims.

Stalking offenders committed identity theft against about 204,000 victims. Over half of these victims had financial accounts opened or closed in their names or money taken from their accounts, and three in ten of these victims had items charged to their credit cards without their consent.

About 16 percent of all victims suffered property damage in conjunction with the stalking. Among stalking victims, the most common type of violent crime experienced in conjunction with stalking was to be hit, slapped, or knocked down (12.3 percent). About 6 percent of the stalking victims had a family member, friend, or co-worker who was attacked.

Weapon involvement and injuries: About 139,000 stalking victims were attacked with a weapon. Stalkers were equally likely to use a knife, blunt instrument, or other object, and 23 percent of the weapons used were handguns. Of the 279,000 victims who were injured in an attack, nearly all (99 percent) of these victims sustained minor bruises and other injuries. About a fifth sustained serious injuries, including gunshot or knife wounds, internal injuries, or broken bones.

Threats: Stalkers made one or more threats to 43 percent of victims. Stalking offenders were most likely to threaten to hit, slap, or otherwise harm the victim (13.6 percent) or to kill the victim (12.1 percent). Somewhat less likely was the stalker threatening to kill him- or herself (9.2 percent). Less than 5 percent of the threats involved harm to a child, friend, co-worker, pet, or the threat of rape or sexual assault.

Notes

1. To place this estimate in perspective, there were about 5.2 million violent crimes—rape/sexual assault, robbery, aggravated assault, and simple assault—committed in 2005.

2. Other races include American Indians, Alaska Natives, Asians, Native Hawaiians, other Pacific Islanders, and persons identifying two or more races.

Chapter 7

Sexual Harassment

Chapter Contents

Section 7.1

What Is Sexual Harassment?

Definition of Sexual Harassment

(The following is based on a definition provided by the Equal Employment Opportunity commission [EEOC]. The underlined portions reflect coverage of students under Title XI of the Educational Amendments of 1971.)

Unwelcome sexual advances, requests for sexual favors, and other verbal or physical conduct of a sexual nature.

When:

1. submission to such conduct is made either explicitly or implicitly as term or condition of person's employment or a student's academic success;

2. submission to or rejection of such conduct by an individual is used as the basis for employment or academic decisions affecting such individuals;

3. such conduct unreasonably interferes with an individual's work or academic performance or creates an intimidating, hostile, or offensive working or learning environment.

Over the years, the courts have used the above definition to define two distinct forms of illegal sexual harassment.

1. Quid pro quo, which means "this for that" or "something for something" and is typified by the first two conditions above.

2. Hostile environment, which is typified by the third condition above.

Yardstick for Evaluating Behaviors That May Be Sexual Harassment

For a common sense, everyday way of looking at behavior to help recognize sexual harassment when it occurs, evaluate the behavior using the following "yardstick."

Sexual harassment is behavior that:

1. is unwanted or unwelcome;

2. is sexual in nature or gender-based;

3. is severe, pervasive, and/or repeated;

4. has an adverse impact on the workplace or academic environment.

It is important to note that sexual harassment often occurs in the context of a relationship where one person has more formal power that the other (such as a supervisor over an employee, or a faculty member over a student) or more informal power (such as one peer over another).

Sexual Harassment Comes in Many Forms

The following are behaviors which could be viewed as sexual harassment when they are unwelcome.

Verbal

- Whistling or making cat calls at someone

- Making sexual comments about a person's clothing or body

- Telling sexual jokes or stories

- Asking personal questions about sexual life, fantasies, preferences, or history

- Repeatedly "asking out" a person who is not interested

- Turning work discussions to sexual topics

- Referring to an adult woman or man as a hunk, doll, babe, or honey

- Telling lies or spreading rumors about a person's personal sex life

Nonverbal

- Paying unwanted attention to someone (i.e., staring, following, blocking a person's path)

- Displaying sexually suggestive visuals

- Making facial expressions such as winking, throwing kisses, or licking

- Giving personal gifts of a sexual nature

- Making sexual gestures with hands or through body movements

Physical

- Hanging around, standing close, or brushing up against a person

- Touching a person's clothing, hair, or body (to include giving a massage around the neck and shoulders)

- Touching or rubbing oneself sexually around another person

- Hugging, kissing, patting, or stroking

What to Do If You Are Sexually Harassed

If you feel you are the victim of sexual harassment, you should try to immediately undertake some course of action. The Affirmative Action/Equal Opportunity (AA/EO) Office can provide advice and/or assistance to you in a timely, professional, and confidential manner. Remember, sexual harassment is against the law, it is not your fault and it does not "come with the job." Here are some specific options that you might want to consider:

1. Talk to the harasser if possible. Tell him or her that you find the behavior offensive. Describe how the harassment negatively affects your work.

2. Continue going to classes/work.

3. Document all sexual harassment incidents or conversations about the incidents. Record the date, time, place, people involved, and who said what to whom.

4. Consider talking to others (co-workers/student) to see if they have experienced sexual harassment.

5. Put your objection to the harassment in writing, sending a copy by registered mail to the harasser and keeping one in you file. Say:

    - On "this date" you did "this."

    - It made me feel "this."

    - I want "this" to happen next (i.e., I want "this" to stop).

Section 7.2

Sexual Harassment in the Workplace and in Schools

"Sexual Harassment," © RAINN (Rape, Abuse and Incest National Network), www.rainn.org. All rights reserved. Reprinted with permission. Immediate crisis help and information is available twenty-four hours per day/seven days per week from the National Sexual Assault Hotline, 800-656-HOPE (4673), or the National Sexual Assault Online Hotline at http://online.rainn.org.

Sexual harassment: unwelcome sexual advances, requests for sexual favors, and other verbal or physical conduct of a sexual nature in which submission to or rejection of such conduct explicitly or implicitly affects an individual's work or school performance or creates an intimidating, hostile, or offensive work or school environment.

Sexual Harassment in the Workplace

Two Types of Sexual Harassment

- **Quid pro quo:** When a perpetrator makes conditions of employment contingent on the victim providing sexual favors. This type of harassment is less common.

- **Hostile environment:** When unwelcome, severe, and persistent sexual conduct on the part of a perpetrator creates an uncomfortable and hostile environment (e.g., jokes, lewd postures, leering, inappropriate touching, rape, etc.). This type of harassment constitutes up to 95 percent of all sexual harassment cases.

Variety of Circumstances

- Survivor and harasser do not have to be of different genders; both can be men, both women, or they can be different genders.

- Similarly, as with sexual assault, women can be perpetrators.

- The harasser can be a supervisor, an agent of the employer, a supervisor in another area, a co-worker, or a nonemployee.

- The survivor does not have to be the person that is directly harassed. It can be anyone affected by the offensive conduct.

- Unlawful sexual harassment may occur without economic injury to or discharge of the survivor.

- The harasser's conduct must be unwelcome.

Common Emotional and Physical Reactions

- Poor concentration at work
- Stress on personal relationships
- Fear/anxiety
- Debilitating depression
- Sleep/weight problems
- Alcohol or drug use
- Staff turnover
- Increased absenteeism
- Tarnished company reputation
- Increased payouts for sick leave and medical benefits
- Vulnerability to hostile confrontations
- Legal and consultant costs
- Lower staff productivity
- Poor staff morale
- Less teamwork

Options for Action

- **Say "No" clearly:** Express in direct language (verbal or written) that behavior must stop.

- **Document the harassment:** Keep a written log, keep track of dates, times, and behavior.

- **Get emotional support:** Friends/family can be good outlets.

- **Document your work:** Keep copies of performance evaluations and memos that attest to the quality of your work.

- **Explore company channels:** Talk to a supervisor and/or contact the personnel officer or human resources department.

- **File a complaint:** If the problem can't be solved through company policy, you may choose to pursue a legal remedy.

Sexual Harassment in the Schools

Sexual harassment is not limited to offices and work arenas. Increasingly, sexual harassment is being displayed in our nation's schools.

It Can Take Milder Forms

- Looks
- Jokes
- Graffiti on bathroom walls
- Comments about body parts

Or More Severe Forms

- Physical intrusion into personal space
- Grabbing
- Brushed up against in a sexual way

Common Reactions

- Less confident
- More self-conscious
- Ashamed
- Embarrassed
- Consequently lower grades

Part Two

Intimate Partner Abuse

Chapter 8

Types of Intimate Partner Abuse

Chapter Contents

Section 8.1

Primary Forms of Intimate Partner Abuse

Excerpted from "Intimate Partner Violence: Definitions,"
U.S. Centers for Disease Control and Prevention, September 20, 2010.

Intimate partner violence (IPV) is a serious, preventable public health problem that affects millions of Americans. The term "intimate partner violence" describes physical, sexual, or psychological harm by a current or former partner or spouse. This type of violence can occur among heterosexual or same-sex couples and does not require sexual intimacy.

IPV can vary in frequency and severity. It occurs on a continuum, ranging from one hit that may or may not impact the victim to chronic, severe battering.

There are four main types of intimate partner violence (Saltzman et al. 2002):

- Physical violence is the intentional use of physical force with the potential for causing death, disability, injury, or harm. Physical violence includes, but is not limited to, scratching; pushing; shoving; throwing; grabbing; biting; choking; shaking; slapping; punching; burning; use of a weapon; and use of restraints or one's body, size, or strength against another person.

- Sexual violence is divided into three categories: (1) use of physical force to compel a person to engage in a sexual act against his or her will, whether or not the act is completed; (2) attempted or completed sex act involving a person who is unable to understand the nature or condition of the act, to decline participation, or to communicate unwillingness to engage in the sexual act, for example, because of illness, disability, or the influence of alcohol or other drugs, or because of intimidation or pressure; and (3) abusive sexual contact.

- Threats of physical or sexual violence use words, gestures, or weapons to communicate the intent to cause death, disability, injury, or physical harm.

- Psychological/emotional violence involves trauma to the victim caused by acts, threats of acts, or coercive tactics. Psychological/emotional abuse can include, but is not limited to, humiliating the victim, controlling what the victim can and cannot do, withholding information from the victim, deliberately doing something to make the victim feel diminished or embarrassed, isolating the victim from friends and family, and denying the victim access to money or other basic resources. It is considered psychological/emotional violence when there has been prior physical or sexual violence or prior threat of physical or sexual violence. In addition, stalking is often included among the types of IPV. Stalking generally refers to "harassing or threatening behavior that an individual engages in repeatedly, such as following a person, appearing at a person's home or place of business, making harassing phone calls, leaving written messages or objects, or vandalizing a person's property" (Tjaden & Thoennes 1998).

References

Saltzman LE, Fanslow JL, McMahon PM, Shelley GA. Intimate partner violence surveillance: uniform definitions and recommended data elements, version 1.0. Atlanta, GA: Centers for Disease Control and Prevention, National Center for Injury Prevention and Control; 2002.

Tjaden P, Thoennes N. *Stalking in America: Findings from the National Violence Against Women Survey.* Washington, DC: Department of Justice (US); 1998. Publication No. NCJ 169592. Available from: http://www.ncjrs.gov/pdf.

Section 8.2

Physical Abuse

Physical abuse is any intentional and unwanted contact with you or something close to your body. Sometimes abusive behavior does not cause pain or even leave a bruise, but it's still unhealthy. Examples of physical abuse are:

- scratching, punching, biting, strangling, or kicking;
- throwing something at you such as a phone, book, shoe, or plate;
- pulling your hair;
- pushing or pulling you;
- grabbing your clothing;
- using a gun, knife, box cutter, bat, mace, or other weapon;
- smacking your bottom;
- forcing you to have sex or perform a sexual act;
- grabbing your face to make you look at them;
- grabbing you to prevent you from leaving or to force you to go somewhere.

Escaping Physical Abuse

Start by learning that you are not alone. More than one in ten high school students have already experienced some form of physical aggression from a dating partner, and many of these teens did not know what to do when it happened. If you are in a similar situation:

- realize this behavior is wrong;
- talk to an adult, friend, or family member that you trust;

- create a safety plan;

- consider getting a restraining order;

- do not accept or make excuses for your partner's abusive behavior;

- remember that physical abuse is never your fault.

Protecting Yourself from Physical Abuse

Unhealthy or abusive relationships usually get worse. It is important to know the warning signs to prevent more serious harm. If you are in an unhealthy or abusive relationship, consider making a safety plan.

Section 8.3

Sexual Abuse

Sexual abuse refers to any action that pressures or coerces someone to do something sexually they don't want to do. It can also refer to behavior that impacts a person's ability to control their sexual activity or the circumstances in which sexual activity occurs, including oral sex, rape, or restricting access to birth control and condoms. Some examples of sexual assault and abuse are:

- unwanted kissing or touching;

- unwanted rough or violent sexual activity;

- rape or attempted rape;

- refusing to use condoms or restricting someone's access to birth control;

- keeping someone from protecting themselves from sexually transmitted infections (STIs).

- sexual contact with someone who is very drunk, drugged, unconscious, or otherwise unable to give a clear and informed "yes" or "no";

- threatening or pressuring someone into unwanted sexual activity.

Keep in Mind

- Everyone has the right to decide what they do or don't want to do sexually. Not all sexual assaults are violent "attacks."

- Most victims of sexual assault know the assailant.

- Both men and women can be victims of sexual abuse.

- Both men and women can be perpetrators of sexual abuse.

- Sexual abuse can occur in same-sex and opposite-sex relationships.

- Sexual abuse can occur between two people who have been sexual with each other before, including people who are married or dating.

What to Do

If you have been sexually assaulted, first get to a safe place away from the attacker. You may be scared, angry, and confused, but remember the abuse was in no way your fault. You have options. You can:

- **Contact someone you trust:** Many people feel fear, guilt, anger, shame, and/or shock after they have been sexually assaulted. Having someone there to support you as you deal with these emotions can make a big difference. It may be helpful to speak with a counselor, someone at a sexual assault hotline, or a support group.

- **Report what happened to the police:** If you do decide to report what happened, you will have a stronger case if you do not alter or destroy any evidence. This means don't shower, wash your hair or body, comb your hair, or change your clothes, even if that is hard to do. If you are nervous about going to the police station, it may help to bring a friend with you. There may also be sexual assault advocates in your area who can assist you and answer your questions.

- **Go to an emergency room or health clinic:** It is very important for you to seek healthcare as soon as you can after being assaulted. You will be treated for any injuries and offered medications to help prevent pregnancy and STIs.

Section 8.4

Emotional Abuse

Emotional abuse is any behavior used to control and mistreat another person.

Many people believe if they're not being physically hurt by their partner, they're not being abused. This is not true.

If you are being treated in a way that makes you upset, ashamed, or embarrassed, you may be experiencing emotional abuse.

Emotional abuse follows a pattern; it happens over and over.

If your partner:

- says mean things to you;

- doesn't let you make decisions;

- threatens you;

- keeps you away from friends, family, and co-workers;

- ignores your feelings;

- puts you down;

- calls you names;

- insults you;

- keeps you from sleeping;

- does things that make you feel crazy;

- tells you and others that you're crazy;

- tells you your decisions are bad;

this is emotional abuse.

Emotional abuse goes with other forms of abuse but may also happen on its own.

If you've ever been told anything like this by your partner:

- "You're so stupid!"
- "Nobody else would ever want you."
- "You look disgusting."
- "You always twist things around."
- "I don't know why I put up with you!"
- "You'll never be good enough to do that."
- "You're crazy!"

this is emotional abuse.

Emotional abuse . . .

- does not get better over time. It only gets worse.
- can be more hurtful than physical abuse.
- can make you feel afraid, vulnerable, powerless, and isolated.
- can cause:
  - depression
  - anxiety
  - constant headaches
  - back, leg, arm, and stomach problems.

Living with verbal abuse such as:

- blaming,
- ridiculing,
- insulting,
- swearing,
- yelling,
- threatening, and/or
- shaming

can lower your self-respect and make you feel useless and worth-less.

Relationship Bill of Rights

I have the right:

- to an equal and healthy relationship with my partner
- to be respected
- to change my mind
- to kindness from my partner
- to emotional support
- to be listened to politely by my partner
- to have my own opinions, even if my partner disagrees
- to have my own feelings
- to clear and honest answers to questions that concern me
- to live free from accusation and blame
- to live free from criticism and judgment
- to have my work and interests spoken of with respect
- to encouragement
- to live free from emotional and physical threat
- to live free from angry outburst and rage
- to be called by no name that hurts, shames, or puts me down
- to be respectfully asked rather than ordered
- to be myself as long as I am respectful of others
- to not have physical or sexual contact with my partner when I choose

If you have been abused:

- you are not alone;
- it is not your fault;
- no one ever deserves to be abused in any way.

Section 8.5

Verbal Abuse

Verbal abuse refers to the use of language as a means to control or subordinate another person for either self-gratification or to impose one's view or will on another or to gain an unfair advantage in resolving a dispute. While both parties subject to a dispute may use inappropriate language with the other, verbal abuse has the distinction of one party typically causing more distress to the other party, and causing insecurities in that party typically for the purpose of exploitation. In other words, the person wielding the verbal abuse does so to gain an advantage over the abused typically to his or her own desire.

Verbal abuse takes several forms, including threats, foul or demeaning language, hostile tone or volume, intensity of delivery whether loud or quiet, and sarcasm.

Threats are meant to scare or intimidate a person into submission. Threats can be of bodily harm to a person or other family, friends, or pets of the person. Threats can also include divulging secrets or making outright lies about a person to either embarrass or cause to look bad in the eyes of others. Threats can also be to property, as in telling a person they will destroy something, and threats can be financial, thus seeking to hold a person hostage by intimating economic hardship. Even the legal system can be used against another and thus threats include telling another person they will unjustly use the legal system to gain an unfair advantage.

Foul or demeaning language refers to using swear words or words like *stupid* or *idiot* to cause a person to feel less about her or himself. Thus language is used to put the other person down and gain a psychological advantage where the abuser thus presents him or herself as superior. Here, one person belittles the other through the use of language.

Hostile tone, volume, or intensity of deliver may appear as shouting, yelling, or screaming or, alternately, talking quietly yet intensely, so as to instill fear. Typically this form of verbal abuse causes the victim to acquiesce for fear of self-harm, particularly scaring the person that matters might escalate to include physical abuse.

Sarcasm refers to the use of humor to mask belittling or threatening language. Thus the information is delivered in such a way so as to provide two distinct messages. The superficial message is that the intention is humor or levity while the deeper message is one that belittles, demeans, or threatens. Because the deliverer uses humor to mask the message, the deliverer will try to deny the deeper message if confronted, thus leaving the receiver somewhat disarmed and unable to defend against the deeper message.

Typically the person using sarcasm denies the deeper message so as to absolve him- or herself from any wrongdoing and more insidiously try to infer there is something wrong with the receiver for their misinterpretation. This obfuscation of the receiver's reality in this scenario is also a form of psychological abuse.

When the receiver gets angry enough at the sarcasm, the person who is sarcastic typically then uses the receiver's display of anger as their evidence that any problem in the relationship originates with the receiver's anger. Thus sarcasm as verbal abuse is a potent form of gaining an advantage in a dispute and is a potent means to control another to one's gain.

Underneath all forms of verbal abuse are issues of power and control. Gaining an advantage to the detriment of the other by abusive means is inherently wrong and can cause significant emotional and psychological distress.

If you are in a lopsided relationship where your partner uses verbal abuse in any form to consistently assert their will over your own, then you may require counseling and other forms of support to end the abuse and either establish an appropriate equilibrium to the relationship or else provide you an opportunity to leave safely and heal from the wounds of the abuse.

Verbal abuse is real and is destructive to relationships and one's well-being. Support and relief can be obtained through local counseling centers. If you are unfamiliar with resources in your area, consult your physician or local child welfare agency, local YWCA/YMCA, women's shelter, or police.

Section 8.6

Economic Abuse

Financial abuse can be very subtle—telling you what you can and cannot buy or requiring you to share control of your bank accounts. At no point does someone with whom you are in a relationship have the right to use money or how you spend it to control you.

Here are some examples of financially abusive behavior:

- Giving you an allowance and closely watching what you buy.

- Placing your paycheck in their account and denying you access to it.

- Keeping you from seeing shared bank accounts or records.

- Forbidding you to work or limiting the hours you do.

- Preventing you from going to work by taking your car or keys.

- Getting you fired by harassing you, your employer, or co-workers on the job.

- Hiding or stealing your student financial aid check or outside financial support.

- Using your social security number to obtain credit without your permission.

- Using your child's social security number to claim an income tax refund without your permission.

- Maxing out your credit cards without your permission.

- Refusing to give you money, food, rent, medicine, or clothing.

- Causing visible bruises and scars so that you are too embarrassed to go to work.

- Using funds from your children's tuition or a joint savings account without your knowledge.

- Spending money on themselves but not allowing you to do the same.

I'm Experiencing Financial Abuse

If your partner does any of these things, you are probably in an unhealthy or abusive relationship. Financial abuse is usually coupled with emotional or physical abuse.

If you are not in control over your finances, or if your partner has removed money from your bank account, it can seem very scary to leave an abusive relationship. There are many organizations who can help you "get back on your feet" and get control over your finances—some even provide short-term loans to cover important expenses as you escape an abusive relationship.

You may also want to talk to someone you trust, like a friend, family member, or legal professional, about getting a protection order. Whether you decide to leave or stay, consider making a safety plan that includes setting aside funds in a secret location.

Section 8.7

Digital Abuse

Digital abuse is the use of technologies such as texting and social networking to bully, harass, stalk, or intimidate a partner. Often this behavior is a form of verbal or emotional abuse perpetrated online.

In a healthy relationship, all communication is respectful, whether in person, online, or by phone. It is never ok for someone to do or say anything that makes you feel bad, lowers your self-esteem, or manipulates you. You may be experiencing digital abuse if your partner:

- tells you who you can or can't be friends with on Facebook and other sites;
- sends you negative, insulting, or even threatening e-mails, Facebook messages, tweets, DMs, or other messages online;
- uses sites like Facebook, Twitter, foursquare, and others to keep constant tabs on you;
- puts you down in their status updates;
- sends you unwanted, explicit pictures and demands you send some in return;
- pressures you to send explicit video;
- steals or insists to be given your passwords;
- constantly texts you and makes you feel like you can't be separated from your phone for fear that you will be punished;
- looks through your phone frequently, checks up on your pictures, texts, and outgoing calls.

You never deserve to be mistreated, online or off. If you're experiencing digital abuse, we encourage you to seek help. Remember:

- Your partner should respect your relationship boundaries.

- It is ok to turn off your phone. You have the right to be alone and spend time with friends and family without your partner getting angry.

- You do not have to text any pictures or statements that you are uncomfortable sending, especially nude or partially nude photos, known as "sexting."

- You lose control of any electronic message once your partner receives it. They may forward it, so don't send anything you fear could be seen by others.

- You do not have to share your passwords with anyone.

- Know your privacy settings. Social networks such as Facebook allow the user to control how their information is shared and who has access to it. These are often customizable and are found in the privacy section of the site. Remember, registering for some applications (apps) require you to change your privacy settings.

- Be mindful when using check-ins like Facebook Places and four-square. Letting an abusive partner know where you are could be dangerous. Also, always ask your friends if it's ok for you to check them in. You never know if they are trying to keep their location secret.

Chapter 9

When Abuse Turns Deadly

Chapter Contents

Section 9.1

Prevalence of Intimate Partner Homicide

Excerpted from "Intimate Partner Violence,"
U.S. Department of Justice, April 2012.

Fatal intimate partner violence includes homicide or murder and non-negligent manslaughter, defined as the willful killing of one human being by another:

- In 2007 intimate partners committed 14 percent of all homicides in the United States. The total estimated number of intimate partner homicide victims in 2007 was 2,340, including 1,640 females and 700 males.

- Females made up 70 percent of victims killed by an intimate partner in 2007, a proportion that has changed very little since 1993.

- Females were killed by intimate partners at twice the rate of males. In 2007 the rate of intimate partner homicide for females was 1.07 per 100,000 female residents, compared to 0.47 per 100,000 male residents.

- Between 1993 and 2007 the total number of homicide victims in the United States fell 31 percent, with a somewhat greater decline for females (-34 percent) than males (-30 percent). Homicide victims killed by intimate partners fell 29 percent, with a greater decline for males (-36 percent) than females (-26 percent).

- Homicide victims killed by an intimate partner declined from an estimated 3,300 in 1993 to an estimated 2,340 in 2007.

- Between 1993 and 2007, female victims killed by an intimate partner declined from 2,200 to 1,640 victims, and male intimate partner homicide victims declined from 1,100 to 700 victims.

Section 9.2

Intimate Partner Strangulation

"Strangulation Assaults in Domestic Violence Cases," by Manisha Joshi, Ph.D., © 2009 Evelyn Jacobs Ortner Center on Family Violence (http://www .sp2.upenn.edu/ortner). All rights reserved. Reprinted with permission.

Strangulation is one of the most lethal forms of violence used by men against their female intimate partners. Strangulation is a form of asphyxia (lack of oxygen) in which blood vessels and air passages are closed as a result of external pressure on the neck.[1] Strangulation can induce the loss of consciousness within about ten seconds and death within four to five minutes.[2] Strangulation is often incorrectly referred to as "choking," which involves internal blocking of the trachea (windpipe) by a foreign object like food.[1] There are three forms of strangulation: hanging, manual (e.g., using one hand, two hands, forearm, kneeling on the victim), and ligature (e.g., using telephone wire, electrical cord, shoelace, piece of clothing).[1] Manual strangulation is the most common form of strangulation used in domestic violence cases.[2]

The act of strangulation symbolizes an abuser's power and control over the victim. The victim is completely overwhelmed by the abuser; she vigorously struggles for air, and is at the mercy of the abuser for her life. Some have asserted that there can be few more frightening experiences than feeling short of breath without any recourse.[3] A single traumatic experience of strangulation or the threat of it may instill so much fear that the victim can get trapped in a pattern of control by the abuser and made vulnerable to further abuse:

- Studies indicate that 23 to 68 percent of women victims of domestic violence have experienced at least one strangulation assault by a male partner during their lifetime;[4,5] and 33 to 47.3 percent of women report that their partner had tried to strangle them in the past year.[6,7]

- Strangulation can be a recurring form of violence in abused women's lives. In a study of sixty-two abused women who came to a shelter or a violence prevention center, 68 percent (n = 42) had a history of strangulation, and on an average, each woman had been strangled 5.3 times in their intimate relationships.[5]

- Strangulation can have substantial physical (e.g., dizziness, nausea, sore throat, voice changes, throat and neck injuries, breathing problems, swallowing problems, ringing in the ears, vision change), neurological (e.g., eyelid droop, facial droop, left or right side weakness, loss of sensation, loss of memory, paralysis), and psychological (e.g., post-traumatic stress disorder [PTSD], depression, suicidal ideation, insomnia) health effects.[1,2,5] And, the higher the number of strangulation attempts experienced, the higher the number of adverse health conditions experienced by victims.[8]

- As compared to other forms of physical violence, strangulation, often leaves no marks or any other external evidence on the skin.[1,2] In a study of police records of three hundred strangulation cases, victims did not have any visible injury in 50 percent of the cases and in 35 percent of the cases the injuries were too minor for the police to photograph.[2] The difficulty in detecting strangulation is a challenge for law enforcement and medical professionals, which helps make it a particularly useful means of intimidation and harm for an abuser.

- Strangulation is a significant risk factor for attempted or completed homicide of women by their male intimates. In a study of fifty-seven women who were killed by a male partner during 1995–96 in Chicago, 53 percent of the victims had experienced strangulation in the preceding year and 18 percent of the victims had been killed by strangulation.[7] In another study of women victims it was found that 45 percent of the attempted homicide victims and 43 percent of the homicide victims had been strangled in the past year by their male partner, as compared to 10%percent of the victims who were abused but were neither a homicide or an attempted homicide victim.[9]

- Strangulation may indicate an ongoing pattern of severe violence in the lives of women victims. In a study of women who came to a Chicago hospital for any health-related reason and had experienced domestic violence in the past year, 210 women were interviewed twice. And, of the 68 women whose partner had tried to strangle them in the year before the initial interview, 65 percent reported in the follow-up interview that they experienced a severe incident in the period after the initial interview (e.g., incident resulting in permanent injury, internal injury, head injury, broken bones; threat or attack with a weapon; being completely "beaten up," strangled, or burned).[7]

- Strangulation might not be the only method of abuse during individual assaults. In a study of women victims who had experienced strangulation, 88 percent of them had also experienced other types of abuse (physical, verbal, sexual) in the same incident.[5]

- In a large proportion of strangulation assaults, children are present during the assault. In the earlier mentioned study of police records of three hundred strangulation cases, children witnessed the strangulation assault in at least 41 percent of the cases. And this number is likely an underestimate because the victim might be reluctant to report that a child was present or because the police might have failed to document the presence of children in some cases.[2]

References

1. Strack, G. B., and McClane, G. E. (1999, May). How to improve your investigation and prosecution of strangulation cases. Retrieved Jan 10, 2008, from http://www.ncdsv.org/images/strangulation_article.pdf

2. Strack, G.B., McClane, G.E., Hawley, D. (2001). A review of 300 attempted strangulation cases: Criminal legal issues. *Journal of Emergency Medicine*, 21, 303–9.

3. Banzett, R. B., and Moosavi, S. H. (2001, March/April). Dyspnea and pain: Similarities and contrasts between two very unpleasant sensations. *APS Bulletin*, 11(1). Retrieved April 1, 2008, from http://www.ampainsoc.org/pub/bulletin/mar01/upda1.htm

4. Berrios, D. C., and Grady, D. (1991). Domestic violence: Risk factors and outcomes. *Western Journal of Medicine*, 155,133–35.

5. Wilbur, L., Highley, M., Hatfield, J., Surprenant, Z., Taliaferro, E., and Smith, D.J., et al. (2001). Survey results of women who have been strangled while in an abusive relationship. *Journal of Emergency Medicine*, 21, 297–302.

6. Roberts, G. L., O'Toole, B. I., Raphael, B., Lawrence, J. M., and Ashby, R. (1996). Prevalence study of domestic violence victims

in an emergency department. *Annals of Emergency Medicine,* 27, 747–53

7. Block, C. R., Devitt, C. O., Fonda, D., Fugate, M., Martin, C., McFarlane, J., et al. (2000). *The Chicago Women's Health Study: Risk of serious injury or death in intimate violence: A collaborative research project.* Washington, DC: U.S. Department of Justice, National Institute of Justice.

8. Smith, D. J., Mills, T., and Taliaferro, E. H. (2001). Frequency and relationship of reported symptomology in victims of intimate partner violence: the effect of multiple strangulation attacks. *Journal of Emergency Medicine,* 21, 323–29.

9. Glass, N., Laughon, K., Campbell, J. C., Block, R. B., Hanson, G., and Sharps, P.S. (2008). Strangulation is an important risk factor for attempted and completed femicides. *Journal of Emergency Medicine,* 35, 329–35.

Section 9.3

Firearms and Domestic Violence

"Intimate Partner Violence and Firearms," reprinted with permission from the Johns Hopkins Center for Gun Policy and Research, Bloomberg School of Public Health (http://www.jhsph.edu/gunpolicy). © 2010 Johns Hopkins University. All rights reserved.

According to the Centers for Disease Control and Prevention (CDC), "intimate partner violence" (IPV) is actual or threatened physical or sexual violence or psychological and emotional abuse directed toward a spouse, ex-spouse, current or former boyfriend or girlfriend, or current or former dating partner. Intimate partners may be heterosexual or of the same sex.[1]

Scope of the Problem

Twenty-two percent of women and 7 percent of men report that they have been physically assaulted by an intimate partner in their lifetime. Among female victims of IPV, 4 percent reported having been threatened with a gun by an intimate partner, and 1 percent sustained firearm injuries in these assaults.[2, a]

In 2007, there were more than eighteen thousand homicides in the United States.[3] While men are more likely to be homicide victims, women are over three and a half times more likely to be killed by an intimate partner, compared to men.[4]

According to federal data collected from police departments, in 2005 approximately 40 percent of female homicide victims ages fifteen to fifty were killed by either a current or former intimate partner.[b] In over half (55 percent) of these cases, the perpetrator used a gun. Among male victims fifteen to fifty years of age, 2 percent were killed by either a current or former intimate partner. About 37 percent of the male intimate partner homicides involved a gun.[4]

Women are at a greater danger of being killed by a current or former intimate partner than by a stranger. More than twice as many women are killed by a husband or intimate acquaintance than are killed by a stranger using a gun, a knife, or any other means.[5]

Firearm Access and Intimate Partner Homicide

Compared to homes without guns, the presence of guns in the home is associated with a threefold increased homicide risk within the home. The risk connected to gun ownership increases to eightfold when the offender is an intimate partner or relative of the victim, and is twenty times higher when previous domestic violence exists.[6]

A study of risk factors for violent death of women in the home found that women living in homes with one or more guns were more than three times more likely to be killed in their homes. The same study concluded that women killed by a spouse, intimate acquaintance, or close relative were seven times more likely to live in homes with one or more guns and fourteen times more likely to have a history of prior domestic violence compared to women killed by nonintimate acquaintances.[7]

Family and intimate assaults with firearms are twelve times more likely to result in death than nonfirearm assaults. This research suggests that limiting access to guns will result in less lethal family and intimate assaults.[8]

A study of women physically abused by current or former intimate partners revealed a fivefold increased risk of the partner murdering the woman when the partner owned a firearm. In fact,[9] homicide risks were found to be 50 percent higher for female handgun purchasers in California compared with licensed drivers matched by sex, race, and age group.[10] Among the women handgun purchasers who were murdered, 45 percent were killed by an intimate partner using a gun. In contrast, 20 percent of all women murdered in California during the study period were killed with a gun by an intimate partner.[11]

Policies to Prevent Batterers' Access to Firearms

Keeping Guns Out of the Hands of Abusers Subject to Restraining Orders

In 1994, Congress enacted the Violent Crime Control and Law Enforcement Act. This law expanded the list of people prohibited from purchasing and possessing firearms to include individuals subject to a court order restraining them from "harassing, stalking, or threatening an intimate partner" or "engaging in other conduct that would place an intimate partner in reasonable fear of bodily injury." This restriction applies only to court orders in which the alleged batterer was present (ex parte orders do not apply). Some states implemented policies to prohibit gun ownership for batterers with restraining orders prior to the passage of federal legislation in 1994.

Prohibiting Firearm Purchase by Domestic Violence Misdemeanants

Under federal law established by the Lautenberg Amendment in 1996,[c] an individual convicted of a domestic violence misdemeanor is prohibited from possessing a firearm.

A recent federal report on the National Instant Criminal Background Check System (NICS) found that from 1998–2001, 14 percent of the two hundred thousand denials for gun purchases generated by NICS were the result of domestic violence misdemeanor convictions. During the same period, the ATF received almost three thousand referrals to retrieve firearms sold to individuals who were ineligible to purchase firearms due to a domestic violence misdemeanor. These sales—representing 26 percent of all referrals to retrieve firearms from proscribed users—occurred because authorities did not complete the background check within the maximum time allowed by federal law (three days). At least a dozen states have laws allowing law enforcement more than the federal three-day limit to complete the background check.[12]

Recent research indicates that laws to restrict firearm purchase for batterers subject to restraining orders are associated with a 10 percent reduction in rates of intimate homicide of women and a 13 percent reduction in rates of intimate homicide of women with firearms.

However, such laws are only effective in reducing intimate partner homicides in states that have implemented a system to screen potential firearms purchasers for restraining orders. No effect on intimate partner homicide was measured for laws that restrict firearm access for domestic violence misdemeanants.[13]

Additional Policy Approaches to the Prevention of Firearm-Related Intimate Partner Violence

State laws vary with regard to firearms and intimate partner violence. Such laws are an important complement to the federal laws discussed above. Some states' laws do not address the topic and rely exclusively on federal law; some states enjoy extensive regulatory systems that far exceed federal law; and other states' laws extend slightly beyond federal protections.

Most state laws that address batterers' access to guns and intimate partner violence fall into one of three categories:

1. Laws that authorize law enforcement officers to seize guns when responding to domestic violence calls;

2. Laws that permit judges to order batterers to surrender their firearms through court protective orders; and

3. Laws that prohibit people with domestic violence offenses from obtaining a permit to carry concealed firearms.

As of mid-2004, eighteen states had a law that authorized police to remove firearms when responding to a domestic violence incident. Sixteen state codes included provisions that allow courts to order firearms removed when issuing a protective order. Ten states had both laws; twenty-six states had neither law. Even within these groups, state laws varied considerably. For example, of the eighteen states that permitted police officers to remove guns when responding to a domestic violence call, eight required police to do so, seven allowed but did not require gun removal, and three others varied by circumstance. States also differ with regard to whether police officers may confiscate ammunition, whether they are authorized to remove the gun if the abuser is not arrested, which guns may be seized (e.g., only those used in the domestic violence incident in question), and whether the time frame for the return of seized firearms is specified.[14]

Notes

a. For these data, "intimate partner" excludes former intimate partners who were never married.

b. For three reasons, it is likely that these figures are lower than the actual prevalence. First, the data represent approximately 85–90 percent of police department reports, and therefore do not offer a complete measure of homicides. Second, Federal Bureau of Investigation (FBI) data do not include a category for former dating relationships (e.g., ex-boyfriend). Third, many relationships reported as "friends" or "acquaintances" may in fact be current or former intimate partners.

c. Section 658 of Public Law 104-208.

References

1. National Center for Injury Prevention and Control. *Injury Fact Book, 2001–2002*. Atlanta, GA: Centers for Disease Control and Prevention; 2001.

2. Tjaden P, Thoennes N. *Full Report of the Prevalence, Incidence, and Consequences of Intimate Partner Violence Against Women: Findings from the National Violence Against Women Survey*. Washington D.C.: U.S. Department of Justice; 2000.

3. Centers for Disease Control and Prevention. Web-based Injury Statistics Query and Reporting System (WISQARS). (2007). National Center for Injury Prevention and Control, Centers for Disease Control and Prevention (producer). Available from: URL: www.cdc.gov/ncipc/wisqars. [2010 Sep 16].

4. Fox JA, Zawitz MW. *Homicide Trends in the United States*. Washington, D.C.: Bureau of Justice Statistics; 2006.

5. Kellermann AL, Mercy JA. Men, women, and murder: Gender-specific differences in rates of fatal violence and victimization. *Journal of Trauma*. 1992;33(1):1–5.

6. Kellermann AL, Rivara FP, Rushforth NB, et al. Gun ownership as a risk factor for homicide in the home. *New England Journal of Medicine*. 1993;329(15):1084–91.

7. Bailey JE, Kellermann AL, Somes GW, Banton JG, Rivara FP, Rushforth NP. Risk factors for violent death of women in the home. *Archives of Internal Medicine*. 1997;157(7):777–82.

8. Saltzman LE, Mercy JA, O'Carroll PW, Rosenberg ML, Rhodes PH. Weapon involvement and injury outcomes in family and intimate assaults. *Journal of the American Medical Association*. 1992;267(22):3043–47.

9. Campbell JC, Webster DW, Koziol-McLain J, et al. Risk factors for femicide in abusive relationships: results from a multisite case control study. *American Journal of Public Health*. 2003;93(7):1089–97.

10. Wintemute GJ, Parham CA, Beaumont JJ, Wright M, Drake C. Mortality among recent purchasers of handguns. *New England Journal of Medicine*. 1999;341(21):1583–90.

11. Wintemute GJ. Increased risk of intimate partner homicide among California women who purchased handguns. *Annals of Emergency Medicine*. 2003;41(2):281–83.

12. United States General Accounting Office. *Gun Control: Opportunities to Close Loopholes in the National Instant Background Check System (GAO 02-720)*. Washington, D.C.; 2002.

13. Vigdor ER, Mercy JA. Do laws restricting access to firearms by domestic violence offenders prevent intimate partner homicide? *Evaluation Review*. 2006;30(3):313–46.

14. Frattaroli S, Vernick JS. Separating batterers and guns: A review and analysis of gun removal laws in 50 states. *Evaluation Review*. 2006;30(3):296–312.

Section 9.4

Assessing Risk of Lethality: Are You in Danger?

All battering is dangerous; one push or shove could result in death. Battering increases in frequency and severity over time. Certain behaviors, actions, and words by an abuser, however, indicate particular danger for you. If you see any of these in your abuser, you should know that your relationship could become deadly.

Signs to look for:

- **Threatens suicide or homicide:** If he says he will kill himself, understand that this likely means he will kill you as well.

- **Fantasizes of homicide or suicide:** If he sees this as a "solution" to his problems, he may attempt it. Beware of your abuser threatening to kill himself. Usually, it means he plans to kill you first.

- **Possesses weapons:** If your abuser owns weapons and has used them or threatened to use them in the past, he has a potential for lethal assault. The use of **guns is a strong predictor of homicide.**

- **Ownership issues:** If your abuser believes you "belong" to him, or "death before divorce," he is more likely to be life endangering.

- **Idolizes you:** If your abuser idolizes you, or depends heavily on you to sustain him, and has isolated himself from others, it is likely he will retaliate against you if you decide to end the relationship.

- **Separation violence:** If your abuser believes you will leave him, and he can't imagine life without you, he may try to kill you. Many homicides occur when a woman is leaving her abusive partner. Please understand how dangerous this time is. Seventy-five percent of women are seriously injured when they leave or try to leave an abusive relationship.

- **Escalating danger:** When your batterer begins to act more and more as if he has no regard for the consequences of his actions—legal or otherwise—you are at extremely increased risk of danger.

Chapter 10

Physical Effects of Domestic Violence

Chapter Contents

Section 10.1

Types of Domestic Violence Injuries

Excerpted from "Investigating Domestic Abuse: Law Enforcement's Role in Homicide Prevention and Ending Intergenerational Violence," Wisconsin Office of Justice Assistance (http://oja.wi.gov), © 2010. Reprinted with permission.

Offensive Injuries to the Victim

- Lacerations, fractures, welts, abrasions, or contusions from being punched, pushed, kicked, slapped, and/or hit with an object

- Injuries and symptoms associated with strangulation (note: not all victims who are strangled will have visible external injuries)

- Fingernail scratches, bite marks, and cigarette, rope, and carpet burns

- Pattern injury to the neck from jewelry being pulled

- Pattern injury to the face from rings during a backhand slap or from a fist

- Wrinkle injuries to the back of the ear from pulling, pinching, or punching

- Clumps of hair or other indications of hair being pulled

- Injury on top or back of head

- Eye injuries (gouging)

Offensive Injuries to the Offender

A person who is being assaulted or in fear of being assaulted may realize they are no match for the violence that is about to be used against them and may use a weapon or other object as an "equalizer":

- Injuries to the hand and/or wrist caused by trauma of striking victim

- Abrasions and cuts on the knuckles

- Injuries caused by a hard object or weapon used to equalize a threat of force

Defensive Injuries to the Victim

A person using self-defense will often admit to using violence, but may not know what to call it:

- Injuries to the back of the arms or palms of hands from blocking blows

- Injuries to the bottoms of the feet from kicking away the assailant

- Injuries to the back, leg, buttocks, or back of head from being struck while in the fetal or other protective position

Defensive Injuries to the Offender

- Scratch marks to the face, hands, and/or arms caused when a victim is defending from attempted frontal strangulation

- Bite marks and/or scratches on chest and arms caused by a victim trying to escape from being straddled or held down

- Bite marks to the hand caused when a victim is trying to avoid having his/her mouth covered

- Bite marks on arms caused when victim is defending an attempted "chokehold"

Section 10.2

Medical Consequences of Domestic Violence

A study released by the U.S. Centers for Disease Control (CDC) in October 2005 found that healthcare costs associated with each incident of domestic violence were $948 in cases where women were the victims and $387 in cases where men were the victims. The study also found that domestic violence against women results in more emergency room visits and inpatient hospitalizations, including greater use of physician services, than domestic violence where men are the victims.

CDC researchers determined healthcare costs by looking at mental health services; the use of medical services such as emergency departments, inpatient hospitals, and physician services; and losses in productivity such as time off from work, childcare, or household duties because of injuries. The average medical cost for women victimized by physical domestic violence was $483 compared to $83 for men; mental health services cost for women was $207 compared to $80 for men; while productivity losses were similar at $257 for women and $224 for men.

Many Colorado doctors do not report their patients' domestic violence–related injuries to police officers, as is required by law in that state. In a study released in the January 2003 issue of the *Annals of Emergency Medicine*, only four in ten doctors said they always reported such injuries.

In the study, nearly all (92 percent) of the 684 doctors surveyed knew that doctors in Colorado are required to immediately notify police if they treat any injuries that resulted from domestic assault or any other crime. But less than half (41 percent) of the doctors that responded to the question said they always followed that law, study findings indicate. In the same study, 30 percent of primary care doctors said they always reported domestic violence–related injuries in comparison to 61 percent of doctors specializing in emergency medicine.

In general, doctors who had received some form of education about the mandatory reporting law, as many did, were more likely to be familiar with the law and were more likely to report domestic violence–related injuries than their less educated peers.

(Source: *Annals of Emergency Medicine* 2003;41:159)

Women who are victims of physical or sexual domestic violence visit their doctors more often than other women. Researchers examined medical records from 1997 to 2002 of several groups of adult female patients of Group Health Cooperative (GHC), a health maintenance organization (HMO) in Seattle. The study found the domestic violence victims averaged more than seventeen doctor visits a year, compared to an average of ten visits for one comparison group, and an average of six visits for another.

The study also found that 27 percent of the domestic violence victims had more than twenty doctor visits a year. Annual healthcare costs were significantly higher for the women who were victims of domestic violence. Their healthcare costs averaged more than $5,000 per year, compared to about $3,400 for those in the second group and $2,400 for those in the third group.

(Source: January 2003 issue of the *American Journal of Preventive Medicine*.)

A study published in 2002 in the *Archives of Internal Medicine* found that abused women experience a 50 percent to 70 percent increase in gynecological, neurological, and stress-related problems either as aftereffects of the abuse or as the result of the high level of stress that the abuse caused. These problems were long term, affecting women even after the relationship was over.

(Source: May 27, 2002, vol. 162, issue 10, *Archives of Internal Medicine*)

Psychological violence coming from an intimate partner can inflict health consequences as serious as physical or sexual violence, according to a study released by the University of Texas at Houston School of Public Health in the November 2002 issue of the *American Journal of Preventive Medicine*. Women and men subjected to abuses of power and control, even if not accompanied by physical or sexual abuse, were more likely to develop physical or mental illnesses or engage in substance abuse than people not abused, the study found.

Violence is cited as a pregnancy complication more often than diabetes, hypertension, or any other serious complication.

(Source: "Battering and Pregnancy," *Midwifery Today*, 19:1998)

Females accounted for 39 percent of the hospital emergency department visits for violence-related injuries in 1994 but 84 percent of the persons treated for injuries inflicted by intimates.

(Source: "Violence by Intimates: Analysis of Data on Crimes by Current or Former Spouses, Boyfriends, and Girlfriends," U.S. Department of Justice, March, 1998)

Thirty-seven percent of all women who sought care in hospital emergency rooms for violence-related injuries in 1994 were injured by a current or former spouse, boyfriend, or girlfriend.

(Source: R. Bachman and L.E. Saltzman, *Violence Against Women: Estimates from the Redesigned Survey*. Washington, DC: Bureau of Justice Statistics, 1995)

In a 1992 study of 691 black, Hispanic, and white pregnant women in public health clinics in Houston, Texas, and Baltimore, Maryland, one in six women reported physical abuse. Participants were invited into the study at the first prenatal visit and were followed up until delivery.

(Source: McFarlane, Parker, Soeken, and Bullock, "Assessing for Abuse during Pregnancy," *Journal of the American Medical Association* 267, no. 23 (1992): 3176–78)

Battered women seek medical attention for injuries sustained as a consequence of domestic violence significantly more often after separation than during cohabitation; about 75 percent of the visits to emergency rooms by battered women occur after separation.

(Source: Stark and Flitcraft, 1988)

Female victims of intimate partner violence are more likely than victims of strangers to experience injuries and to require medical treatment.

(Source: Bureau of Justice Statistics, "Female Victims of Violent Crime," NCJ 1626021996)

Section 10.3

Domestic Abuse and Traumatic Brain Injury

"Domestic Abuse and Traumatic Brain Injury Information Guide," reprinted with permission from the New York State Office for the Prevention of Domestic Violence (www.opdv.ny.gov), © 2012. The complete text of this document is available at http://www.opdv.ny.gov/professionals/tbi/dvandtbi_infoguide.html.

Domestic violence (DV) is a common cause of brain injury in women, who constitute the vast majority of victims of severe physical violence by an intimate partner.

The head and face are common targets of intimate partner assaults, and victims often suffer head, neck, and facial injuries. One study of women in shelters found that the vast majority had been hit in the head or severely shaken by their partners, most more than once. The more times they had been hit in the head or shaken, the more severe, and the more frequent, were their symptoms.[1]

What Is Traumatic Brain Injury?

Traumatic brain injury (TBI) is an injury to the brain that is caused by external physical force:

- Penetrating injuries are caused when a foreign object (such as a bullet, knife, or blunt object) pierces the skull. This type of injury causes focal damage, limited to the specific parts of the brain that lie along the path that the object travels.

- Closed head injuries occur from blows to the head that do not fracture the skull, or from severe shaking. They can cause both localized damage and diffuse or widespread damage, due to bleeding, and to stretching, tearing, and swelling of brain tissue—which can continue to damage the brain for hours or days after they originally occur. A DV victim can suffer a closed head injury when her partner hits her on the head with an object, smashes her head against a wall, pushes her downstairs, or violently shakes her.

133

- Cutting off oxygen, as happens in strangulation, also injures the brain.

A victim of domestic violence may suffer a TBI without knowing it if she had no severe trauma or obvious symptoms at first, or if she did not lose consciousness or received no medical care.

Note: While a TBI can lead to aggressive behavior, it does not cause or excuse the targeted pattern of coercive control usually seen in DV. If a woman thinks her partner is violent because he has suffered a TBI, she might want to try and get an evaluation for him, but she should also be helped to plan for safety.

Difficulties Caused by Traumatic Brain Injury

TBI can lead to impairments, ranging from mild to severe, in cognition (thinking), emotions, behavior, and physical functioning. The person with a TBI may or may not recognize that he or she is having problems. The most common symptoms reported are headaches, severe fatigue, memory loss, depression, and difficulty communicating. Other problems experienced by people who have brain injuries include:

- Cognitive difficulties, such as decreased ability to concentrate, pay attention, and solve problems, and communication difficulties.

- Difficulty with executive functioning, such as difficulty making decisions, considering long-term consequences, taking initiative, feeling motivated, and starting and finishing actions; disinhibition and impulsiveness.

- Changes in behavior, personality, or temperament, such as irritability, difficulty tolerating frustration, and emotional expression that doesn't fit the situation.

- Physical effects, such as vision problems, insomnia, loss of coordination, and seizures.

Information for Service Providers

TBI service providers: Living with domestic violence can make it harder to recover from a brain injury. You can more effectively serve your clients if you routinely screen for DV. Screening can help you identify clients who have been assaulted by intimate partners. Some may have suffered multiple brain injuries due to multiple assaults, and some may have partners who still assault them on an ongoing basis.

Others may have partners who try to prevent them from accessing services, which is common among batterers.

When a victim discloses that she is being abused, support her right to make her own decisions as far as possible, even if living independently is not a realistic possibility for her. Don't try to take control or tell her what to do. Connect her with domestic violence services. If she wishes, reach out to the domestic violence agency with information about TBI, what support she needs, and what services are available to her. Look for ways that you can work together to provide effective advocacy for both problems.

Brain injury can make it harder for a victim of domestic violence to:

- Assess danger and defend herself against assaults.

- Make and remember safety plans.

- Go to school or hold a job (increasing her financial dependency on the abuser).

- Leave her abusive partner and live on her own.

- Access services.

- Adapt to living in a shelter. She may become stressed, anxious and confused or disruptive, or have trouble understanding or remembering shelter rules and procedures.

- Retain custody of her children.

Domestic violence service providers: Screen everyone who seeks DV services for TBI. A brief screening tool that was designed to be used by professionals who are not TBI experts is the HELPS.[2] HELPS is an acronym for the most important questions to ask:

H = Were you hit in the head?

E = Did you seek emergency room treatment?

L = Did you lose consciousness? (Not everyone who suffers a TBI loses consciousness.)

P = Are you having problems with concentration and memory?

S = Did you experience sickness or other physical problems following the injury?

If you suspect a victim has a brain injury, or she answers "yes" to any of these questions, help her get an evaluation by a medical or

neuropsychological professional—especially if she has suffered repeated brain injuries, which may decrease her ability to recover and
increase her risk of death. If she wishes, reach out to the TBI service
provider with information about DV, what support she needs, and what
services are available to her. Look for ways to work together.

Working with Abused Women Who Have a TBI

The following strategies can help when a victim has difficulties
with attention, concentration, information processing, memory, and
executive functioning:

- Minimize distractions, such as phone calls, interruptions, and
  bright lights.

- Meet with her alone, unless she wants someone else included.

- Keep meetings short and build in breaks.

- Work on one task at a time and stick to the topic at hand.

- Be factual and concrete; break information down into small
  pieces.

- Double-check to be sure she has understood you—repeat, repeat,
  repeat.

- If safety allows, write important information down in a journal
  or calendar, such as court dates, contact numbers, directions, order of protection information, to-do lists, etc.

- Develop checklists.

- Help her prioritize goals and break them into small, tangible
  steps.

- Break tasks down into sequential steps; write out steps to
  problem-solving tasks.

- Help her fill out forms and make important phone calls.

- Allow extra time for her to complete tasks (e.g., to fill out a
  form).

- Point out possible consequences of decisions, short- and
  long-term.

- Provide respectful feedback on problem areas that affect her
  safety, if she thinks she is functioning better than she is.

Safety Planning

Safety planning is a concrete, specific process. When working with a victim who has a TBI, you may need to:

- Break plans down into even smaller steps and put the steps in sequence: first do A, then B, then C, etc.

- Review plans frequently and in detail, to help compensate for problems with memory, motivation, initiative, and follow-through.

- Find out what she needs in order to manage her life. Incorporate benefits, rehabilitation and support services, assistive devices (voice recorders, timers, personal digital assistants (PDAs), post-its, etc.) service animals, and her ability to drive, work, and live on her own into safety planning.

- Be realistic about how much—or how little—she may be able to do in a given day. Depression and fatigue are common for people with TBIs.

- Provide extra support and coaching when she has to deal with the justice system or Family Court. Role-play upcoming stressful situations, such as going to court.

Notes

1. Jackson, H., et al. (2002). Traumatic Brain Injury: A Hidden Consequence for Battered Women. *Professional Psychology: Research and Practice*, 33, 1, 39–45.

2. International Center for the Disabled, HELPS Screening Tool, 1992.

Section 10.4

Domestic Violence and HIV Risk

"Violence against Women and HIV Risk," U.S. Department of Health and
Human Services Office on Women's Health, July 1, 2011

Violence against women plays a big role in causing human immunodeficiency virus (HIV) infection among women. In date rape or sexual assault, forced sex can cause cuts that allow easy entry of HIV. This is especially true for young girls, whose reproductive tracts are less fully developed.

If you are currently in an abusive relationship, you are more likely to get HIV. That's partly because abusive men are more likely to have sexual partners other than their wife. Women in violent relationships often lack any control. Either partner may have other sexual relationships going on at the same time.

Fear of violence keeps some women from insisting on condom use. Fear of violence also keeps some women from seeking treatment for HIV or other sexually transmitted infections (STIs). Women may delay being tested for HIV or not get the results because they are afraid that sharing their HIV-positive status may result in physical violence.

Women with HIV may be at risk of violence when they tell a partner about their HIV status. If you have HIV, take these steps to lower the risk that your partner will react violently when you reveal your status:

- Tell your partner that you have HIV before you get sexually involved.

- Break the news in a semi-public place. A public park is a good place because it gives you some privacy, but make sure other people are around in case you need help.

- If you feel at all threatened by your partner's reaction, stop seeing him or her. If you must meet, do so only in public.

- Find a domestic violence service in your community and ask for help.

Chapter 11

Emotional and Socioeconomic Effects of Domestic Violence

Chapter Contents

Section 11.1

Violence against Women Can Take Lifelong Toll

Women who've suffered from gender-based violence are more likely to develop anxiety disorders or other mental woes, experience physical and mental disabilities, and have worse quality of life than other women, new research shows.

Gender-based violence includes rape and other forms of sexual assault, intimate-partner violence (such as spouse abuse), and stalking.

Risks for these long-term problems rose with the intensity of abuse. For example, women who'd experienced three or four types of gender-based violence had ten times the odds of developing an anxiety disorder than women who haven't experienced such violence, the study found. The odds of a woman who'd been subjected to such violence developing a substance abuse problem were almost six times higher than for a woman who hasn't experienced gender-based violence.

"Gender-based violence is a public health problem and occurs to many women. Women need to recognize that the social and psychological problems they are experiencing may be related to their past or current exposure to violence and not pass these reactions off to other causes," said the study's lead author, Susan Rees, a senior research fellow at the University of New South Wales in Sydney, Australia.

Results of the study are published in the August 3, 2011, issue of the *Journal of the American Medical Association*.

In the United States, more than 20 percent of women have experienced intimate-partner violence, stalking, or both. A full 17 percent have reported rape or attempted rape, according to background information in the study.

The data for Rees's study came from a national survey done in Australia on mental health and well-being. The survey included over 4,400 women between the ages of sixteen and eighty-five years old.

In that group, 1,218 women (27 percent) reported experiencing at least one form of gender-based violence, while 139 had been exposed to three or more forms of gender-based violence.

The average age that women were first raped was thirteen years old, and twelve years old for sexual assault. The average age that women were beaten by a partner or stalked was twenty-two years old.

The more violence a woman was exposed to, the greater her risk of developing mental illnesses, according to the study.

For example, about 15 percent of women who had been subjected to one form of gender-based violence experienced post-traumatic stress disorder (PTSD). But, if women were subjected to three or more forms of gender-based violence, that number jumped to more than 56 percent, the investigators found.

Suicide rates were significantly higher for women who'd experienced gender-based violence. The average rate of attempted suicide was 1.6 percent for all women in the study, but it was 6.6 percent for women who'd experienced one form of violence, and 34.7 percent for women exposed to three or more types of violence.

Rates of physical and mental disabilities were also much higher for women who had experienced gender-based violence. These women also tended to report an impaired quality of life.

Even though the study team had expected the findings, "the extent and strength of the associations we found was surprising and very concerning," Rees said.

She noted that "the nature of gender-based violence is particularly insidious because it occurs in the very situations where the victim/survivor usually expects to enjoy conditions of safety, security, and love, particularly the home."

Furthermore, this type of aggression, "often occurs repeatedly, unlike other traumas such as exposure to natural disasters, so you get a compounding effect. Gender-based violence is unfortunately still largely considered a personal and private matter, making help-seeking very difficult for many women, so they rarely received the support trauma survivors need to assist recovery," Rees noted.

One U.S. expert said the findings need to be heeded closely.

"This study really demonstrated the extent of gender-based violence and the long-term consequences of violence against women," said Andrea Gielen, director of the Center for Injury Research and Policy at the Johns Hopkins Bloomberg School of Public Health in Baltimore. "There are huge implications for health services; this is not just a one-time treatment in the ER for a broken bone. People who treat women for any health-related issues need to think about the extent that such violence can affect women," Gielen said.

Gielen added that in the United States, a measure of help is on the way. The federal government recently adopted recommendations from the Institute of Medicine on preventive services for women's health, and one new rule is that healthcare insurers must cover the cost of screening and counseling for domestic violence.

"Any woman who is experiencing gender-based violence needs to realize that there are things she can do, there are hotlines she can call, there are resources available," Gielen said. "Talking about the experience with an informed and supportive health professional is a good thing to do to move on."

Sources

Susan Rees, Ph.D., Australian Research Council QE-11 Senior Research Fellow, Psychiatry Research and Teaching Unit, University of New South Wales, Sydney, Australia; Andrea Gielen, Sc.D., director, Center for Injury Research and Policy, Johns Hopkins Bloomberg School of Public Health, Baltimore; Aug. 3, 2011, *Journal of the American Medical Association.*

Section 11.2

Domestic Violence and Homelessness

Background

Domestic violence is defined as emotionally and/or physically controlling an intimate partner, often involving tactics such as physical assault, stalking, and sexual assault (Domesticviolence.org). Approximately one out of every four women will experience domestic violence in her lifetime and 1.3 million women are victims of domestic violence each year. Victims of domestic violence lost about eight million days of paid work because of the violence that they experienced. 4.1 million dollars is spent directly on mental health and medical services for domestic violence victims (National Coalition Against Domestic Violence). Considering the cost and prevalence, as well as the direct relationship between housing and domestic violence, a majority of homeless women are victims of domestic violence. Twenty-eight percent of families were homeless because of domestic violence in 2008 (U.S. Conference of Mayors, 2008). Thirty-nine percent of cities cited domestic violence as the primary cause of family homelessness (U.S. Conference of Mayors, 2007).

Domestic Violence as a Contributing Factor to Homelessness

When a woman decides to leave an abusive relationship, she often has nowhere to go. This is particularly true of women with few resources. Lack of affordable housing and long waiting lists for assisted housing mean that many women and their children are forced to choose between abuse at home and life on the streets. Approximately 63 percent of homeless women have experienced domestic violence in their adult lives (National Network to End Domestic Violence). Moreover, shelters are frequently filled to capacity and must turn away battered women and their children. In 2008, a majority of cities saw an increase in family homelessness, though a large number of foreclosures has also influenced this number. Yet, cities have been responsive. Barely any homeless families were found living on the streets in 2008, compared to 2007, when 25 percent of people living on the streets were families (U.S. Conference of Mayors, 2008).

Some cities have decided to combat the increase of homeless families by providing motel vouchers for the nights when the shelters are full. But, because of the nature of being a homeless family, it takes a longer period of time to find permanent housing. Compared with single men and women, families remained in emergency shelter, transitional housing, and permanent supportive housing longer (U.S. Conference of Mayors, 2008). There are a number of reasons for this finding, but domestic violence victims in particular have difficulty. Victims often have poor credit records and employment histories because of the violence they have experienced. Landlords often discriminate against victims if they have a protection order or any other indicator of domestic violence. If violence occurs in the home, landlords can evict their tenants, resulting in a victim becoming homeless because she was abused.

Policy Issues

Currently, victims of domestic abuse have unmet needs for both short and long-term housing. On a given day, 1,740 people could not be provided emergency shelter and 1,422 could not be provided transitional shelter (National Network to End Domestic Violence, 2007).

Shelters provide immediate safety to battered women and their children and help women gain control over their lives. The provision of safe emergency shelter is a necessary first step in meeting the needs of women fleeing domestic violence.

A sizable portion of the welfare population experiences domestic violence at any given time. Thus, without significant housing support, many welfare recipients are at risk of homelessness or continued violence. In the absence of cash assistance, women who experience domestic violence may be at increased risk of homelessness or compelled to live with a former or current abuser in order to prevent homelessness. Welfare programs must make every effort to assist victims of domestic violence and to recognize the tremendous barrier to employment that domestic violence presents.

In 2005, the "Violence Against Women Act" was passed. This bill mandated that programs receiving funds from the McKinney Vento Homelessness Assistance Act and data collected by the Homeless

Management Information Services (HMIS) could not give identifying information about the victims.

Long-term efforts to address homelessness must include increasing the supply of affordable housing, ensuring adequate wages and income supports, and providing necessary supportive services.

References

American Civil Liberties Union, Women's Rights Project. "Domestic Violence and Homelessness," 2004. Available atwww.aclu.org

DeSimone, Peter et al. Homelessness in Missouri: Eye of the Storm? 1998. Available for $6.00 from the Missouri Association for Social Welfare, 308 E. High St., Jefferson City, MO 65101; 573-634-2901.

Douglass, Richard. The State of Homelessness in Michigan: A Research Study, 1995. Available, free, from the Michigan Interagency Committee on Homelessness, c/o Michigan State Housing Development Authority, P.O. Box 30044, Lansing, MI 48909; 517-373-6026.

Homes for the Homeless. Ten Cities 1997–1998: A Snapshot of Family Homelessness Across America. Available from Homes for the Homeless & the Institute for Children and Poverty, 36 Cooper Square, 6th Floor, New York, NY 10003; 212-529-5252.

Institute for Women's Policy Research. "Domestic Violence and Welfare Receipt," 1997. *IWPR Welfare Reform Network News*, Issue No. 4. April. Available from the Institute for Women's Policy Research, 1400 20th Street, NW, Suite 104, Washington DC 20036; 202-785-5100

Mullins, Gretchen. "The Battered Woman and Homelessness," in *Journal of Law and Policy*, 3 (1994) 1:237–55. Entire issue available for $30.00 from William S. Hein & Co., Inc., 1285 Main St., Buffalo, NY 14209; 800-828-7571.

National Alliance to End Homelessness. 2007. "Fact Checker: Domestic Violence." Washington, DC: National Alliance to End Homelessness. Available at: http://www.naeh.org.

National Network to End Domestic Violence. 2007. "Domestic Violence Counts: A 24-hour census of domestic violence shelters and services across the United States." Washington, DC: National Network to End Domestic Violence.

Owen, Greg et al. *Minnesota Statewide Survey of Persons Without Permanent Shelter; Volume I: Adults and Their Children*, 1998. Available for $20.00 from the Wilder Research Center, 1295 Bandana Blvd., North, Suite 210, St. Paul, MN 55108-5197; 612-647-4600.

U.S. Conference of Mayors. *A Status Report on Hunger and Homelessness in America's Cities: 2005, 2006, 2007, 2008*. Available for $15.00 from the U.S. Conference of Mayors, 1620 Eye Street, NW, 4th Floor, Washington, DC, 20006-4005, 202-293-7330.

Virginia Coalition for the Homeless. 1995 Shelter Provider Survey, 1995. Out of Print. Virginia Coalition for the Homeless, P.O. Box 12247, Richmond, VA 23241; 804-644-5527.

Zorza, Joan. "Woman Battering: A Major Cause of Homelessness," in *Clearinghouse Review*, vol. 25, no. 4, 1991. Available for $6.00 from the National Clearinghouse for Legal Services, 205 W. Monroe St., 2nd Floor, Chicago, IL 60606-5013; 800-621-3256.

Chapter 12

Children and Exposure to Domestic Violence

Chapter Contents

Section 12.1

Effects of Domestic Violence on Children

Children living in families where domestic violence occurs may be exposed to intimate partner violence and abuse in a number of ways. They may be direct witnesses to abuse, may suffer harm incidental to the domestic abuse, may have their lives disrupted by moving or being separated from parents, may be used by the batterer to manipulate or gain control over the victim, and they themselves are more likely to be abused. Exposure to domestic violence is widespread internationally and it is associated with other forms of child maltreatment, according to a 2006 UNICEF World Report on Violence Against Children.

Children may be direct witnesses to domestic violence, often seeing abusive incidents or hearing violence as it happens in their homes and families. As witnesses, children may be considered secondary victims and can be harmed psychologically and emotionally. According to a study published in 2003, over 15 million children in the United States lived in families where intimate partner violence had occurred at least once in the past year, and seven million children live in families in which severe partner violence occurred.[1]

A 2007 study in the United States found that in 38 percent of incidents of intimate partner violence which involve female victims, children under age twelve were residents of the household.[2]

Children can be displaced by the domestic violence when they seek shelter along with their abused parent. While statistics are not available globally, many shelters take in children as well as their abused parent. According to a study of domestic violence shelters and services in the United States, in a single day in 2008, 16,458 children were living in a domestic violence shelter or transitional housing facility, while an additional 6,430 children sought services at a nonresidential program.[3]

The U.S. government's Child Welfare Information Gateway provides a review of some research about the effects of domestic violence on children. Studies indicate that child witnesses, on average, are more aggressive and fearful and more often suffer from anxiety, depression, and other trauma-related symptoms when compared to children who have not witnessed abuse or been abused. Children growing up in violent homes often feel they are responsible for the abuse and may feel guilty because they think they caused it or because they are unable to stop it. They live with constant anxiety that another beating will occur or that they will be abandoned. They may feel guilty or confused for loving the abuser or getting mad at the victim. Children may be at a higher risk of alcohol or drug abuse, experience cognitive problems or stress-related ailments (headaches, rashes), and have difficulties in school. The Family Violence Prevention Fund offers a good overview of facts related to how children can be affected by domestic violence, and provides many additional resources.

A 2005 study of low-income preschool children in the U.S. state of Michigan found that nearly half of the children in the study had been exposed to at least one incident of mild or severe violence in the family. Those children who had been exposed to violence suffered symptoms of post-traumatic stress disorder, such as bed-wetting or nightmares, and were at greater risk than their peers of having allergies, asthma, gastrointestinal problems, headaches and flu.[4]

The effects of witnessing domestic violence appear to diminish with time, as long as the violence ends or they are no longer exposed to it, but the impact can continue through adulthood. As adults, child witnesses may continue to suffer from depression, anxiety, and trauma-related symptoms, such as post-traumatic stress disorder. Even two decades ago, research by Strauss and colleagues indicated that boys who witness domestic violence were more likely to batter their partners as adults and abuse their own children.[5]

In *Problems Associated with Children's Witnessing of Domestic Violence*, Jeff Edleson (1999), an expert on children and domestic violence and batterers' intervention programs, provides a more in-depth discussion of some of the ways in which children's health can be affected by witnessing domestic violence. Edleson reviewed nearly one hundred studies that reported behavioral, emotional, cognitive, and long-term problems that are statistically associated with a child's witnessing of domestic violence.

Research has also shown that there is a strong correlation or overlap between child abuse and domestic abuse. Additional reviews of the research by Edleson (1999) and others have indicated that there is approximately a 50 percent overlap between domestic violence and child maltreatment. Children may be inadvertently or accidentally hurt through incidents of domestic violence. They may be hit by items thrown by the batterer, and older children, in particular, may be hurt trying to protect their mother. At least one study, published in 2003, indicated that the more severe the abuse against the mother, the more likely a child is to attempt to intervene in an incident.[6]

A 1998 literature review reported that between 45 percent and 70 percent of children who are exposed to domestic violence are also victims of abuse, and that 40 percent of child victims of abuse are also exposed to domestic violence.[7]

Babies are also impacted by domestic violence, especially when violence happens to women during pregnancy. For example, a 2005 multicountry study on domestic violence against women conducted by the World Health Organization (WHO) found that 11 to 44 percent of ever-abused ever-pregnant women reported being assaulted during pregnancy.

According to Lundy Bancroft, among others, children are sometimes used by batterers to manipulate or spy on their victims, becoming a tool for the abusive partner. A batterer may threaten to take custody of or kidnap the children if the victim reports the abuse; he may also threaten to harm or kill the children. In addition, a batterer often insults and demeans his victim's parenting of the children. He may also tell her that she will lose custody if she seeks help or tries to get a divorce because she "allowed" the abuse to happen. He may even harm the children in order to control their mother. During and after separation, batterers continue to use these tactics. Unsupervised visitation and joint custody, in particular, provide the batterer with opportunities to abuse, threaten, and intimidate their former partners even when no longer living with them. Mothers' and children's human rights are violated by state actors in the United States such as the court system and child protection workers, which have been documented in Massachusetts and Arizona.

The connections between child maltreatment and abuse of women indicates a strong need for coordination between child welfare advocates and domestic abuse agencies and advocates. In particular, it is critical that agencies that work with abused children are trained to recognize signs of domestic violence and to respond appropriately. In the 2002 U.S. District Court case, *Nicolson v. Williams* (U.S. District Court, East District of New York, Case #00-CV2229), the judge concluded that the New York City agency for child protection had overstepped its authority when it removed several children from their abused mothers due solely to their mothers having been victims of domestic violence. Expert testimony concluded that while children exposed to domestic violence may be at greater risk of experiencing emotional and behavioral difficulties, there are a wide range of responses and many negative outcomes seem to diminish over time when the child and mother's safety is restored.

Because of the correlation between intimate partner violence and child abuse, and the potential impact that exposure to such violence can have on children, it is important that the laws governing child abuse and child custody do not have unintended effects on battered women. It is important to ensure that the legal and social responses to cases of domestic violence involving children do not blame or revictimize the abused parent or further traumatize the children. Advocates and all those responding must carefully consider the options available and strive to do what is best to help make all victims more safe, while holding the perpetrators of the abuse accountable for their behavior.

Notes

1. From: Whitfield, Anda, Dube, & Felittle (2003), Violent Childhood Experiences and the Risk of Intimate Partner Violence in Adults: Assessment in a Large Health Maintenance Organization.

2. From: Catalano & Shannan (2007). Intimate Partner Violence in the United States.

3. From: The National Network to End Domestic Violence, (2009). Domestic Violence Counts 2008: A 24-hour Census of Domestic Violence Shelters and Services.

4. From: Graham-Bermann & Seng (2005).Violence Exposure and Traumatic Stress Symptoms as Additional Predictors of Health Problems in High-Risk Children.

5. From: Strauss, Gelles, & Smith, (1990). Physical Violence in American Families: Risk Factors and Adaptations to Violence in 8,145 Families. [out of print]

6. From: Edleson, Mbilinyi, Beeman, & Hagemeister. (2003). How children are involved in adult domestic violence: Results from a four city telephone survey.

7. From: Levey, Steketee & Keilitz (2000) Lessons Learned in Implementing an Integrated Domestic Violence Court: The District of Columbia Experience.

Compiled From

UNICEF (2006). World Report on Violence Against Children.

Whitfield, Anda, Dube, & Felittle (2003). Violent Childhood Experiences and the Risk of Intimate Partner Violence in Adults: Assessment in a Large Health Maintenance Organization. *Journal of Interpersonal Violence*, 18(2): 166–85.

Catalano & Shannan (2007). Intimate Partner Violence in the United States. U.S. Department of Justice, Bureau of Justice Statistics. (http://bjs.ojp.usdoj.gov/content/pub/pdf/ipvus.pdf)

The National Network to End Domestic Violence (2009). Domestic Violence Counts 2009: A 24-hour Census of Domestic Violence Shelters and Services. (Available at http://www.nnedv.org/resources/census/375-census-2009-report.html.)

Sandra Graham-Bermann & Julie Seng (2005).Violence Exposure and Traumatic Stress Symptoms as Additional Predictors of Health Problems in High-Risk Children, 146, *J. of Pediatrics* 309.

Edleson, J. L. (1999). Problems Associated with Children's Witnessing of Domestic Violence. (Available at http://new.vawnet.org/category/Main_Doc.php?docid=392.)

Edleson, J. L., Mbilinyi, L. F., Beeman, S. K. & Hagemeister, A. K. (2003). How children are involved in adult domestic violence: Results from a four city telephone survey. *Journal of Interpersonal Violence*, 18(1) 18–32.

Levey, Steketee & Keilitz (2000). Lessons Learned in Implementing an Integrated Domestic Violence Court: The District of Columbia Experience (Available at http://contentdm.ncsconline.org/cgi-bin/showfile.exe?CISOROOT=/famct&CISOPTR=7.)

World Health Organization. (2005). Multi-country study on women's health and domestic violence against women. (Chapter 2). (Available at: http://www.who.int/gender/violence/who_multicountry_study/en/.)

Bancroft with Silverman. The Batterer as parent: Addressing the impact of domestic violence on family dynamics. http://www.lundybancroft.com/art_custody_visitation.html

Slote, K. Y., Cuthber, C., Mesh, C. J., Driggers, M. G., Bancroft L. & Silverman, J. G. (2005). Battered Mothers Speak Out: Participatory Human Rights Documentation as a Model for Research and Activism in the U.S., *Violence Against Women*, 11, 11.

Battered Mothers' Testimony Project (BMTP) (2003). Battered Mothers Fight to Survive the Family Court System, Research & Action Report, Wellesley College. http://www.stopfamilyviolence.org/sites/documents/0000/0035/AZ_bmtp_report.pdf.

Arizona Coalition Against Domestic Violence (June 2003). "Battered mothers testimony project: A human rights approach to child custody and domestic violence."

U.K. Home Office Report. (undated). Tackling Domestic violence: Providing support for children who have witnessed domestic violence. (Home Office Practice and Development Report #33). Available online from http://rds.homeoffice.gov.uk/rds/pdfs04/dpr33.pdf.

Section 12.2

Domestic Abuse and Childhood Obesity

Reprinted with permission from SLACK Incorporated, © 2010.
Intimate partner violence connected to obesity in young children.
Endocrine Today. News: In the Journals. June 10, 2010.

Children whose mothers experienced chronic abuse at the hands of their partners were more likely to be obese at age 5 years, recent data indicated.

To evaluate the effect that domestic violence has on obesity in preschool-aged children, researchers at Boston University School of Medicine assessed data collected during the Fragile Families and Child Well-being Study —a prospective cohort study that involved children born between 1998 and 2000 and was conducted in 20 cities throughout the United States.

For their analysis, the researchers examined a subset of 1,595 children whose mothers completed interviews at birth and follow-up via telephone or in-home assessment at 12, 36 and 60 months. Children's height and weight were also measured at the 3- and 5-year evaluations.

Results revealed that 16.5% of these children were obese at age 5, and 49.4% of mothers reported physical, sexual or restrictive partner violence at some point during the study period. Chronic abuse was experienced by 16.8%. After adjusting for potential confounders, such as maternal age and obesity, children of these mothers were 80% more likely to be obese at age 5 compared with children whose mothers reported no domestic violence (adjusted OR=1.80; 95% CI, 1.24-2.61).

The researchers noted that girls whose mothers reported chronic intimate partner violence had a higher risk for obesity (adjusted OR=2.21; 95% CI, 1.30-3.75) when compared with boys (adjusted OR=1.66; 95% CI, 0.94-2.93). This risk increased for both boys and girls if the mother perceived the neighborhood in which they lived as unsafe (adjusted OR=1.56; 95% CI, 1.03-2.36). Analyses indicated, however, that these numbers were not statistically significant.

Several factors could explain the link between chronic abuse and elevated risk of childhood obesity, the researchers said. For instance, domestic violence may influence maternal responsiveness to the socioemotional needs of the child and cause stress that leads to emotional eating. Furthermore, they point out that a child's neuroendocrine, serotonin and cortisol systems may be altered by witnessing traumatic events.

Section 12.3

Child Abuse and Intimate Partner Violence: How Prevalent Is Co-Occurrence?

Excerpted from "Child Protection in Families Experiencing Domestic Violence," U.S. Department of Health and Human Services, 2003. Reviewed by David A. Cooke, M.D., FACP, May 2012.

Over the past few decades, there has been a growing awareness of the co-occurrence of domestic violence and child maltreatment. Studies report that there are between 750,000 and 2.3 million victims of domestic violence each year. Many of these victims are abused several times, so the number of domestic violence incidents is even greater. According to a national study by the U.S. Department of Health and Human Services, approximately 903,000 children were identified by child protective services (CPS) as victims of abuse or neglect in 2001. Increasingly, service providers and researchers have recognized that some of these adult and child victims are from the same families.

Research suggests that in an estimated 30 to 60 percent of the families where either domestic violence or child maltreatment is identified, it is likely that both forms of abuse exist. Studies show that for victims who experience severe forms of domestic violence, their children also are in danger of suffering serious physical harm. In a national survey of over six thousand American families, researchers found that 50 percent of men who frequently assaulted their wives also abused their children. Other studies demonstrate that perpetrators of domestic violence who were abused as children are more likely to physically harm their children.

Rates of Domestic Violence

Domestic violence measured by the National Crime Victimization Survey (NCVS) includes rape or sexual assault, robbery, and aggravated and simple assault committed by a current or former spouse, boyfriend, or girlfriend. In 2000, about one in every two hundred households acknowledged that someone in the household experienced some

155

form of domestic violence. There is no statistically significant difference in this rate over the prior six years.

Table 12.1. Rates of Domestic Violence by Household Characteristics

Characteristic of the Household	Percentage of Households that Experienced Domestic Violence
Caucasian	0.4%
African American	0.5%
Hispanic	0.5%
Other	0.5%
Urban	0.5%
Suburban	0.4%
Rural	0.4%
Northeast	0.3%
Midwest	0.7%
South	0.4%
West	0.5%

Table 12.2. Rates of Domestic Violence by Household Size

Household Size	Percentage of Households that Experienced Domestic Violence
1 person	0.4%
2 to 3 persons	0.4%
4 to 5 persons	0.5%
6 or more persons	1.0%

Table 12.3. Domestic Violence by Type of Crime and Gender in 2001

Type of Crime	Female	Male	Total
Rape or Sexual Assault	41,740		41,740
Robbery	44,060	16,570	60,630
Aggravated Assault	81,140	36,350	117,490
Simple Assault	421,550	50,310	471,860
Overall Violent Crime	588,490	103,230	691,720

As with other crimes measured using the NCVS, a household counted as experiencing domestic violence was counted only once, regardless of the number of times that a victim experienced violence and regardless of the number of victims in the household during the year. The following statistics represent reported cases.

The Co-Occurrence of Child Maltreatment and Domestic Violence

An estimated 3.3 to 10 million children a year are at risk for witnessing or being exposed to domestic violence, which can produce a range of emotional, psychological, and behavioral problems for children. This estimate is derived from an earlier landmark study that found approximately 3 million American households experienced at least one incident of serious violence each year. The broad range of this estimate highlights the fact that the exact number of domestic violence incidents is unknown, and there sometimes is incongruence or a lack of agreement about exactly what constitutes "domestic violence."

One study estimates that as many as 10 million teenagers are exposed to parental violence each year. This estimate comes from a survey in which adults were asked "whether, during their teenage years, their father had hit their mother and how often" and vice versa for the mother. The survey found that about one in eight, 12.6 percent of the sample, recalled such an incident. In these cases, 50 percent remembered their father hitting the mother, 19 percent recalled their mother hitting the father, and 31 percent recalled the parents hitting each other.

These estimates are based on research that identified maltreated children who accompanied victims of domestic violence to shelters and identified adult victims via CPS caseloads. Additionally, research examining the relationship between victims and their own use of violence indicate that they are more likely to perpetrate physical violence against their children than caretakers who are not abused by a partner or spouse. Children who witness domestic violence and are victimized by abuse exhibit more emotional and psychological problems than children who only witness domestic violence.

Current data regarding the co-occurrence between domestic violence and child maltreatment compel child welfare and programs that address domestic violence to reevaluate their existing philosophies, policies, and practice approaches towards families experiencing both forms of violence. The overlap of these issues may be particularly critical in identifying cases with a high risk of violence, such as the relationship between domestic violence and child fatalities in CPS cases. A review of CPS cases in two states identified domestic violence in approximately 41 to 43 percent of cases resulting in the critical injury or death of a child. A number of protocols and practice guidelines have surfaced over the past decade to provide child welfare and service providers with specific assessment and intervention procedures aimed at enhancing the safety of children and victims of domestic violence.

Part Three

Abuse in Specific Populations

Chapter 13

Child Abuse

Chapter Contents

Section 13.1

Types of Child Abuse

"Physical Abuse" is reprinted from "Child Abuse: Physical," "Neglect and Psychological Abuse" is reprinted from "Child Neglect and Psychological Abuse," and "Sexual Abuse" is reprinted from "Child Abuse: Sexual," © 2012 A.D.A.M., Inc.

Physical Abuse

Physical child abuse or non-accidental child trauma refers to fractures and other signs of injury that occur when a child is hurt in anger.

The physical signs of child abuse used to be called battered child syndrome. This syndrome referred to many fractures that occurred at different times in children too young to have received them from an accident. The definition of child abuse has since been expanded.

Causes

Physical abuse tends to occur at moments of great stress. Many people who commit physical abuse were abused themselves as children. As a result, they often do not realize that abuse is not appropriate discipline.

Often people who commit physical abuse also have poor impulse control. This prevents them from thinking about what happens as a result of their actions.

The rate of child abuse is fairly high. The most common form is neglect.

The major risk factors for child abuse include:

- alcoholism;
- domestic violence;
- drug abuse;
- being a single parent;
- lack of education;
- poverty.

However, it is important to note that cases of child abuse are found in every racial or ethnic background and social class. It is impossible to tell abusers from non-abusers by looking at their appearance or background.

Symptoms

An adult may bring an injured child to an emergency room with a strange explanation of the cause of the injury. The child's injury may not be recent.

Symptoms include:

- black eyes;
- broken bones that are unusual and unexplained;
- bruise marks shaped like hands, fingers, or objects (such as a belt);
- bruises in areas where normal childhood activities would not usually result in bruising;
- bulging fontanelle (soft spot) or separated sutures in an infant's skull;
- burn (scalding) marks, usually seen on the child's hands, arms, or buttocks;
- choke marks around the neck;
- cigarette burns on exposed areas or on the genitals;
- circular marks around the wrists or ankles (signs of twisting or tying up);
- human bite marks;
- lash marks;
- unexplained unconsciousness in an infant.

Exams and Tests

Typical injuries in abused children include:

- any fracture in an infant too young to walk or crawl;
- Bleeding in the back of the eye, seen with shaken baby syndrome or a direct blow to the head;
- Collection of blood in the brain (subdural hematoma) without good explanation;

- Evidence of fractures at the tip of long bones or spiral-type fractures that result from twisting;

- Evidence of skull fracture;

- Fractured ribs, especially in the back;

- Internal damage, such as bleeding or rupture of an organ from blunt trauma;

- Multiple bruises that occurred at different times—especially in unusual areas of the body or in patterns that suggest choking, twisting, or severe beating with objects or hands;

- Other unusual skin damage, including burns or burn scars.

The following tests can reveal physical injuries:

- Bone x-ray: All of the child's bones, including the skull, are x-rayed to look for unseen fractures or old, healing fractures.

- Magnetic resonance imaging (MRI) or computed tomography (CT) scan of the head or abdomen are done if there is a skull fracture; bleeding in the eye; unexplained vomiting; severe bruising of the face, skull, or abdomen; unexplained nervous system (neurological) symptoms; headaches; or loss of consciousness.

The following medical conditions have symptoms similar to those of physical abuse:

- Osteogenesis imperfecta: Almost all children with this condition have an abnormal (blue) coloring of the whites of the eyes. These children may have spontaneous fractures or break bones after accidents that would not harm the bones of a normal child.

- Undetected bleeding disorders such as hemophilia, Von Willebrand disease, or liver disease can lead to abnormal bruising patterns. The doctor can test for these disorders.

- Unusual bruising and scarring patterns can also be caused by folk medicine or Oriental medicine practices such as coin rubbing, cupping, and burning herbs on the skin over acupuncture points (called moxibustion). The doctor should always ask about alternative healing practices.

Treatment

If you think a child is in immediate danger because of abuse or neglect, you should call 911.

If you suspect a child is being abused, report it immediately. Most states have a child abuse hotline. You may also use the Childhelp National Child Abuse Hotline (800-4-A-CHILD).

Physical injuries are treated as appropriate.

The parents will need counseling or an intervention of some type. In some cases, the child may be temporarily or permanently removed from the home to prevent further danger. Life-threatening abuse, or abuse resulting in permanent damage to the infant or child may result in legal action.

Counseling, including play therapy, is also necessary for abused children over age two. The child will need help dealing with the fear and pain of abuse caused by adults, who should be trusted figures. Failing to get this help can lead to significant psychological problems, such as post-traumatic stress disorder (PTSD).

The appropriate government agency usually makes decisions about placing the child with an outside caregiver or returning the child to the home. This is typically done through the court system. The structure of these agencies varies from state to state.

Support Groups

Support groups are available for survivors of abuse and for abusive parents who want to get help.

Outlook (Prognosis)

The child's physical recovery depends on the severity of the injuries. Psychological recovery depends on the results of therapy, and whether the child can develop trusting relationships with adult caregivers.

The authorities will determine whether the abuser gets psychiatric help, such as parenting training and impulse/anger management training.

Child protection agencies generally make every effort to reunite families when possible.

Possible Complications

Because adults are so much stronger and bigger than children, an abused child can be severely injured or killed by accident. Physical abuse of a child can lead to severe brain damage, disfigurement, blindness, crippling, and death. Abused individuals may carry emotional scars for a lifetime.

Children can be permanently removed from the parents' custody if the parents are abusive enough. However, this experience can also cause the child psychological problems. The child may feel rejected, or the placement may not lead to a strong, long-term attachment to the new caregivers.

When to Contact a Medical Professional

All states require that you report any known or suspected child abuse. Call your healthcare provider, Child Protective Services, or local police if you suspect or know that someone is being abused.

Prevention

Recognize the warning signs of abuse. The caregiver may:

- have alcohol or drug problems;
- have a history of abuse or was abused as a child;
- have emotional problems or mental illness;
- have high stress factors, including poverty;
- not look after the child's hygiene or care;
- not seem to love or have concern for the child.

Counseling or parenting classes may prevent abuse when any of these factors are present. Watchful guidance and support from the extended family, friends, clergy, or other supportive persons may prevent abuse or allow early intervention in cases of abuse.

References

Johnson CF. Abuse and neglect of children. In: Kliegman RM, Behrman RE, Jenson HB, Stanton BF, eds. *Nelson Textbook of Pediatrics. 18th ed*. Philadelphia, Pa: Saunders Elsevier; 2007: chap 36.

Berkowitz CD, Stewart ST. Child maltreatment. In: Marx JA, Hockberger RS, Walls RM, et al, eds. *Rosen's Emergency Medicine: Concepts and Clinical Practice. 7th ed*. Philadelphia, Pa: Mosby Elsevier; 2009: chap 63.

Neglect and Psychological Abuse

Child neglect (also called psychological abuse) is a form of child abuse that occurs when someone intentionally does not provide a child with food, water, shelter, clothing, medical care, or other necessities.

Other forms of child neglect include:

- allowing the child to witness violence or severe abuse between parents or adults;
- ignoring, insulting, or threatening the child with violence;
- not providing the child with a safe environment and adult emotional support;
- showing reckless disregard for the child's well-being.

Causes

The rate at which children are physically and emotionally neglected is difficult to define.

Risk factors may include:

- mental illness;
- poverty;
- stresses in the family;
- substance abuse by parents or caregivers.

Abused children are at risk of becoming abusers themselves as adults.

Symptoms

Symptoms of psychological abuse may include:

- difficulties in school;
- eating disorders, leading to weight loss or poor weight gain;
- emotional issues such as low self-esteem, depression, and anxiety;
- rebellious behavior;
- sleep disorders;
- vague physical complaints.

Exams and Tests

Children with suspected emotional abuse should be examined by a trained mental health professional. All neglected or psychologically abused children should be examined for other forms of physical abuse.

Treatment

If you think a child is in immediate danger because of abuse or neglect, you should call 911.

If you suspect that a child is being abused, report it right away. Most states have a child abuse hotline. You may also use the Childhelp National Child Abuse Hotline (800-4-A-CHILD).

The law requires healthcare workers, school employees, and child care professionals to report suspected abuse.

Treatment of the abused child may include nutritional and mental health therapy.

It may be necessary to remove the child from the home to prevent further abuse.

Treatment for abusers may involve parenting classes and treatment for mental illness, alcohol, or drug abuse.

Outlook (Prognosis)

With treatment, many children and parents can be reunited as a family. The long-term outcome depends on:

- how severe the abuse was;

- for how long the child was abused;

- the success of therapy and parenting classes.

Possible Complications

As in all forms of child abuse, severe injury or death is possible. Other long-term problems may include:

- becoming an abuser in adulthood;

- depression;

- lack of self-confidence;

- rebellious behavior.

When to Contact a Medical Professional

Call your health care provider if a child has:

- physical changes, such as unexplained injuries, weight loss, or severe tiredness;

- unexplained behavior changes.

Suspected child abuse of any form must be reported to the authorities.

Prevention

Community programs, such as home visits by nurses and social workers, can help families change behaviors or prevent the start of abuse in high-risk families.

School-based programs to improve parenting, communication, and self-image can help prevent future abuse and may help to identify abused children.

Parenting classes are very helpful. Newlywed adults without children should be encouraged to take these classes before they have each child. The dynamics in the home change when each new child is born.

References

Johnson CF. Abuse and neglect of children. In: Kliegman RM, Behrman RE, Jenson HB, Stanton BF, eds. *Nelson Textbook of Pediatrics. 18th ed*. Philadelphia, Pa: Saunders Elsevier; 2007: chap 36.

Sexual Abuse

Child sexual abuse is the deliberate exposure of minor children to sexual activity. This means a child is forced or talked into sex or sexual activities by another person. Such abuse includes:

- oral sex;
- pornography;
- sexual intercourse;
- touching (fondling).

Causes

Society was reluctant to deal with child sexual abuse a few decades ago. Today, it is considered a serious issue.

It is difficult to determine how often child sexual abuse occurs, because it is more secret than physical abuse. Children are often scared to tell anyone about the abuse. Many cases of abuse are not reported.

Abusers are usually men. They tend to know the person they are abusing. The abuser violates the trust of the younger person, which makes the sexual abuse even more devastating.

Child sexual abuse occurs in all social and economic classes of people. It has the same type of risk factors as physical child abuse, including:

- alcohol and drug abuse;
- family troubles;
- poverty.

Abusers often have a history of physical or sexual abuse themselves.

A small group of repeated abusers have the psychiatric disorder, pedophilia. Their preferred sexual contact is with children.

Symptoms

Symptoms of sexual abuse in children are similar to those of depression or severe anxiety and nervousness. They can include:

- bowel disorders, such as soiling oneself (encopresis);
- eating disorders, such as anorexia nervosa;
- genital or rectal symptoms, such as pain during a bowel movement or urination, or vaginal itch or discharge;
- repeated headaches;
- sleep problems;
- stomach aches (vague complaints).

Children who are abused may:

- display disruptive behaviors such as using alcohol and street drugs or engaging in high-risk sexual behaviors;
- do poorly in school;
- have excessive fears;
- withdraw from normal activities.

Exams and Tests

If you suspect a child has been sexually abused, the child should be examined as soon as possible by a trained healthcare professional. Most pediatricians, many family medicine doctors, and most emergency room (ER) doctors have been trained to examine cases involving sexual abuse.

Do not delay a doctor's exam for any reason. Many signs of injury related to sexual abuse are temporary. The exam should be done within seventy-two hours of the event or discovery.

A complete physical exam must always be performed, so that the examiner can look for any signs of physical and sexual abuse. The two forms of abuse may exist together.

Affected areas may include the mouth, throat, penis, anus, and vagina, including the hymen. The hymen is a thin piece of tissue covering the opening of the vagina. It can be affected by abuse.

Your doctor may also order blood tests to check for sexually transmitted diseases, such as syphilis and human immunodeficiency virus (HIV), and pregnancy in females. These tests can help determine treatment.

Photographs of injuries may help establish what happened. It is extremely important to write down symptoms due to any form of child abuse.

An exam will automatically be scheduled when suspected child sexual abuse is reported to police or child protection agencies. A second exam with an expert abuse examiner should be scheduled after the first exam. A doctor or nurse specialist can be found through Child Protective Services programs anywhere in the United States.

Treatment

Treatment for the physical signs of sexual abuse is the same as for any types of cuts, bruises, or scrapes. The patient may need medicines to prevent or treat sexually transmitted diseases. Older females may receive medicines to prevent pregnancy.

All children who have been sexually abused or traumatized in any way should receive mental health counseling.

Any suspicion of child sexual abuse must be reported to Child Protective Services and the police. Medical professionals, teachers, and child care professionals are required by law to make a report.

Once a case is reported, child protection agencies and the police must investigate. If the report is considered true, the child must be protected from further abuse. The child may be placed with a non-abusing parent, another relative, or a foster home.

Support Groups

Support groups for abused children, their parents, and caretakers are available and strongly recommended.

Outlook (Prognosis)

The biggest issue is the child's mental health. The outcome depends on:

- family and social support;
- the child's personality;
- the length of time the child was abused and the type of abuse;
- therapy.

Possible Complications

- Anxiety disorders
- Depression
- Eating disorders
- Post-traumatic stress disorder (PTSD)
- Sleep disorders
- Unsafe sexual activities

Those who have been abused as children have an increased risk of becoming abusers themselves when they reach adulthood.

When to Contact a Medical Professional

If you suspect child abuse in any form, immediately call your health-care provider, Child Protective Services, or police.

Prevention

Prevention involves teaching children never to keep secrets and the difference between "good" and "bad" touches. Parents need to begin this work at home. Most schools now have programs to teach young school-aged children about sexual abuse and its prevention.

Teenagers also need to be taught how to avoid rape and date rape.

Constant supervision and vigilance by adults is essential to preventing all forms of child abuse.

References

Johnson CF. Abuse and neglect of children. In: Kliegman RM, Behrman RE, Jenson HB, Stanton BF, eds. *Nelson Textbook of Pediatrics. 18th ed*. Philadelphia, Pa: Saunders Elsevier; 2007: chap 36.

Section 13.2

Recognizing Child Abuse and Neglect

"Recognizing Child Abuse and Neglect: Signs and Symptoms," U.S. Department of Health and Human Services, 2007. Adapted with permission from "Recognizing Child Abuse: What Parents Should Know," © Prevent Child Abuse America. Reviewed by David A. Cooke, M.D., FACP, May 2012.

The first step in helping abused or neglected children is learning to recognize the signs of child abuse and neglect. The presence of a single sign does not prove child abuse is occurring in a family, but a closer look at the situation may be warranted when these signs appear repeatedly or in combination.

If you do suspect a child is being harmed, reporting your suspicions may protect the child and get help for the family. Any concerned person can report suspicions of child abuse and neglect. Some people (typically certain types of professionals) are required by law to make a report of child maltreatment under specific circumstances—these are called mandatory reporters.

For more information about where and how to file a report, contact your local child protective services agency or police department.

Recognizing Child Abuse

The following signs may signal the presence of child abuse or neglect.

The child:

- shows sudden changes in behavior or school performance;

- has not received help for physical or medical problems brought to the parents' attention;

- has learning problems (or difficulty concentrating) that cannot be attributed to specific physical or psychological causes;

- is always watchful, as though preparing for something bad to happen;

- lacks adult supervision;

- is overly compliant, passive, or withdrawn;
- comes to school or other activities early, stays late, and does not want to go home.

The parent:

- shows little concern for the child;
- denies the existence of—or blames the child for—the child's problems in school or at home;
- asks teachers or other caregivers to use harsh physical discipline if the child misbehaves;
- sees the child as entirely bad, worthless, or burdensome;
- demands a level of physical or academic performance the child cannot achieve;
- looks primarily to the child for care, attention, and satisfaction of emotional needs.

The parent and child:

- rarely touch or look at each other;
- consider their relationship entirely negative;
- state that they do not like each other.

Types of Abuse

The following are some signs often associated with particular types of child abuse and neglect: physical abuse, neglect, sexual abuse, and emotional abuse. It is important to note, however, that these types of abuse are more typically found in combination than alone. A physically abused child, for example, is often emotionally abused as well, and a sexually abused child also may be neglected.

Signs of Physical Abuse

Consider the possibility of physical abuse when the child:

- has unexplained burns, bites, bruises, broken bones, or black eyes;
- has fading bruises or other marks noticeable after an absence from school;
- seems frightened of the parents and protests or cries when it is time to go home;

- shrinks at the approach of adults;
- reports injury by a parent or another adult caregiver.

Consider the possibility of physical abuse when the parent or other adult caregiver:

- offers conflicting, unconvincing, or no explanation for the child's injury;
- describes the child as "evil," or in some other very negative way;
- uses harsh physical discipline with the child;
- has a history of abuse as a child.

Signs of Neglect

Consider the possibility of neglect when the child:

- is frequently absent from school;
- begs or steals food or money;
- lacks needed medical or dental care, immunizations, or glasses;
- is consistently dirty and has severe body odor;
- lacks sufficient clothing for the weather;
- abuses alcohol or other drugs;
- states that there is no one at home to provide care.

Consider the possibility of neglect when the parent or other adult caregiver:

- appears to be indifferent to the child;
- seems apathetic or depressed;
- behaves irrationally or in a bizarre manner;
- is abusing alcohol or other drugs.

Signs of Sexual Abuse

Consider the possibility of sexual abuse when the child:

- has difficulty walking or sitting;
- suddenly refuses to change for gym or to participate in physical activities;

- reports nightmares or bedwetting;
- experiences a sudden change in appetite;
- demonstrates bizarre, sophisticated, or unusual sexual knowledge or behavior;
- becomes pregnant or contracts a venereal disease, particularly if under age fourteen;
- runs away;
- reports sexual abuse by a parent or another adult caregiver.

Consider the possibility of sexual abuse when the parent or other adult caregiver:

- is unduly protective of the child or severely limits the child's contact with other children, especially of the opposite sex;
- is secretive and isolated;
- is jealous or controlling with family members.

Signs of Emotional Maltreatment

Consider the possibility of emotional maltreatment when the child:

- shows extremes in behavior, such as overly compliant or demanding behavior, extreme passivity, or aggression;
- is either inappropriately adult (parenting other children, for example) or inappropriately infantile (frequently rocking or head-banging, for example);
- is delayed in physical or emotional development;
- has attempted suicide;
- reports a lack of attachment to the parent.

Consider the possibility of emotional maltreatment when the parent or other adult caregiver:

- constantly blames, belittles, or berates the child;
- is unconcerned about the child and refuses to consider offers of help for the child's problems;
- overtly rejects the child.

This section was adapted, with permission, from *Recognizing Child Abuse: What Parents Should Know*, Prevent Child Abuse America, © 2003.

Section 13.3

Recession Tied to Rise in Child Abuse

"Incidence of Child Abuse Skyrocketed During Recent Recession,"
May 1, 2010, © 2010 Children's Hospital of Pittsburgh (www.chp.edu).
All rights reserved. Reprinted with permission.

The number of cases of abusive head trauma in children has increased dramatically since the beginning of the recession in December 2007, according to a multicenter study led by Children's Hospital of Pittsburgh of the University of Pittsburgh Medical Center (UPMC).

Results of the study were presented by lead researcher Rachel Berger, MD, MPH, on Saturday, May 1, 2010, at the Pediatric Academic Societies (PAS) annual meeting in Vancouver, British Columbia. Dr. Berger is a child abuse specialist and researcher at Children's Hospital's Child Advocacy Center.

The study involved 512 patients with abusive head trauma who ranged in age from nine days to six years. It addition to Pittsburgh, the patients were treated at children's hospitals in Cincinnati, Columbus, and Seattle.

The number of cases of abusive head trauma (shaken baby syndrome) rose from 6.0 per month before December 1, 2007, to 9.3 per month after that date. Researchers collected demographic and clinical data for all cases of unequivocal abusive head trauma before the recession (January 1, 2004, through November 30, 2007) and cases during the recession (December 1, 2007, through December 31, 2009).

"Our results show that there has been a rise in abusive head trauma, that it coincided with the economic recession, and that it's not a phenomenon isolated to our region but happening on a much more widespread level," Dr. Berger said. "This suggests we may need to dramatically increase our child abuse prevention efforts now and in future times of economic hardship."

Of the children studied, 63 percent had injuries severe enough that they had to be admitted to pediatric intensive care units, and 16 percent died.

Dr. Berger said that the impetus for the study was that in 2008, more patients at Children's Hospital of Pittsburgh of UPMC died from abusive head trauma than from non-inflicted brain injury.

"To think that more children died from abusive head trauma than from any other type of brain injury that year is really remarkable and highly concerning," Dr. Berger said.

Dr. Berger and colleagues said a possible reason for the increase in abuse is that important programs such as social services are often cut during a recession and the loss of those programs can increase family stress. An increase in family stress is a known risk factor for abuse, according to Dr. Berger.

In addition to Children's Hospital, other centers participating in the study were Nationwide Children's Hospital in Columbus, Ohio, Seattle Children's Hospital, and Cincinnati Children's Hospital Medical Center.

Section 13.4

Long-Term Consequences of Child Abuse and Neglect

Excerpted from the U.S. Department of Health and Human Services, 2008.

An estimated 905,000 children were victims of child abuse or neglect in 2006 (U.S. Department of Health and Human Services, 2008). While physical injuries may or may not be immediately visible, abuse and neglect can have consequences for children, families, and society that last lifetimes, if not generations.

The impact of child abuse and neglect is often discussed in terms of physical, psychological, behavioral, and societal consequences. In reality, however, it is impossible to separate them completely. Physical consequences, such as damage to a child's growing brain, can have psychological implications such as cognitive delays or emotional difficulties. Psychological problems often manifest as high-risk behaviors. Depression and anxiety, for example, may make a person more likely to smoke, abuse alcohol or illicit drugs, or overeat. High-risk behaviors, in turn, can lead to long-term physical health problems such as sexually transmitted diseases, cancer, and obesity.

This section provides an overview of some of the most common physical, psychological, behavioral, and societal consequences of child abuse and neglect, while acknowledging that much crossover among categories exists.

Factors Affecting the Consequences of Child Abuse and Neglect

Not all abused and neglected children will experience long-term consequences. Outcomes of individual cases vary widely and are affected by a combination of factors, including the following:

- The child's age and developmental status when the abuse or neglect occurred.
- The type of abuse (physical abuse, neglect, sexual abuse, etc.).
- The frequency, duration, and severity of abuse.
- The relationship between the victim and his or her abuser (English et al., 2005; Chalk, Gibbons, & Scarupa, 2002).

Researchers also have begun to explore why, given similar conditions, some children experience long-term consequences of abuse and neglect while others emerge relatively unscathed. The ability to cope, and even thrive, following a negative experience is sometimes referred to as "resilience." A number of protective and promotive factors may contribute to an abused or neglected child's resilience. These include individual characteristics, such as optimism, self-esteem, intelligence, creativity, humor, and independence, as well as the acceptance of peers and positive individual influences such as teachers, mentors, and role models. Other factors can include the child's social environment and the family's access to social supports. Community well-being, including neighborhood stability and access to safe schools and adequate healthcare, are other protective and promotive factors (Fraser & Terzian, 2005).

Physical Health Consequences

The immediate physical effects of abuse or neglect can be relatively minor (bruises or cuts) or severe (broken bones, hemorrhage, or even death). In some cases the physical effects are temporary; however, the pain and suffering they cause a child should not be discounted. Meanwhile, the long-term impact of child abuse and neglect on physical health is just beginning to be explored. According to the National Survey of Child and Adolescent Well-Being (NSCAW), more than one-quarter of children who had been in foster care for longer than twelve months had some lasting or recurring health problem (Administration for Children and Families, Office of Planning, Research, and Evaluation [ACF/OPRE], 2004a). Below are some outcomes researchers have identified.

Shaken baby syndrome: Shaking a baby is a common form of child abuse. The injuries caused by shaking a baby may not be immediately noticeable and may include bleeding in the eye or brain, damage to the spinal cord and neck, and rib or bone fractures (National Institute of Neurological Disorders and Stroke, 2007).

Impaired brain development: Child abuse and neglect have been shown, in some cases, to cause important regions of the brain to fail to form or grow properly, resulting in impaired development (De Bellis & Thomas, 2003). These alterations in brain maturation have long-term consequences for cognitive, language, and academic abilities (Watts-English, Fortson, Gibler, Hooper, & De Bellis, 2006). NSCAW found more than three-quarters of foster children between one and two years of age to be at medium to high risk for problems with brain development, as opposed to less than half of children in a control sample (ACF/OPRE, 2004a).

Poor physical health: Several studies have shown a relationship between various forms of household dysfunction (including childhood abuse) and poor health (Flaherty et al., 2006; Felitti, 2002). Adults who experienced abuse or neglect during childhood are more likely to suffer from physical ailments such as allergies, arthritis, asthma, bronchitis, high blood pressure, and ulcers (Springer, Sheridan, Kuo, & Carnes, 2007).

Psychological Consequences

The immediate emotional effects of abuse and neglect—isolation, fear, and an inability to trust—can translate into lifelong consequences, including low self-esteem, depression, and relationship difficulties. Researchers have identified links between child abuse and neglect and the following things.

Difficulties during infancy: Depression and withdrawal symptoms were common among children as young as three who experienced emotional, physical, or environmental neglect (Dubowitz, Papas, Black, & Starr, 2002).

Poor mental and emotional health: In one long-term study, as many as 80 percent of young adults who had been abused met the diagnostic criteria for at least one psychiatric disorder at age twenty-one. These young adults exhibited many problems, including depression, anxiety, eating disorders, and suicide attempts (Silverman, Reinherz, & Giaconia, 1996). Other psychological and emotional conditions associated with abuse and neglect include panic disorder, dissociative disorders, attention-deficit/hyperactivity disorder, depression, anger, post-traumatic stress disorder, and reactive attachment disorder (Teicher, 2000; De Bellis & Thomas, 2003; Springer, Sheridan, Kuo, & Carnes, 2007).

Cognitive difficulties: NSCAW found that children placed in out-of-home care due to abuse or neglect tended to score lower than the general population on measures of cognitive capacity, language development, and academic achievement (U.S. Department of Health and Human Services, 2003). A 1999 LONGSCAN study also found a relationship between substantiated child maltreatment and poor academic performance and classroom functioning for school-age children (Zolotor, Kotch, Dufort, Winsor, & Catellier, 1999).

Social difficulties: Children who experience rejection or neglect are more likely to develop antisocial traits as they grow up. Parental neglect is also associated with borderline personality disorders and violent behavior (Schore, 2003).

Behavioral Consequences

Not all victims of child abuse and neglect will experience behavioral consequences. However, behavioral problems appear to be more likely among this group, even at a young age. An NSCAW survey of children ages three to five in foster care found these children displayed clinical or borderline levels of behavioral problems at a rate of more than twice that of the general population (ACF, 2004b). Later in life, child abuse and neglect appear to make the following things more likely.

Difficulties during adolescence: Studies have found abused and neglected children to be at least 25 percent more likely to experience problems such as delinquency, teen pregnancy, low academic achievement, drug use, and mental health problems (Kelley, Thornberry, & Smith, 1997). Other studies suggest that abused or neglected children are more likely to engage in sexual risk-taking as they reach adolescence, thereby increasing their chances of contracting a sexually transmitted disease (Johnson, Rew, & Sternglanz, 2006).

Juvenile delinquency and adult criminality: According to a National Institute of Justice study, abused and neglected children were 11 times more likely to be arrested for criminal behavior as a juvenile, 2.7 times more likely to be arrested for violent and criminal behavior as an adult, and 3.1 times more likely to be arrested for one of many forms of violent crime (juvenile or adult) (English, Widom, & Brandford, 2004).

Alcohol and other drug abuse: Research consistently reflects an increased likelihood that abused and neglected children will smoke cigarettes, abuse alcohol, or take illicit drugs during their lifetime (Dube et al., 2001). According to a report from the National Institute on Drug Abuse, as many as two-thirds of people in drug treatment programs reported being abused as children (Swan, 1998).

Abusive behavior: Abusive parents often have experienced abuse during their own childhoods. It is estimated approximately one-third of abused and neglected children will eventually victimize their own children (Prevent Child Abuse New York, 2003).

Societal Consequences

While child abuse and neglect almost always occur within the family, the impact does not end there. Society as a whole pays a price for child abuse and neglect, in terms of both direct and indirect costs.

Direct costs: Direct costs include those associated with maintaining a child welfare system to investigate and respond to allegations of child abuse and neglect, as well as expenditures by the judicial, law enforcement, health, and mental health systems. A 2001 report by Prevent Child Abuse America estimates these costs at $24 billion per year.

Indirect costs: Indirect costs represent the long-term economic consequences of child abuse and neglect. These include costs associated with juvenile and adult criminal activity, mental illness, substance abuse, and domestic violence. They can also include loss of productivity due to unemployment and underemployment, the cost of special education services, and increased use of the health care system. Prevent Child Abuse America estimated these costs at more than $69 billion per year (2001).

Summary

Much research has been done about the possible consequences of child abuse and neglect. The effects vary depending on the circumstances of the abuse or neglect, personal characteristics of the child, and the child's environment. Consequences may be mild or severe;

disappear after a short period or last a lifetime; and affect the child physically, psychologically, behaviorally, or in some combination of all three ways. Ultimately, due to related costs to public entities such as the health care, human services, and educational systems, abuse and neglect impact not just the child and family, but society as a whole.

References

Administration for Children and Families, Office of Planning, Research and Evaluation. (2004a). Who are the children in foster care? NSCAW Research Brief No. 1. Retrieved August 9, 2007, from the National Data Archive on Child Abuse and Neglect website: www.ndacan.cornell.edu/ NDACAN/Datasets/Related_Docs/NSCAW_Research_Brief_1.

Administration for Children and Families, Office of Planning, Research and Evaluation. (2004b). Children ages 3 to 5 in the child welfare system. NSCAW Research Brief No. 5. Washington, DC: Author.

Chalk, R., Gibbons, A., & Scarupa, H. J. (2002). The multiple dimensions of child abuse and neglect: New insights into an old problem. Washington, DC: Child Trends. Retrieved April 27, 2006, from www .childtrends.org/Files/ChildAbuseRB.

De Bellis, M., & Thomas, L. (2003). Biologic findings of post-traumatic stress disorder and child maltreatment. *Current Psychiatry Reports*, 5, 108–17.

Dube, S. R., Anda, R. F., Felitti, V. J., Chapman, D., Williamson, D. F., & Giles, W. H. (2001). Childhood abuse, household dysfunction and the risk of attempted suicide throughout the life span: Findings from the Adverse Childhood Experiences Study. *Journal of the American Medical Association*, 286, 3089–96.

Dubowitz, H., Papas, M. A., Black, M. M., & Starr, R. H., Jr. (2002). Child neglect: Outcomes in high-risk urban preschoolers. *Pediatrics*, 109, 1100–1107.

English, D. J., Upadhyaya, M. P., Litrownik, A. J., Marshall, J. M., Runyan, D. K., Graham, J. C., & Dubowitz, H. (2005). Maltreatment's wake: The relationship of maltreatment dimensions to child outcomes. *Child Abuse and Neglect*, 29, 597–619.

English, D. J., Widom, C. S., & Brandford, C. (2004). Another look at the effects of child abuse. *NIJ journal*, 251, 23–24.

Felitti, V. J. (2002). The relationship of adverse childhood experiences to adult health: Turning gold into lead. *Zeitschrift für Psychosomatische*

Medizin und Psychotherapie 48(4), 359–69. Retrieved June 18, 2007, from www.acestudy.org/docs/GoldintoLead.pdf

Flaherty, E. G., et al. (2006). Effect of early childhood adversity on health. *Archives of Pediatrics and Adolescent Medicine*, 160, 1232–38.

Fraser, M. W., & Terzian, M. A. (2005). Risk and resilience in child development: principles and strategies of practice. In G. P. Mallon & P. M. Hess (Eds.), *Child welfare for the 21st century: A handbook of practices, policies, and programs* (pp. 55–71). New York, NY: Columbia University Press.

Johnson, R., Rew, L., & Sternglanz, R. W. (2006). The relationship between childhood sexual abuse and sexual health practices of homeless adolescents. *Adolescence*, 41(162), 221–34.

Kelley, B. T., Thornberry, T. P., & Smith, C. A. (1997). In the wake of childhood maltreatment. Washington, DC: National Institute of Justice. Retrieved April 27, 2006, from www.ncjrs.gov/pdffiles1/165257.pdf.

National Institute of Neurological Disorders and Stroke. (2007). Shaken baby syndrome. Retrieved June 4, 2007, from www.ninds.nih.gov/disorders/shakenbaby/shakenbaby.htm

Prevent Child Abuse America. (2001). Total estimated cost of child abuse and neglect in the United States. Retrieved April 27, 2006, from http://member.preventchildabuse.org/site/DocServer/cost_analysis.pdf?docID=144

Prevent Child Abuse New York. (2003). The costs of child abuse and the urgent need for prevention. Retrieved April 27, 2006, from http://pca-ny.org/pdf/cancost.pdf

Schore, A. N. (2003). Early relational trauma, disorganized attachment, and the development of a predisposition to violence. In M. F. Solomon & D. J. Siegel (Eds.), *Healing trauma: Attachment, mind, body, and brain*. New York, NY: Norton.

Silverman, A. B., Reinherz, H. Z., & Giaconia, R. M. (1996). The long-term sequelae of child and adolescent abuse: A longitudinal community study. *Child Abuse and Neglect*, 20(8), 709–23.

Springer, K. W., Sheridan, J., Kuo, D., & Carnes, M. (2007). Long-term physical and mental health consequences of childhood physical abuse: Results from a large population-based sample of men and women. *Child Abuse & Neglect*, 31, 517–30.

Swan, N. (1998). Exploring the role of child abuse on later drug abuse: Researchers face broad gaps in information. *NIDA Notes*, 13(2). Retrieved April 27, 2006, from the National Institute on Drug Abuse website: www.nida.nih.gov/NIDA_Notes/NNVol13N2/exploring.html

Teicher, M. D. (2000). Wounds that time won't heal: The neurobiology of child abuse. *Cerebrum: The Dana Forum on brain science*, 2(4), 50–67.

U.S. Department of Health and Human Services. (2003). National Survey of Child and Adolescent Well-Being: One year in foster care wave 1 data analysis report. Retrieved April 27, 2006, from www.acf.hhs.gov/programs/opre/abuse_neglect/nscaw/reports/nscaw_oyfc/oyfc_title.html

U.S. Department of Health and Human Services. (2008). *Child maltreatment 2006*. Washington, DC: Government Printing Office. Retrieved April 1, 2008, from www.acf.hhs.gov/programs/cb/pubs/cm06/index.htm

Watts-English, T., Fortson, B. L., Gibler, N., Hooper, S. R., & De Bellis, M. (2006). The psychobiology of maltreatment in childhood. *Journal of Social Sciences* 62(4) 717–36.

Zolotor, A., Kotch, J., Dufort, V., Winsor, J., Catellier, D., & Bou-Saada I. (1999). School performance in a longitudinal cohort of children at risk of maltreatment. *Maternal and Child Health Journal*, 3(1), 19–27.

Section 13.5

Child Maltreatment Statistics

"Child Maltreatment: Facts at a Glance," U.S. Centers
for Disease Control and Prevention, 2010.

Child Maltreatment

- In 2008, U.S. state and local child protective services (CPS) received 3.3 million reports of children being abused or neglected.[1]

- CPS estimated that 772,000 (10.3 per 1,000) of children were victims of maltreatment. Approximately three-quarters of them had no history of prior victimization.

- Seventy-one percent of the children were classified as victims of child neglect; 16 percent as victims of physical abuse; 9 percent as victims of sexual abuse; and 7 percent as victims of emotional abuse.

A non-CPS study estimated that one in five U.S. children experience some form of child maltreatment: approximately 1 percent were victims of sexual assault; 4 percent were victims of child neglect; 9 percent were victims of physical abuse; and 12 percent were victims of emotional abuse.[2]

Note: A child is counted each time she or he is a subject of a report, which means a child may be counted more than once as a victim of child maltreatment.

Gender and Race Disparities among Children

In 2008, some children had higher rates of victimization:

- African-American (16.6 per 1,000 children)

- American Indian or Alaska Native (13.9 per 1,000 children)

- Multiracial (13.8 per 1,000 children)[1]

Overall, rates of victimization were slightly higher for girls (10.8 per 1,000 children) than boys (9.7 per 1,000 children).[1]

Characteristics of Perpetrators

- Most children are maltreated by their parents versus other relatives or caregivers.[1]

- Perpetrators are typically less than thirty-nine years of age.[1]

- Female perpetrators, mostly mothers, are typically younger than male perpetrators.[1]

Nonfatal Cases of Child Maltreatment

In 2008, CPS reported the approximate rates of child maltreatment victims:

- 21.7 per 1,000 for infants less than one year old;

- 12.9 per 1,000 for one-year-olds;

- 12.4 per 1,000 for two-year-olds;

- 11.7 per 1,000 for three-year-olds;

- 11.0 per 1,000 for four- to seven-year-olds;

- 9.2 per 1,000 for eight- to eleven-year-olds;

- 8.4 per 1,000 for twelve- to fifteen-year-olds; and

- 5.5 per 1,000 for sixteen- to seventeen-year-olds.[1]

Non-CPS studies have reported higher rates of nonfatal child maltreatment cases, ranging from 15 to 43 per 1,000 children.[3,4]

Deaths from Child Maltreatment

In 2008, an estimated 1,740 children ages birth to seventeen died from abuse and neglect (rate of 2.3 per 100,000 children)[1]:

- Eighty percent of deaths occurred among children younger than age four; 10 percent among four- to seven-year-olds; 4 percent among eight- to eleven-year-olds; 4 percent among twelve- to fifteen-year-olds; and 2 percent among sixteen- to seventeen-year-olds.

- Thirty-nine percent of deaths were non-Hispanic white children.

- Thirty percent of deaths were African-American children.

- Sixteen percent of deaths were Hispanic children.

Note: Some numbers in this section have been rounded.

References

1. U.S. Department of Health and Human Services, Administration on Children, Youth and Families. Child Maltreatment 2008 [Washington, DC: U.S. Government Printing Office, 2010] available at: http://www.acf.hhs.gov.

2. Finkelhor D, Turner H, Ormond R, Hamby SL. Violence, abuse, and crime exposure in a national sample of children and youth. *Pediatrics* 2009; 124:1411–23.

3. Theodore AD, Chang JJ, Runyan DK, Hunter WM, Bangdewala SI, Agans R. Epidemiologic features of the physical and sexual maltreatment of children in the Carolinas. *Pediatrics* 2005; 115: e331–e337.

4. Finkelhor D, Ormrod H, Turner H, Hamby S. The victimization of children and youth: a comprehensive national survey. *Child Maltreatment* 2005; 10: 5–25.

Chapter 14

Teen Dating Violence

Chapter Contents

Section 14.1

What Is Teen Dating Violence?

"Teen Dating Violence," U.S. Centers for Disease
Control and Prevention, October 7, 2010.

Unhealthy relationships can start early and last a lifetime. Dating violence often starts with teasing and name calling. These behaviors are often thought to be a "normal" part of a relationship. But these behaviors can lead to more serious violence like physical assault and rape.

Teen dating violence is defined as physical, sexual, or psychological/emotional violence within a dating relationship. You may have heard several different words used to describe teen dating violence. Here are just a few:

- Relationship abuse

- Intimate partner violence

- Relationship violence

- Dating abuse

- Domestic abuse

- Domestic violence

Adolescents and adults are often unaware how regularly dating violence occurs. In a nationwide survey, 9.8 percent of high school students report being hit, slapped, or physically hurt on purpose by their boyfriend or girlfriend in the twelve months prior to the survey (Centers for Disease Control and Prevention, 2009 Youth Risk Behavior Survey).

What are the consequences of dating violence?

As teens develop emotionally, they are heavily influenced by their relationship experiences. Healthy relationship behaviors can have a positive effect on a teen's emotional development. Unhealthy, abusive, or violent relationships can cause short-term and long-term negative effects or consequences to the developing teen. Victims of teen dating

190

violence are more likely to do poorly in school, and report binge drinking, suicide attempts, and physical fighting. Victims may also carry the patterns of violence into future relationships.

Why does dating violence happen?

Treat others with respect. This idea may seem like common sense but the truth is, quite a few teens are involved in violent relationships. And many think it's justified. After all, society seems to be okay with it; just look at all the TV shows and listen to popular songs these days. Violence is never acceptable. But there are reasons why it happens.

Violence is related to certain risk factors. Risks of having unhealthy relationships increase for teens who do the following things:

- Believe it's okay to use threats or violence to get their way or to express frustration or anger

- Use alcohol or drugs

- Can't manage anger or frustration

- Hang out with violent peers

- Have a friend involved in dating violence

- Have low self-esteem or are depressed

- Have learning difficulties and other problems at school

- Don't have parental supervision and support

- Witness violence at home or in the community

- Have a history of aggressive behavior or bullying

Dating violence can be prevented when teens, families, organizations, and communities work together to implement effective prevention strategies.

Section 14.2

Who Perpetrates Teen Dating Violence?

National Institute of Justice, U.S. Department
of Justice, October 27, 2008.

The authors reviewed the findings from three studies that examined who (boys, girls, or both) commits violence in teen dating relationships.

In the Toledo adolescent relationship study, which interviewed more than 1,300 seventh-, ninth- and eleventh-graders, 13 percent of girls in physically aggressive relationships reported that boys were the sole perpetrators, 36 percent said they were the sole perpetrators, and 51 percent reported both they and their partner committed aggressive acts during the relationship. Six percent of the boys in physically aggressive relationships said they were the sole perpetrators, 47 percent said girls were the sole perpetrators, and 47 percent reported mutual aggression.

In the Suffolk County study of dating aggression in Long Island, New York, high schools, 5 percent of girls in physically aggressive relationships reported that boys were the sole perpetrators, 28 percent said they were the sole perpetrators, and 65 percent reported both they and their partner committed aggressive acts during the relationship. Five percent of the boys in physically aggressive relationships said they were the sole perpetrators, 27 percent said girls were the sole perpetrators, and 66 percent reported mutual aggression.

In the Oregon youth couples study, which videotaped teen couples while they performed problem-solving tasks, researchers observed that in 8 percent of the physically aggressive relationships, boys were the sole perpetrators; in 33 percent of the physically aggressive relationships, girls were the sole perpetrators; and in 58 percent there was mutual aggression.

Section 14.3

What to Do If Someone Is Pressuring You

If you need to get out of an uncomfortable or scary situation here are some things that you can try:

1. Remember that being in this situation is not your fault. You did not do anything wrong; it is the person who is making you uncomfortable that is to blame.

2. Be true to yourself. Don't feel obligated to do anything you don't want to do. "I don't want to" is always a good enough reason. Do what feels right to you and what you are comfortable with.

3. Have a code word with your friends or family so that if you don't feel comfortable you can call them and communicate your discomfort without the person you are with knowing. Your friends or family can then come to get you or make up an excuse for you to leave.

4. Lie. If you don't want to hurt the person's feelings it is better to lie and make up a reason to leave than to stay and be uncomfortable, scared, or worse. Some excuses you could use are: needing to take care of a friend or family member, not feeling well, having somewhere else that you need to be, etc.

5. Try to think of an escape route. How would you try to get out of the room? Where are the doors? Windows? Are there people around who might be able to help you? Is there an emergency phone nearby?

6. If you and/or the other person have been drinking, you can say that you would rather wait until you both have your full judgment before doing anything you may regret later.

What Should I Do If I Am sexually Assaulted?

Sexual assault is a crime of motive and opportunity. Ultimately, there is no surefire way to prevent an attack. If you or someone you know has been affected by sexual violence, it's not your fault. You are not alone. Help is available 24/7 through the National Sexual Assault Hotlines at 800-656-HOPE.

Section 14.4

What to Do If You or a Friend Are a Victim of Teen Dating Violence

"Teen Dating Violence," © 2006 National Crime Prevention
Council (www.ncpc.org). All rights reserved. Reprinted with permission.
Reviewed by David A. Cooke, M.D., FACP, July 2012.

Dating violence or abuse affects one in four teens. Abuse isn't just hitting. It's yelling, threatening, name calling, saying "I'll kill myself if you leave me," obsessive phone calling or paging, and extreme possessiveness.

Are You Going Out With Someone Who . . .

- is jealous and possessive, won't let you have friends, checks up on you, or won't accept breaking up?

- tries to control you by being bossy, giving orders, making all the decisions, or not taking your opinion seriously?

- puts you down in front of friends or tells you that you would be nothing without him or her?

- scares you? Makes you worry about reactions to things you say or do? Threatens you? Uses or owns weapons?

- is violent? Has a history of fighting, loses his or her temper quickly, brags about mistreating others? Grabs, pushes, shoves, or hits you?

- pressures you for sex or is forceful or scary about sex? Gets too serious about the relationship too fast?

- abuses alcohol or other drugs and pressures you to use them?

- has a history of failed relationships and always blames the other person for all of the problems?

- believes that he or she should be in control of the relationship?

- makes your family and friends uneasy and concerned for your safety?

If you answered yes to any of these questions, you could be a victim of dating abuse. Both males and females can be victims of dating violence, as can partners in heterosexual and homosexual relationships.

What if Your Partner Is Abusing You and You Want Out?

- Don't put up with abuse. You deserve better.

- Know that you are not alone. Teens from all different backgrounds across the country are involved in or have been involved in a violent relationship.

- Understand that you have done nothing wrong. It is not your fault.

- Know that the longer you stay in the abusive relationship, the more intense the violence will become.

- Recognize that being drunk is not an excuse for someone to become abusive.

- Talk with your parents, a friend, a counselor, a faith leader or spiritual leader, or someone else you trust. The more isolated you are from friends and family, the more control the abuser has over you.

- Know that you can get help from professionals at rape crisis centers, health services, counseling centers, or your family's healthcare provider.

- Alert a school counselor or security officer about the abuse.

- Keep a daily log of the abuse for evidence.

- Remember that no one is justified in attacking you just because he or she is angry.

- Do not meet him or her alone. Do not let him or her in your home or car when you are alone.

- Avoid being alone at school, your job, or on the way to and from places.

- Always tell someone where you are going and when you plan to be back.

- Plan and rehearse what you will do if he or she becomes abusive.

How to Be a Friend to a Victim of Dating Violence

Most teens talk to other teens about their problems. If a friend tells you things that sound like his or her relationship is abusive, these suggestions can help.

- Don't ignore signs of abuse. Talk to your friend.

- Express your concerns. Tell your friend you're worried. Support, don't judge.

- Point out your friend's strengths—many people in abusive relationships are no longer capable of seeing their own abilities and gifts.

- Encourage your friend to confide in a trusted adult. Offer to go with your friend for professional help.

- Find out what laws in your state may protect your friend from the abuser.

- Never put yourself in a dangerous situation with the victim's partner. Don't try to mediate or otherwise get involved directly.

- Call the police if you witness an assault. Tell an adult—school principal, parent, guidance counselor, or school resource officer—if you suspect the abuse but don't witness it.

Take Action

- Educate your community. Start a peer education program on teen dating violence.

- Encourage your school or a community organization to start a program to help abusers conquer their behavior. Teaching how to be in a relationship without resorting to violence will help break the cycle.

- Read up on healthy relationships and dating violence. Ask your school library to purchase books about living without violence and the cycle of domestic violence.

- Inquire about having health, social studies, contemporary living, and other classes incorporate discussions of teen dating violence and its prevention.

Section 14.5

Safety Planning for Teens

Why Do I Need a Safety Plan?

Everyone deserves a relationship that is healthy, safe, and supportive. If you are in a relationship that is hurting you, it is important for you to know that the abuse is not your fault. It is also important for you to start thinking of ways to keep yourself safe from the abuse, whether you decide to end the relationship or not. While you can't control your partner's abusive behavior, you can take action to keep yourself as safe as possible.

What Is a Safety Plan?

A safety plan is a practical guide that helps lower your risk of being hurt by your abuser. It includes information specific to you and your life that will help keep you safe. A good safety plan helps you think through lifestyle changes that will help keep you as safe as possible at school, at home, and other places that you go on a daily basis.

How Do I Make a Safety Plan?

Take some time for yourself to go through each section of this safety planning section. You can complete it on your own, or you can work through it with a friend or an adult you trust.

Keep in Mind

- In order for this safety plan to work for you, you'll need to fill in personalized answers, so you can use the information when you most need it.

- Once you complete your safety plan, be sure to keep it in an accessible but secure location. You might also consider giving a copy of your safety plan to someone that you trust.

- Getting support from someone who has experience working with teens in abusive relationships can be very useful.

My Safety Workbook

If I live with my abuser, I will have a bag ready with these important items in case I need to leave quickly:

- Cell phone and charger
- Spare money
- Keys
- Driver's license or other form of identification
- Copy of restraining order
- Birth certificate, social security card, immigration papers, and other important documents
- Change of clothes
- Medications
- Special photos or other valuable items
- If I have children—anything they may need (important papers, formula, diapers)

I could talk to the following people at school if I need to rearrange my schedule in order to avoid my abuser, or if I need help staying safe at school:

- School counselor:
- Coach:
- Teachers:
- Principal:

- Assistant/vice principal:
- School security:
- Other:

The safest way for me to get to and from school is:

_____

_____.

If I need to leave school in an emergency, I can get home safely by:

_____

_____.

I can make sure that a friend can walk with me between classes. I will ask:

_____and/or

_____.

I will eat lunch and spend free periods in an area where there are school staff or faculty nearby. These are some areas on campus where I feel safe:

_____,_____

_____, and_____.

Figure 14.1. Staying Safe at School

These Are Things I Can Do to Help Keep Myself Safe Everyday

- I will carry my cell phone and important telephone numbers with me at all times.

- I will keep in touch with someone I trust about where I am or what I am doing.

- I will stay out of isolated places and try to never walk around alone.

- I will avoid places where my abuser or his or her friends and family are likely to be.

- I will keep the doors and windows locked when I am at home, especially if I am alone.

- I will avoid speaking to my abuser. If it is unavoidable, I will make sure there are people around in case the situation becomes dangerous.

- I will call 911 if I feel my safety is at risk.

- I can look into getting a protective order so that I'll have legal support in keeping my abuser away.

- I will remember that the abuse is not my fault and that I deserve a safe and healthy relationship.

These Are Things I Can Do to Help Keep Myself Safe in My Social Life

- I will ask my friends to keep their cell phones with them while they are with me in case we get separated and I need help.

I can tell this family member about what is going on in my relationship:
_____

There may be times when no one else is home. During those times, I can have people stay with me. I will ask:
_____

The safest way for me to leave my house in an emergency is:
_____.

If I have to leave in an emergency, I should try to go to a place that is public, safe and unknown by my abuser. I could go here:
_____
and/or here:_____.

I will use a code word so I can alert my family, friends, and neighbors to call for help without my abuser knowing about it. My code word is:
_____.

Figure 14.2. *Staying Safe at Home*

My abuser often tries to make me feel bad about myself by saying or doing this:

_____

_____.

When he/she does this, I will think of these things I like about myself:

_____,

_____ and

_____.

I will do things I enjoy, like:

_____,

_____ and

_____.

I will join clubs or organizations that interest me, like:

_____ or _____.

Figure 14.3. *Staying Safe Emotionally*

If I feel down, depressed or scared, I can call the following friends or family members:

Name:_____

  Phone #: _____

Name:_____

  Phone #: _____

Name:_____

  Phone #: _____

Name:_____

  Phone #: _____

Figure 14.4. *People You Can Call If You're Depressed*

- If possible, I will go to different malls, banks, grocery stores, movie theaters, etc. than the ones my abuser goes to or knows about.

- I will not go out alone, especially at night.

- No matter where I go, I will be aware of how to leave safely in case of an emergency.

- I will leave if I feel uncomfortable in a situation, no matter what my friends are doing.

- I will spend time with people who make me feel safe, supported, and good about myself.

During an emergency, I could call the following friends or family members at any time of day or night:

Name:_____

  Phone #: _____

Name:_____

  Phone #: _____

Name:_____

  Phone #: _____

Name:_____

  Phone #: _____

Figure 14.5. People You Can Call in an Emergency

These Are Things I Can Do to Stay Safe Online and With My Cell Phone

- I will not say or do anything online that I wouldn't in person.

- I will set all my online profiles to be as private as they can be.

- I will save and keep track of any abusive, threatening, or harassing comments, posts, or texts.

- I will never give my password to anyone other than my parents or guardians.

- If the abuse and harassment does not stop, I will change my usernames, email addresses, and/or cell phone number.

- I will not answer calls from unknown, blocked, or private numbers.

- I can see if my phone company can block my abuser's phone number from calling my phone.

- I will not communicate with my abuser using any type of technology if unnecessary, since any form of communication can be recorded and possibly used against me in the future.

For emergencies: 911

Break the Cycle: 888.988.TEEN or www.thesafespace.org

National Teen Dating Violence Hotline: 866.331.9474

Local police station:_____

   Phone #:_____

   Address:_____

Local domestic violence organization:_____

   Phone #:_____

   Address:_____

Local free legal assistance:_____

   Phone #:_____

   Address:_____

Nearest youth shelter:_____

   Phone #:_____

   Address:_____

Figure 14.6. Getting Help in Your Community

Section 14.6

Teen Dating Violence Statistics

What Is It?

According to the National Center for Injury Prevention and Control and the U.S. Department of Health and Human Services, dating
violence is defined as the physical, sexual, or psychological/emotional
violence within a dating relationship. Dating abuse occurs in both
casual and serious relationships, and in both heterosexual and same-
sex relationships.[1]

Teen Dating Violence Prevalence

- Based on the 2009 Youth Risk Behavior Survey (YRBS), 9.8
  percent of high school students nationwide reported being the
  victim of physical violence at the hands of a romantic partner
  during the previous year.[2]

  *2009 YRBS surveyed 16,410 students in grades nine to twelve
  from 158 public and private high schools across the country.*

- In a study of gay, lesbian, and bisexual adolescents, youths involved in same-sex dating are just as likely to experience dating
  violence as youths involved in opposite sex dating.[3]

  *Analyses focused on 117 adolescents aged twelve to twenty-one years
  (50 percent female) from Wave II of the National Longitudinal Study
  of Adolescent Health who reported exclusively same-sex romantic or
  sexual relationships in the eighteen months before interview.*

- A study published in the November 2007 issue of the *Journal of
  Pediatrics* found that as many as one in five adolescent females
  and one in ten adolescent males have been abused physically or
  sexually by a dating partner.[4]

Study compared 23 boys and 102 girls who reported having experienced dating violence with 671 male and 720 female adolescents with no history of intimate partner abuse in 1999 and in 2004.

- The 2009 YRBS found that black non-Hispanic students were the most likely to be victims of dating violence (14.2 percent), followed by Hispanic students (11.5 percent) and white non-Hispanic students (8 percent).[5]

2009 YRBS surveyed 16,410 students in grades nine to twelve from 158 public and private high schools across the country.

- A 2009 study published in the *Journal of Early Adolescence* found that half of all sixth graders surveyed said they are dating and 42.1 percent of these children reported being victims of "dating" physical violence.[6]

Survey interviewed 5,404 sixth-grade students from four diverse U.S. sites.

- Analysis of longitudinal data from the Welfare, Children, and Families: A Three-City Study (Boston, Chicago, and San Antonio), indicated that early involvement with antisocial peers at ages ten to fifteen years was linked to dating violence perpetration for Hispanic and African American males and females.[7]

Survey interviewed 765 people ages sixteen to twenty years old.

Health and Education Impacts

- Girls and boys experiencing teen dating violence are more likely to suffer long-term negative behavioral and health consequences, including suicide attempts, depression, cigarette smoking, and marijuana use.[8]

Survey interviewed a nationally representative sample of eight hundred teens age twelve to seventeen years old and their parents living in the continental United States and in nine focus groups conducted in four U.S. cities with teens between twelve and eighteen years old.

- Teen victims of physical dating violence are more likely than their non-abused peers to engage in unhealthy diet behaviors (taking diet pills or laxatives and vomiting to lose weight) and engage in risky sexual behaviors (first intercourse before the age of fifteen years old, not using a condom during last intercourse).[9]

According to a study of 4,163 female ninth- to twelfth-grade students who participated in the 1997 and 1999 Massachusetts Youth Risk Behavior Surveys.

Being physically or sexually abused by a dating partner leaves teen girls up to six times more likely to become pregnant and more than two times as likely to report a sexually transmitted disease (STD).[10]

A study of 1,641 ninth- to twelfth-grade female students who reported to have had sexual intercourse and completed the 1999 and 2001 Massachusetts Youth Risk Behavior Surveys.

- The Unintentional Injury and Violence-Related Behaviors and Academic Achievement report of the 2009 YRBS found that 20 percent of students surveyed who were hit, slapped, or physically hurt on purpose by their boyfriend or girlfriend during the twelve months before the survey received mostly D's/ and F's in school.[11]

2009 YRBS surveyed 16,410 students in grades nine to twelve from 158 public and private high schools across the country.

- The 4th R, a twenty-one-lesson, school-based curriculum that addresses healthy relationships, sexual health, and substance abuse, was evaluated with 1,722 Canadian ninth-grade students in a cluster randomized trial. At the 2.5-year follow-up (end of eleventh grade), the prevalence of physical dating violence perpetration was higher among students who did not receive the curriculum versus students who did receive it. (9.8 percent vs. 7.4 percent).[12]

Survey interviewed a total of 1,722 students aged fourteen to fifteen from twenty public schools (52.8 percent girls).

Abusive Digital Behaviors

- A 2009 MTV and Associated Press survey found that 50 percent of fourteen- to twenty-four-year-olds have experienced some type of digital abuse, and over 10 percent have had a boyfriend or girlfriend call them names, put them down, or say mean things to them on the internet or via cell phone.[13]

Survey interviewed 600 teens and 647 adults from across the country.

- According to the 2010 Pew Research Center Teens and Mobile Phones survey[14]:

- One in four (26 percent) twelve- to seventeen-year-old cell phone users have been bullied or harassed through text messages and phone calls.

- Fifteen percent of teens say they have received a sexually suggestive nude or nearly nude image of someone they know by text, but only 4 percent of teens have sent such a message.

- Seventy-five percent of all twelve- to seventeen-year-olds now own cell phones, up from 45 percent in 2004, and 88 percent of teen cell phone users are text messagers.

Survey interviewed a nationally representative sample of eight hundred teens age twelve to seventeen years old and their parents living in the continental United States and in nine focus groups conducted in four U.S. cities with teens between twelve and eighteen years old.

References

1. National Center for Injury Prevention and Control. Available at http://www.cdc.gov/ncipc/dvp/DatingViolence.htm. U.S. Dept. of Health & Human Services. Available at http://www.womens health.gov/violence/types/dating.cfm.

2. Centers for Disease Control and Prevention, Youth Risk Behavior Surveillance- United States, 2009. Available at http://www.cdc.gov/mmwr/pdf/ss/ss5905.pdf.

3. Young ML, Waller MW, Martin SL, Kupper LL. "Prevalence of Partner Violence in Same-Sex Romantic and Sexual Relationships in a National Sample of Adolescents." *Journal of Adolescent Health*, Vol. 35, Issue 2 (124–31). August 2004.

4. Ackard, D.M., M.E., Eisenberg, and D. Neumark-Sztainer, "Long-Term Impact of Adolescent Dating Violence on the Behavioral and Psychological Health of Male and Female Youth," *Journal of Pediatrics* 151 (2007): 476–81 (http://www.jpeds.com/article/S0022-3476(07)00362-9/abstract); http://www.reuters.com/article/idUSCOL06795220071210.

5. Centers for Disease Control and Prevention, Youth Risk Behavior Surveillance- United States, 2009. Available at http://www.cdc.gov/mmwr/pdf/ss/ss5905.pdf.

6. Simon, Thomas R., Shari Miller, Deborah Gorman-Smith, Pamela Orpinas and Terri Sullican, "Physical Dating Violence Norms and Behavior Among Sixth-Grade Students From Four U.S. Sites," *The Journal of Early Adolescence* (2009).

7. Schnurr M.P., and Lohman B.J., 2008. "How much does school matter? An examination of adolescent dating violence perpetration." *Journal of Youth and Adolescence, Special Issue on Aggression in Romantic Relationships*, 37, 266–83.

8. Ackard, D.M., M.E., Eisenberg, and D. Neumark-Sztainer, "Long-Term Impact of Adolescent Dating Violence on the Behavioral and Psychological Health of Male and Female Youth," *Journal of Pediatrics* 151 (2007): 482–87 (http://www.jpeds.com/article/S0022-3476(07)00362-9/abstract); and Olshen, E. K.H. McVeigh, R.A. Wunsch-Hitzig, and V.I. Rickert, "Dating Violence, Sexual Assault, and Suicide Attempts Among Urban Teenagers," *Archives of Pediatrics and Adolescent Medicine* 161 (2007): 539–45 (http://archpedi.ama-assn.org/cgi/content/full/161/6/539).

9. Silverman, J, Raj A, et al. 2001. "Dating Violence Against Adolescent Girls and Associated Substance Use, Unhealthy Weight Control, Sexual Risk Behavior, Pregnancy, and Suicidality." *JAMA.* 286:572 015079. Available at http://jama.ama-assn.org/cgi/reprint/286/5/572.

10. Decker M, Silverman J, Raj A. 2005. "Dating Violence and Sexually Transmitted Disease/HIV Testing and Diagnosis Among Adolescent Females." *Pediatrics.* 116: 272–76. http://pediatrics.aappublications.org/cgi/reprint/116/2/e272.

11. Unintentional Injury and Violence-Related Behaviors and Academic Achievement report. Centers for Disease Control and Prevention, Youth Risk Behavior Surveillance-United States, 2009. Available at http://www.cdc.gov/healthyyouth/health_and_academics/pdf/unintentional_injury_violence.pdf.

12. Wolfe, David A, Crooks, Claire, Jaffe, Peter, Chiodo, Debbie, Hughes, Ray, et al. "A School-Based Program to Prevent Adolescent Dating Violence." *Archives of Pediatrics & Adolescent Medicine*, 2009. http://archpedi.ama-assn.org/cgi/contect/abstract/163/8/69

13. MTV and the Associated Press, 2009. Digital Abuse Survey. Available at: http://www.athinline.org/MTV-AP_Digital_Abuse_Study_Full.pdf and http://www.athinline.org/MTV-AP_Digital_Abuse_Study_Executive_Summary.pdf.

14. Lenhart, Amanda. Teens, Cell Phones and Texting. Pew Internet & American Life Project, April 20, 2010. http://pewresearch.org/pubs/1572/teens-cell-phones-text-messages.

Chapter 15

Date Rape

Chapter Contents

Section 15.1

What Is Date Rape?

"Date Rape," February 2009, reprinted with permission from
www.kidshealth.org. This information was provided by Kids
Health ®, one of the largest resources online for medically reviewed health information written for parents, kids, and teens.
For more articles like this, visit www.KidsHealth.org, or www
.TeensHealth.org. Copyright © 1995–2012 The Nemours Foundation. All rights reserved.

When people think of rape, they might think of a stranger jumping
out of a shadowy place and sexually attacking someone. But it's not
only strangers who rape. In fact, about half of all people who are raped
know the person who attacked them. Girls and women are most often
raped, but guys also can be raped.

Most friendships, acquaintances, and dates never lead to violence,
of course. But, sadly, sometimes it happens. When forced sex occurs
between two people who already know each other, it is known as date
rape or acquaintance rape.

Even if the two people know each other well, and even if they were
intimate or had sex before, no one has the right to force a sexual act
on another person against his or her will.

Although it involves forced sex, rape is not about sex or passion.
Rape has nothing to do with love. Rape is an act of aggression and
violence.

You may hear some people say that those who have been raped
were somehow "asking for it" because of the clothes they wore or
the way they acted. That's wrong: The person who is raped is not to
blame. Rape is always the fault of the rapist. And that's also the case
when two people are dating—or even in an intimate relationship.
One person never owes the other person sex. If sex is forced against
someone's will, that's rape.

Healthy relationships involve respect—including respect for the
feelings of others. Someone who really cares about you will respect
your wishes and not force or pressure you to have sex.

Alcohol and Drugs

Alcohol is often involved in date rapes. Drinking can loosen inhibitions, dull common sense, and—for some people—allow aggressive tendencies to surface.

Drugs may also play a role. You may have heard about "date rape" drugs like Rohypnol ("roofies"), gamma-hydroxybutyrate (GHB), and ketamine. Drugs like these can easily be mixed in drinks to make a person black out and forget things that happen. Both girls and guys who have been given these drugs report feeling paralyzed, having blurred vision, and lack of memory.

Mixing these drugs with alcohol is highly dangerous and can kill.

Protecting Yourself

The best defense against date rape is to try to prevent it whenever possible. Here are some things both girls and guys can do:

- Avoid secluded places (this may even mean your room or your partner's) until you trust your partner.

- Don't spend time alone with someone who makes you feel uneasy or uncomfortable. This means following your instincts and removing yourself from situations that you don't feel good about.

- Stay sober and aware. If you're with someone you don't know very well, be aware of what's going on around you and try to stay in control. Also, be aware of your date's ability to consent to sexual activity—you may become guilty of committing rape if the other person is not in a condition to respond or react.

- Know what you want. Be clear about what kind of relationship you want with another person. If you are not sure, then ask the other person to respect your feelings and to give you time. Don't allow yourself to be subject to peer pressure or encouraged to do something that you don't want to do.

- Go out with a group of friends and watch out for each other.

- Don't be afraid to ask for help if you feel threatened.

- Take self-defense courses. These can build confidence and teach valuable physical techniques a person can use to get away from an attacker.

Getting Help

Unfortunately, even if someone takes every precaution, date rape can still happen. If you're raped, here are some things that you can do:

- If you're injured, go straight to the emergency room—most medical centers and hospital emergency departments have doctors and counselors who have been trained to take care of someone who has been raped.

- Call or find a friend, family member, or someone you feel safe with and tell them what happened.

- If you want to report the rape, call the police right away. Preserve all the physical evidence. Don't change clothes or wash.

- Write down as much as you can remember about the event.

- If you aren't sure what to do, call a rape crisis center. If you don't know the number, your local phone book will have hotline numbers.

Don't be afraid to ask questions and get information. You'll have lots of questions as you go through the process—such as whether to report the rape, who to tell, and the kinds of reactions you may get from others.

Rape isn't just physically damaging—it can be emotionally traumatic as well. It may be hard to think or talk about something as personal as being raped by someone you know. But talking with a trained rape crisis counselor or other mental health professional can give you the right emotional attention, care, and support to begin the healing process. Working things through can help prevent lingering problems later on.

Section 15.2

Date Rape Drugs

Excerpted from "Date Rape Drugs Fact Sheet,"
U.S. Department of Health and Human Services Office on
Women's Health, December 5, 2008.

What are date rape drugs?

These are drugs that are sometimes used to assist a sexual assault. Sexual assault is any type of sexual activity that a person does not agree to. It can include touching that is not okay; putting something into the vagina; sexual intercourse; rape; and attempted rape. These drugs are powerful and dangerous. They can be slipped into your drink when you are not looking. The drugs often have no color, smell, or taste, so you can't tell if you are being drugged. The drugs can make you become weak and confused—or even pass out—so that you are unable to refuse sex or defend yourself. If you are drugged, you might not remember what happened while you were drugged. Date rape drugs are used on both females and males.

The three most common date rape drugs are:

- **Rohypnol (roh-HIP-nol):** Rohypnol is the trade name for flunitrazepam (FLOO-neye-TRAZ-uh-pam). Abuse of two similar drugs appears to have replaced Rohypnol abuse in some parts of the United States. These are: clonazepam (marketed as Klonopin in the United States and Rivotril in Mexico) and alprazolam (marketed as Xanax). Rohypnol is also known as:

  - Circles

  - Forget Pill

  - LA Rochas

  - Lunch Money

  - Mexican Valium

  - Mind Erasers

  - Poor Man's Quaalude

- R-2
- Rib
- Roach
- Roach-2
- Roches
- Roofies
- Roopies
- Rope
- Rophies
- Ruffies
- Trip-and-Fall
- Whiteys

- **GHB, which is short for gamma hydroxybutyric (GAM-muh heye-DROX-ee-BYOO-tur-ihk) acid:** GHB is also known as:
  - Bedtime Scoop
  - Cherry Meth
  - Easy Lay
  - Energy Drink
  - G
  - Gamma 10
  - Georgia Home Boy
  - G-Juice
  - Gook
  - Goop
  - Great Hormones
  - Grievous Bodily Harm (GBH)
  - Liquid E
  - Liquid Ecstasy
  - Liquid X
  - PM
  - Salt Water

- Soap
- Somatomax
- Vita-G
- Ketamine (KEET-uh-meen), also known as:
  - Black Hole
  - Bump
  - Cat Valium
  - Green
  - Jet
  - K
  - K-Hole
  - Kit Kat
  - Psychedelic Heroin
  - Purple
  - Special K
  - Super Acid

These drugs also are known as "club drugs" because they tend to be used at dance clubs, concerts, and "raves."

What do the drugs look like?

Rohypnol comes as a pill that dissolves in liquids. Some are small, round, and white. Newer pills are oval and green-gray in color. When slipped into a drink, a dye in these new pills makes clear liquids turn bright blue and dark drinks turn cloudy. But this color change might be hard to see in a dark drink, like cola or dark beer, or in a dark room. Also, the pills with no dye are still available. The pills may be ground up into a powder.

GHB has a few forms: a liquid with no odor or color, white powder, and pill. It might give your drink a slightly salty taste. Mixing it with a sweet drink, such as fruit juice, can mask the salty taste.

Ketamine comes as a liquid and a white powder.

What effects do these drugs have on the body?

These drugs are very powerful. They can affect you very quickly and without your knowing. The length of time that the effects last varies.

It depends on how much of the drug is taken and if the drug is mixed with other drugs or alcohol. Alcohol makes the drugs even stronger and can cause serious health problems—even death.

Rohypnol: The effects of Rohypnol can be felt within thirty minutes of being drugged and can last for several hours. If you are drugged, you might look and act like someone who is drunk. You might have trouble standing. Your speech might be slurred. Or you might pass out.

Rohypnol can cause these problems:

- Muscle relaxation or loss of muscle control

- Difficulty with motor movements

- Drunk feeling

- Problems talking

- Nausea

- Can't remember what happened while drugged

- Loss of consciousness (black out)

- Confusion

- Problems seeing

- Dizziness

- Sleepiness

- Lower blood pressure

- Stomach problems

- Death

GHB: GHB takes effect in about fifteen minutes and can last three or four hours. It is very potent: A very small amount can have a big effect. So it's easy to overdose on GHB. Most GHB is made by people in home or street "labs." So, you don't know what's in it or how it will affect you.

GHB can cause these problems:

- Relaxation

- Drowsiness

- Dizziness

- Nausea

- Problems seeing

- Loss of consciousness (black out)
- Seizures
- Can't remember what happened while drugged
- Problems breathing
- Tremors
- Sweating
- Vomiting
- Slow heart rate
- Dream-like feeling
- Coma
- Death

Ketamine: Ketamine is very fast acting. You might be aware of what is happening to you, but unable to move. It also causes memory problems. Later, you might not be able to remember what happened while you were drugged.

Ketamine can cause these problems:

- Distorted perceptions of sight and sound
- Lost sense of time and identity
- Out of body experiences
- Dream-like feeling
- Feeling out of control
- Impaired motor function
- Problems breathing
- Convulsions
- Vomiting
- Memory problems
- Numbness
- Loss of coordination
- Aggressive or violent behavior
- Depression
- High blood pressure
- Slurred speech

Are these drugs legal in the United States?

Some of these drugs are legal when lawfully used for medical purposes. But that doesn't mean they are safe. These drugs are powerful and can hurt you. They should only be used under a doctor's care and order.

Rohypnol is not legal in the United States. It is legal in Europe and Mexico, where it is prescribed for sleep problems and to assist anesthesia before surgery. It is brought into the United States illegally.

Ketamine is legal in the United States for use as an anesthetic for humans and animals. It is mostly used on animals. Veterinary clinics are robbed for their ketamine supplies.

GHB was recently made legal in the United States to treat problems from narcolepsy (a sleep disorder). Distribution of GHB for this purpose is tightly restricted.

How can I protect myself from being a victim?

- Don't accept drinks from other people.

- Open containers yourself.

- Keep your drink with you at all times, even when you go to the bathroom.

- Don't share drinks.

- Don't drink from punch bowls or other common, open containers. They may already have drugs in them.

- If someone offers to get you a drink from a bar or at a party, go with the person to order your drink. Watch the drink being poured and carry it yourself.

- Don't drink anything that tastes or smells strange. Sometimes, GHB tastes salty.

- Have a nondrinking friend with you to make sure nothing happens.

- If you realize you left your drink unattended, pour it out.

- If you feel drunk and haven't drunk any alcohol—or, if you feel like the effects of drinking alcohol are stronger than usual—get help right away.

Are there ways to tell if I might have been drugged and raped?

It is often hard to tell. Most victims don't remember being drugged or assaulted. The victim might not be aware of the attack until eight or twelve hours after it occurred. These drugs also leave the body very quickly. Once a victim gets help, there might be no proof that drugs were involved in the attack. But there are some signs that you might have been drugged:

- You feel drunk and haven't drunk any alcohol—or, you feel like the effects of drinking alcohol are stronger than usual.

- You wake up feeling very hung over and disoriented or having no memory of a period of time.

- You remember having a drink, but cannot recall anything after that.

- You find that your clothes are torn or not on right.

- You feel like you had sex, but you cannot remember it.

What should I do if I think I've been drugged and raped?

- **Get medical care right away:** Call 911 or have a trusted friend take you to a hospital emergency room. Don't urinate, douche, bathe, brush your teeth, wash your hands, change clothes, or eat or drink before you go. These things may give evidence of the rape. The hospital will use a "rape kit" to collect evidence.

- **Call the police from the hospital:** Tell the police exactly what you remember. Be honest about all your activities. Remember, nothing you did—including drinking alcohol or doing drugs—can justify rape.

- **Ask the hospital to take a urine (pee) sample that can be used to test for date rape drugs:** The drugs leave your system quickly. Rohypnol stays in the body for several hours, and can be detected in the urine up to seventy-two hours after taking it. GHB leaves the body in twelve hours. Don't urinate before going to the hospital.

- **Don't pick up or clean up where you think the assault might have occurred:** There could be evidence left behind—such as on a drinking glass or bed sheets.

- **Get counseling and treatment:** Feelings of shame, guilt, fear, and shock are normal. A counselor can help you work through these emotions and begin the healing process. Calling a crisis center or a hotline is a good place to start.

219

Chapter 16

Digital Dating Abuse

Chapter Contents

Section 16.1

Texting
and Sexting

Next to talking one-on-one, texting is currently one of the most instant forms of communication. While texting might be the perfect platform to say a quick "hi," there are some things to watch out for in a textual relationship with your partner.

Texting Too Much

If your partner texts too much, it's not only irritating, but unnecessary. Keeping in touch with your significant other throughout the day can be thoughtful, but constant contact is probably overdoing it. Consider talking to your partner about giving you a little bit of space. Remember, if they're using text messaging to monitor everywhere you go, that is a warning sign of abuse.

Sexting

Does your partner ask for inappropriate pictures of you? Or send them to you? Even if you trust that your partner will be the only one to ever see the pictures, you can never guarantee that they won't end up on someone else's phone or online. Seriously consider playing it safe and making a policy of not sending and instantly deleting inappropriate photos. The same goes for webcams and instant messaging, too. Remember you never have to do anything you aren't comfortable with, no matter how much your partner pressures you.

Sexting can also have legal consequences. Any nude photos or video of someone under eighteen could be considered child pornography, which is always illegal. Even if whoever sent the image did so willingly, the recipient can still get in a lot of trouble.

Reading Someone Else's Texts

Does your partner ask to read your texts? Or read them behind your back? Healthy relationships are built on trust, not jealousy. You have the right to privacy and the ability to talk to whomever you like. You may want to explain to your partner that you have nothing to hide, but don't like them going through your phone or deciding who your friends are. If your partner refuses to change, you could be in an unhealthy relationship.

Threats over Text

Threats over text should be taken seriously—try not to write them off as angry venting. Keep track of threatening texts and think about talking to someone you trust about what is happening. Being in a violent relationship is dangerous—don't go through it alone.

What Can I Do?

Whether you feel like your partner is already using their cell phone in an abusive way or you're trying to prevent it, here are tips to keep you safe and healthy:

- Remember, it's ok to turn off your phone. Just be sure your parent or guardian knows how to contact you in an emergency.

- Don't answer calls from unknown or blocked numbers. Your abuser can easily call you from another line if they suspect you are avoiding them.

- Don't respond to hostile, harassing, abusive, or inappropriate texts or messages. Responding can encourage the person who sent the message and won't get them to stop. Your messages might also get you in trouble and make it harder to get a restraining order or file a criminal report.

- Save or document troublesome texts, as you may need them later for evidence in case you file a criminal report or ask for a restraining order.

- Many phone companies can block up to ten numbers from texting or calling you. Contact your phone company or check their website to see if you can do this on your phone.

- If you are in or coming out of a dangerous relationship, avoid using any form of technology to contact your abuser. It can be dangerous and may be used against you in the future.

- It may seem extreme, but if the abuse and harassment don't stop, changing your phone number may be your best option.

If you are feeling threatened or suffocated by your partner's constant calls or texts, it may be a sign that you are in an unhealthy and potentially abusive relationship. When your partner says or does things that make you afraid, lowers your self-esteem, or manipulates you, it is called verbal or emotional abuse. You have the right to be in a safe and healthy relationship free from all types of abuse.

Section 16.2

Technology Use and Digital Dating Abuse among Teens

Excerpted from Hinduja, S. and Patchin, J. W. (2011), *Electronic Dating Violence: A Brief Guide for Educators and Parents*, Cyberbullying Research Center (www.cyberbullying.us). © 2011 Cyberbullying Research Center. All rights reserved. Reprinted with permission.

What Does Research Tell Us About Electronic Dating Violence?

Recent studies have shown that dating violence among youthful populations remains a significant social problem, and a few studies sponsored in part by private sector corporations indicate that the internet and cell phones serve a contributing role (CDC 2006; Connolly & Friendlander 2009; Giordano 2007; Mulford & Giordano 2008; O'Leary, et al. 2008). For example, an online survey of teens sponsored by the Liz Claiborne company revealed that 36 percent of teens say their boyfriend or girlfriend checked up on them as many as thirty times per day and 17 percent reported that their significant other made them afraid not to respond to cell phone calls, e-mail, or text messages (Picard 2007). Another recent poll found that 22 percent of youth between the ages of fourteen and twenty-four who were involved in a romantic relationship said that their partner wrote something about them online or in a text message that wasn't true (MTV-AP 2009). This same survey reported that 22 percent of youth felt that their significant other checked up on them too often online or via cell phone.

In research based on a random sample of approximately 4,400 eleven- to eighteen-year-old youth from a large school district in the southern United States from 2010, we found that about 12 percent of students had been the victim of some form of electronic dating violence. More specific results are summarized below.

Victimization

- 10 percent of youth said a romantic partner has prevented them from using a computer or cell phone.

- 6 percent of boys and girls say their romantic partner posted something publicly online to make fun of, threaten, or embarrass them.

- Among boys, 10.4 percent, and among girls, 9.8 percent said they received a threatening cell phone message from their romantic partner.

- Among boys, 5.4 percent, and among girls, 3.4 percent said their romantic partner uploaded or shared a humiliating or harassing picture of them online or through their cell phone.

Offending

- Seven percent of youth admitted that they prevented their romantic partner from using a computer or cell phone.

- Six percent of boys and 4 percent of girls say they posted something publicly online to make fun of, threaten, or embarrass their romantic partner.

- About 7 percent of youth said they sent a threatening cell phone message to their romantic partner.

- Five percent of boys and 3 percent of girls said they uploaded or shared a humiliating of harassing picture of their romantic partner online or through their cell phone.

Relationships

- Victims of traditional (offline) dating violence are significantly more likely to be victims of electronic forms of dating violence (r = .75) than those who have not experienced offline bullying. [Ed.

Note: R values represent a statistical measure called the correlation coefficient. Numbers shown in this list are between 0 and 1. Numbers closer to 0 represent a lesser relationship, and numbers closer to 1indicate a greater relationship.]

- Those who admit to engaging in traditional dating violence also report engaging in electronic forms of dating violence (r = .77).

- Victims of dating violence (r = .51) and specifically electronic forms of dating violence (r = .64) are significantly more likely to also be victims of cyberbullying.

- Youth who are cyberbullied are 3.6 times as likely to experience electronic teen dating violence as those who are not cyberbullied.

- Youth who admit to engaging in dating violence (r = .52) and specifically electronic forms of dating violence (r = .65) also admit to engaging in cyberbullying.

- Youth who share their passwords with their significant other are nearly three times as likely to be victims of electronic dating violence.

- All forms of dating violence increase as youth get older.

Notes

CDC. (2006). Physical dating violence among high school students - United States, 2003. *Morbidity and Mortality Weekly Report*, 55.

Connolly, J., & Friendlander, L. (2009). Peer Group Influences on Adolescent Dating Aggression. *The Prevention Researcher*, 16(1), 8–11.

Giordano, P. (2007, December 4, 2007). Recent Research on Gender and Adolescent Relationships: Implications for Teen Dating Violence Research/Prevention. Paper presented at the Workshop on Teen Dating Violence: Developing a Research Agenda to Meet Practice Needs, Crystal City, VA.

MTV-AP. (2009). Digital Abuse Study. Retrieved from http://www.athin line.org/MTV-AP_Digital_Abuse_Study_Executive_Summary.pdf.

Mulford, C., & Giordano, P. C. (2008). Teen Dating Violence: A Closer Look at Adolescent Romantic Relationships. *NIJ Journal*(261), 34–40.

O'Leary, K. D., Smith-Slep, A. M., Avery-Leaf, S., & Cascardi, M. (2008). Gender Differences in Dating Aggression Among Multiethnic High School Students. *Journal of Adolescent Health*, 42(5), 473–79.

Picard, P. (2007). Tech Abuse in Teen Relationships Study. Retrieved from www.loveisnotabuse.com/pdf/06-208_Tech_Relationship_Abuse_TPL.pdf.

Section 16.3

Cyberbullying

Reprinted from "What Is Cyberbullying?"
and "Report Cyberbullying," U.S. Department of
Health and Human Services, stopybullying.gov, 2012.

What Is Cyberbullying?

Cyberbullying is bullying that takes place using electronic technology. Electronic technology includes devices and equipment such as cell phones, computers, and tablets as well as communication tools including social media sites, text messages, chat, and websites.

Examples of cyberbullying include mean text messages or e-mails, rumors sent by e-mail or posted on social networking sites, and embarrassing pictures, videos, websites, or fake profiles.

Why Cyberbullying Is Different

Kids who are being cyberbullied are often bullied in person as well. Additionally, kids who are cyberbullied have a harder time getting away from the behavior:

- Cyberbullying can happen twenty-four hours a day, seven days a week, and reach a kid even when he or she is alone. It can happen any time of the day or night.

- Cyberbullying messages and images can be posted anonymously and distributed quickly to a very wide audience. It can be difficult and sometimes impossible to trace the source.

- Deleting inappropriate or harassing messages, texts, and pictures is extremely difficult after they have been posted or sent.

Effects of Cyberbullying

Cell phones and computers themselves are not to blame for cyberbullying. Social media sites can be used for positive activities, like connecting kids with friends and family, helping students with school, and for entertainment. But these tools can also be used to hurt other people. Whether done in person or through technology, the effects of bullying are similar.

Kids who are cyberbullied are more likely to do the following:

- Use alcohol and drugs

- Skip school

- Experience in-person bullying

- Be unwilling to attend school

- Receive poor grades

- Have lower self-esteem

- Have more health problems

Frequency of Cyberbullying

The 2008–2009 School Crime Supplement (National Center for Education Statistics and Bureau of Justice Statistics) indicates that 6 percent of students in grades six to twelve experienced cyberbullying.

The 2011 Youth Risk Behavior Surveillance Survey finds that 16 percent of high school students (grades nine to twelve) were electronically bullied in the past year.

Research on cyberbullying is growing. However, because kids' technology use changes rapidly, it is difficult to design surveys that accurately capture trends.

Report Cyberbullying

When cyberbullying happens, it is important to document and report the behavior so it can be addressed.

Steps to Take Immediately

- Don't respond to and don't forward cyberbullying messages.

- Keep evidence of cyberbullying. Record the dates, times, and descriptions of instances when cyberbullying has occurred. Save and print screenshots, e-mails, and text messages. Use this evidence to report cyberbullying to web and cell phone service providers.

- Block the person who is cyberbullying.

Report Cyberbullying to Online Service Providers

Cyberbullying often violates the terms of service established by social media sites and internet service providers:

- Review their terms and conditions or rights and responsibilities sections. These describe content that is or is not appropriate.

- Visit social media safety centers to learn how to block users and change settings to control who can contact you.

- Report cyberbullying to the social media site so they can take action against users abusing the terms of service.

Report Cyberbullying to Law Enforcement

When cyberbullying involves these activities it is considered a crime and should be reported to law enforcement:

- Threats of violence

- Child pornography or sending sexually explicit messages or photos

- Taking a photo or video of someone in a place where he or she would expect privacy

- Stalking and hate crimes

Some states consider other forms of cyberbullying criminal. Consult your state's laws and law enforcement for additional guidance.

Report Cyberbullying to Schools

Cyberbullying can create a disruptive environment at school and is often related to in-person bullying. The school can use the information to help inform prevention and response strategies.

In many states, schools are required to address cyberbullying in their anti-bullying policy. Some state laws also cover off-campus behavior that creates a hostile school environment.

Section 16.4

Some Statistics on Internet Aggression

Excerpted from "Electronic Media and Youth Violence:
A CDC Issue Brief for Educators and Caregivers," Centers for
Disease Control and Prevention, 2008.

How common is electronic aggression?

Because electronic aggression is fairly new, limited information is available, and those researching the topic have asked different questions about it. Thus, information cannot be readily compared or combined across studies, which limits our ability to make definitive conclusions about the prevalence and impact of electronic aggression.

What we know about electronic aggression is based upon a few studies that measure similar but not exactly the same behaviors. For example, in their studies, some of the panelists use a narrow definition of electronic aggression (e.g., aggression perpetrated through e-mail or instant messaging),[1] while others use a broader definition (e.g., aggression perpetrated through e-mail, instant messaging, on a website, or through text messaging).[2] In addition to different definitions, in their research the panelists also asked young people to report about their experiences over different time periods (e.g., over the past several months, since the beginning of school, in the past year), and surveyed youth of different ages (e.g., sixth- to eighth-graders, ten- to fifteen-year-olds, ten- to seventeen-year-olds). As a result, the most accurate way to describe the information we have is to give ranges that include the findings from all of the studies.

We know that most youth (65 to 91 percent) report little or no involvement in electronic aggression.[1,2,3] However, 9 to 35 percent of young people say they have been the victim of electronic aggression.[2,3] As with face-to-face bullying, estimates of electronic aggression perpetration are lower than victimization, ranging from 4 to 21 percent.[1] In some cases, the higher end of the range (e.g., 21 percent and 35 percent) reflects studies that asked about electronic aggression over a longer time period (e.g., a year as opposed to two months). In other cases, the higher percentages reflect studies that defined electronic aggression more broadly (e.g., spreading rumors, telling lies, or making threats as opposed to just telling lies).

When we look at data across all of the panelists' studies, the percentage of young people who report being electronic aggression victims has a fairly wide range (9 to 35 percent). However, if we look at victimization over a similar time frame, such as "monthly or more often" or "at least once in the past two months," the range is much narrower, from 8 to 11 percent.[1,2]

Similarly, although the percentage of young people who admit they perpetrate electronic aggression varies considerably across studies (4 to 21 percent),[5] the range narrows if we look at similar time periods. Approximately 4 percent of surveyed youth report behaving aggressively electronically "monthly or more often," or "at least once in the past two months."[3,5]

We currently know little about whether certain types of electronic aggression are more common than other forms. A study that looked at electronic aggression victimization "over the past year," found that making rude or nasty comments was the type of electronic aggression most frequently experienced by victims (32 percent), followed by rumor spreading (13 percent), and then by threatening or aggressive comments (14 percent).[2]

Who is at risk?

Whether the rates of electronic aggression perpetration and victimization differ for boys and girls is unknown. Research examining differences by sex is limited, and findings are conflicting. Some studies have not found any differences, while others have found that girls perpetrate electronic aggression more frequently than do boys.[1,3]

There is also little information about whether electronic aggression decreases or increases as young people age. As with other forms of aggression, there is some evidence that electronic aggression is less common in fifth grade than in eighth grade, but is higher in eighth grade than eleventh grade, suggesting that electronic aggression may peak around the end of middle school/beginning of high school.[1,3]

Current studies on electronic aggression have focused primarily on white populations. We have no information on how electronic aggression varies by race or ethnicity.

It is important to note that there is an overlap between victims and perpetrators of electronic aggression. As with many types of violence, those who are victims are also at increased risk for being perpetrators. Across the studies conducted by our panelists, between 7 and 14 percent of surveyed youth reported being both a victim and a perpetrator of electronic aggression.[3,5]

Although the news media has recently devoted a lot of attention to the potential dangers of technology, face-to-face verbal and physical aggression are still far more common than electronic aggression. Verbal bullying is the type of bullying most often experienced by young people, followed by physical bullying, and then by electronic aggression.[1] However, electronic aggression is becoming more common. In 2000, 6 percent of internet users ages ten to seventeen said they had been the victim of "online harassment," defined as threats or other offensive behavior [not sexual solicitation] sent online to someone or posted online. By 2005, this percentage had increased by 50 percent, to 9 percent.[4] As technology becomes more affordable and sophisticated, rates of electronic aggression are likely to continue to increase, especially if appropriate prevention and intervention policies and practices are not put into place.

What is the relationship between victims and perpetrators of electronic aggression?

Electronic technology allows adolescents to hide their identity, by sending or posting messages anonymously, by using a false name, or by assuming someone else's on-screen identity. So, unlike the aggression or bullying that occurs in the schoolyard, victims and perpetrators of electronic aggression may not know the person with whom they are interacting. Between 13 and 46 percent of young people who were victims of electronic aggression report not knowing their harasser's identity.[3,4] Similarly, 22 percent of young people who admit they perpetrate electronic aggression report they do not know the identity of their victim. In the schoolyard, the victim can respond to the bully or try to get a teacher or peer to help. In contrast, in the electronic world a victim is often alone when responding to aggressive e-mails or text messages, and his or her only defense may be to turn off the computer, cell phone, or personal digital assistant (PDA). If the electronic aggression takes the form of posting of a message or an embarrassing picture of the victim on a public website, the victim may have no defense.

As for the victims and perpetrators who are not anonymous, in one study, almost half of the victims (47 percent) said the perpetrator was another student at school.[3] In addition, aggression between siblings is no longer limited to the backseat of the car: 12 percent of victims reported their brother or sister was the perpetrator, and 10 percent of perpetrators reported being electronically aggressive toward a sibling.[3]

Do certain types of electronic technology pose a greater risk for victimization?

The news media often carry stories about young people victimized on social networking websites. Young people do experience electronic aggression in chat rooms: 25 percent of victims of electronic aggression said the victimization happened in a chat room and 23 percent said it happened on a website. However, instant messaging appears to be the most common way electronic aggression is perpetrated.[3] Fifty-six percent of perpetrators of electronic aggression and 67 percent of victims said the aggression they experienced or perpetrated was through instant messaging. Victims also report experiencing electronic aggression through e-mail (25 percent) and text messages (16 percent).

The way electronic aggression is perpetrated (e.g., through instant messaging, the posting of pictures on a website, sending an e-mail) is also related to the relationship between the victim and the perpetrator. Victims are significantly more likely to report receiving an aggressive instant message when they know the perpetrator from in-person situations (64 percent of victims), than they are if they only know the perpetrator online (34 percent).[4] Young people who are victimized by people they only know online are significantly more likely than those victimized by people they know from in-person situations to be victimized through e-mail (18 percent vs. 5 percent), chat rooms (18 percent vs. 4 percent), and online gaming websites (14 percent vs. 0 percent).[4]

In terms of frequency, electronic aggression perpetrated by young people who know each other in person appears to be more similar to face-to-face bullying than does aggression perpetrated by young people who only know each other online. For example, like in-person bullying, electronic aggression between young people who know each other in person is more likely to consist of a series of incidents. Fifty-nine percent of the incidents perpetrated by young people who knew each other in person involved a series of incidents by the same harasser, compared to 27 percent of incidents perpetrated by on-line-only contacts. In addition, 59 percent of the incidents perpetrated by young people who knew each other in person involved sending or posting messages for others to see, versus 18 percent of those perpetrated by young people the victims only knew on-line.[4]

References

1. Williams KR, Guerra NG. Prevalence and predictors of internet bullying. *J Adolesc Health* 2007; 41 (6 Suppl 1):S14–S21.

2. Ybarra ML, Diener-West M, Leaf PJ. Examining the overlap in internet harassment and school bullying: implications for school intervention. *J Adolesc Health* 2007; 41(6 Suppl 1):S42–S50.

3. Kowalski RM, Limber SP. Electronic bullying among middle school students. *J Adolesc Health* 2007; 41 (6 Suppl 1):S22–S30.

4. Wolak J, Mitchell KJ, Finkelhor D. Does on-line harassment constitute bullying? An exploration of on-line harassment by known peers and on-line only contacts. *J Adolesc Health* 2007; 41(6 Suppl 1):S51–58.

5. Ybarra ML, Espelage DL, Mitchell KJ. The co-occurrence of Internet harassment and unwanted sexual solicitation victimization and perpetration: associations with psychosocial indicators. *J Adolesc Health* 2007; 41(6 Suppl 1):S31–S41.

Chapter 17

Abuse in Pregnancy

Chapter Contents

Section 17.1

Domestic Violence during Pregnancy: Prevalence and Consequences

"The Facts on Reproductive Health and Violence Against Women," © 2008 Futures Without Violence. All rights reserved. Reprinted with permission. For additional information, visit www.futureswithoutviolence.org.

Violence against women is a costly and pervasive problem, and women of reproductive age—in particular, those ages sixteen to twenty-four—are at greatest risk. Violence limits women's ability to manage their reproductive health and exposes them to sexually transmitted diseases. Abuse during pregnancy can have lasting harmful effects for a woman, the developing fetus, and newborns:

- On average, almost five hundred women (483) are raped or sexually assaulted each day in this country.[1]

- One in five Boston public high school girls report physical or sexual abuse by a dating partner.[2]

- According to the World Health Organization, 6 to 59 percent of women in countries around the world experience sexual violence (being physically forced to have sex against their will, having sex because they were afraid of what their partners might do, or being forced to do something sexual that was humiliating or degrading) from an intimate partner sometime in their lives.[3]

Contraception

- Some women have trouble getting prompt access to emergency contraception—a safe, effective back-up birth control method that can prevent pregnancy when taken within days of unprotected intercourse.

- A study of 474 adolescent mothers on public assistance found that 51 percent, and two in three of those who experienced domestic violence at the hands of their boyfriends, experienced some form of birth control sabotage by a dating partner.[4]

Teen and Adult Unintended Pregnancy

- As many as two-thirds of adolescents who become pregnant were sexually or physically abused sometime in their lives.[5]

- Some 25 to 50 percent of adolescent mothers experience partner violence before, during, or just after their pregnancy.[6]

- Forty percent of pregnant women who have been exposed to abuse report that their pregnancy was unintended, compared to just 8 percent of non-abused women.[7]

Sexually Transmitted Infections

- Violence is linked to a wide range of reproductive health issues including sexually transmitted disease (STD) and human immunodeficiency virus (HIV) transmission, miscarriages, risky sexual health behavior, and more.[8]

- Women disclosing physical violence are nearly three times more likely to experience a sexually transmitted infection than women who don't disclose physical abuse.[9]

- One in three adolescents tested for sexually transmitted infections and HIV have experienced domestic violence.[10]

Violence during Pregnancy

- Homicide is the second leading cause of traumatic death for pregnant and recently pregnant women in the U.S., accounting for 31 percent of maternal injury deaths.[11]

- Women experiencing abuse in the year prior to and/or during a recent pregnancy are 40 to 60 percent more likely than non-abused women to report high blood pressure, vaginal bleeding, severe nausea, kidney or urinary tract infections, and hospitalization during pregnancy and are 37 percent more likely to deliver preterm. Children born to abused mothers are 17 percent more likely to be born underweight and more than 30 percent more likely than other children to require intensive care upon birth.[12]

- Few doctors screen their patients for abuse,[13] even though up to one in twelve pregnant women are battered.[14]

- Women who were screened for abuse and given a wallet sized referral reported fewer threats of violence, assaults, or even harassment at work.[15]

Notes

1. National Crime Victimization Survey: Criminal Victimization, 2005. U.S. Department of Justice, Bureau of Justice Statistics. Retrieved September 2006. Available at http://www.ojp.usdoj.gov/bjs/pub/pdf/cv05.pdf.

2. Silverman JG, Raj A, Mucci LA, Hathaway JE. Dating Violence Against Adolescent Girls and Associated Substance Use, Unhealthy Weight control, Sexual Risk Behavior, Pregnancy and Suicidality. *JAMA*. 2001:286(5)572–79.

3. Garcia-Moreno C. 2005. Multi-Country Study on Women's Health and Domestic Violence Against Women. World Health Organization. Geneva, Switzerland. Countries studied include: Bangladesh, Brazil, Ethiopia, Japan, Namibia, Peru, Samoa, Serbia and Montenegro, Thailand and the United Republic of Tanzania. Available at http://www.who.int/gender/violence/who_multicountry_study/en/.

4. Domestic Violence and Birth Control Sabotage: A Report from the Teen Parent Project. 2000. Center for Impact Research. Chicago, IL. Available at http://www.impactresearch.org/documents/dvandbirthcontrol.pdf.

5. Leiderman, Sally and Cair Almo. 2001. Interpersonal Violence and Adolescent Pregnancy: Prevalence and Implications for Practice and Policy. Center for Assessment and Policy Development and the National Organization on Adolescent Pregnancy, Parenting, and Prevention. Available at http://capd.traininghelpdesk.com/pubfiles/pub-2001-10-01.pdf.

6. Ibid.

7. Hathaway JE; Mucci, LA, Silverman JG, Brooks DR, Mathews R, Pavlos CA, Health Status and Health Care Use of Massachusetts Women Reporting Partner Abuse. *American Journal of Preventive Medicine*. 2000; 19(4); 318–21.

8. Violence Against Women: Effects on Reproductive Health. *Outlook* 20(1). 2002. Available at http://www.path.org/files/EOL20_1.pdf.

9. Coker, AL, Smith PH, Bethea L, King MR, McKeown RE. Physical Health Consequences of Physical and Psychological Intimate Partner Violence. *Archives of Family Medicine*. 2000; 9 451–57.

10. Decker, MR, Silverman, JG and Raj, A; 2005 *Pediatrics*: Vol. 116 No. 2 August 2005, pp. e272–e276.

11. Chang J, Berg C, Saltzman L, Herndon J. 2005. Homicide: A Leading Cause of Injury Deaths Among Pregnant and Postpartum Women in the United States, 1991–1999. *American Journal of Public Health*. 95(3): 471–77.

12. Silverman, JG, Decker, MR, Reed, E, Raj, A. Intimate Partner Violence Victimization Prior to and During Pregnancy Among Women Residing in 26 U.S. States: Associations with Maternal and Neonatal Health. *American Journal of Obstetrics and Gynecology* 2006; 195(1): 140–48.

13. Parsons, L., et. al. 2000. Violence Against Women and Reproductive Health: Toward Defining a Role for Reproductive Health Care Services. *Maternal and Child Health Journal*. 4(2): 135.

14. Gazmararian JA, Petersen R, Spitz AM, Goodwin MM, Saltzman LE, Marks JS. Violence and reproductive health: current knowledge and future research directions. *Maternal and Child Health Journal* 2000;4(2): 79–84.

15. McFarlane, Judith M.; Groff, Janet Y.; O'Brien, Jennifer A.; Watson, Kathy; 2006. *Nursing Research*. 55(1):52–61.

Section 17.2

How to Help a Pregnant Woman Who Is in an Abusive Relationship

Pregnancy, birth and the postpartum period represent particularly high-risk times for women experiencing interpersonal abuse. The birth of a baby brings about new, at times unanticipated challenges beyond those she may have previously faced as they are unique to childbearing (e.g. growing fetus, newborn care). Family and friends may find it particularly challenging to remain supportive in these situations and the stigma of experiencing abuse in pregnancy may further reduce a pregnant woman's fear of disclosing on-going abuse. It is important to be aware that isolation at the hands of an abusive partner is a major contributing factor to why women are unable to leave, and abusers often use this as a strategy (to maintain power and control in the relationship.

Manifestations of Abuse during the Childbearing Years

In pregnancy, woman abuse tactics may include, but are not limited to the following:

- Limiting the partner's access to prenatal care

- Increasing physical assaults aimed at abdominal area

- Derogatory/insulting comments directed at the woman's changing body

- Restricting her choice of caregiver

- Preventing partner from obtaining information related to pregnancy and birth or forcing her to consent to tests against her will

- Threatening to leave her if she does/doesn't terminate pregnancy

The 1993 Violence Against Women survey (twelve thousand women) found that 21 percent of the women who had been abused by their partners had been assaulted during pregnancy. Of these women, 40 percent stated that the abuse began when they became pregnant. Why?

- He may not want the pregnancy.
- The abuse may be an attempt(s) to cause a miscarriage.
- He may feel that he will lose the "spotlight" to the new baby.
- He may be uncomfortable with the woman's changing body and resent her for it.
- He may want to ensure that he will maintain control over her when more people are likely to be involved with their lives.
- He may resent the increase in responsibilities that a new baby will bring.

However, the strongest predictor that a woman will be abused during her pregnancy is prior abuse in the relationship.

What You Should Not Do

If a friend or family member tells you that she is being abused, there are certain things you should *never* do:

- Never insist that she leave her abusive partner.
- Never make comments that suggest she is responsible for the abuse.
- Never judge her reasons for remaining in the relationship.
- Never endanger her by providing information in an unsafe way (e.g. in a joint mailbox or leave a phone message).
- Never force her to do what you think is best for her or her unborn baby or child(ren).

Never Insist That the Woman Leave Her Abusive Partner

Understandably, it is very difficult not to insist that a loved one leave her abusive partner. Remember, a woman who is experiencing abuse often is very fearful of what will happen to her if she tries to leave an abusive partner. This may be because of threats the partner may have made to harm her, her family, and/or her property should she try to leave. There is also the hope that women maintain, that the abuse will end once the baby arrives. Many women are harmed by their estranged partners once they leave an abusive relationship, and harassment can be ongoing. However, if you can remain open to supporting her and respecting without judgment her decision to stay, you will establish yourself as a caring and sensitive ally that she can turn to if and when she is able to leave her abusive partner. Women must be ready to leave on their own terms—coercion and ultimatums by family, friends, or outside agencies attempting to force them to leave often cause women to become more isolated and disconnected from potential supports. It is essential that any woman leaving an abusive relationship have an opportunity to make a safety plan with the appropriate woman abuse service providers, so that in the even that needs to leave in an emergency, she knows where she is going and how she will get there.

Never Make Comments That Suggest She Is Responsible for the Abuse

Women in abusive relationships are often told by their abusive partners that they are to blame for the abuse they experience. Comments like "you pushed my buttons," "if only you hadn't . . .," "I wouldn't have had to do that if you would have just . . .," "You are making such a big deal out of this," "I only . . .," "It wasn't as bad as you are making it out to be," "you exaggerate," and "you're crazy/stupid," said repeatedly to a woman, cause her to start believing them. Women internalize these messages and start to hold themselves responsible, when in fact the abusive partner needs to be held solely accountable for his/her choices, including the choice to engage in hurtful and damaging expressions of anger, fear, sadness, or frustration. Blaming a woman who has been abused further erodes her self-esteem, making it that much more difficult for her to seek support to leave the abusive partner. She will likely not turn to you for comfort, reassurance, or assistance in the future if you display an attitude of judgment against her.

Never Judge Her Reasons for Remaining in the Relationship

Maintaining a clear focus on who is responsible for the abuse helps us to assist the woman from a caring and understanding space. It is important to recognize the complex dynamics of abuse and how they work to skew a woman's sense of reality of her self, her relationship, and her partner. As we mentioned above, there are ongoing risks for women and children when they attempt to leave an abusive relationship. Her reasons for staying may include an awareness of how real those risks are, especially if she has attempted to leave an abusive relationship in the past.

There is also a lack of affordable housing options, inadequate protection from the estranged partner from law enforcement, limited daycare spots, and wait-lists for counseling and shelters, not to mention social and cultural expectations that perpetuate stigma and shame for the woman experiencing abuse. We need to look at how many barriers a woman can face attempting to leave an abusive relationship and how immensely difficult to overcome they can appear to be for a woman in the childbearing year.

Never Endanger Her by Providing Information in an Unsafe Way (e.g., Mailing It to Her)

Abusive partners may take mail, search purses, or erase email/phone messages. It is advisable to ask her in private what would be the best way for her to receive information. Sometimes pamphlets and important phone numbers can be kept at a workplace or a friend's house. For some women they may need to memorize the number to a local shelter or be advised to call 911 in the case of an emergency.

Never Force Her to Do What Anyone Else Thinks Is Best for Her or Her Unborn Baby

Well-meaning friends, family, and healthcare providers often give abused women advice on what they should or shouldn't be doing to care for themselves. It can be difficult to understand that sometimes the best thing that you can do is just be there. It sounds so simple, but women who are abused have often lost many friends or have never felt comfortable enough to tell others about their abuse. If she has shared her story with you, reward her courage and ask her how she would like you to help . . . if at all.

How You Can Help

Just as the transition to mothering can present unique risks for women, experiencing abuse it is, for some, a time when they are finally able to reach out for help for the safety of themselves and their child(ren) to be. Asking for help to leave an abusive relationship is a tremendous act of courage, and should be taken seriously. Be there to listen, care, and refer to the most appropriate community service. If you do not know who to contact, call your local police department or women's shelter.

Section 17.3

Stress of Domestic Violence Can Be Passed to Unborn Children

A new study provides evidence that stress from domestic violence during pregnancy may make offspring more prone to stress as an adult.

However, the research doesn't directly prove a cause-and-effect relationship.

It may be difficult to ever prove that stress affecting the bodies of stressed-out pregnant mothers disrupts the inner chemistry of their children. The study does point to the importance of a low-stress pregnancy, however.

"Healthy development starts in the womb, and it is not only nutritional," said study co-author Axel Meyer, an evolutionary biologist at the University of Konstanz in Germany. "Behavioral and emotional factors are important, and the effects are long-lasting."

In recent years, scientists have tried to understand how stress during pregnancy affects the fetus, possibly by altering genes. Research has suggested that anxious and stressed mothers are more likely to have children who develop attention and behavior problems and other issues, said Thomas G. O'Connor, director of the Wynne Center for Family Research at the University of Rochester Medical Center in new York.

It's challenging to figure out whether there's a direct link because many factors other than maternal stress—such as the environment in which a child is raised—could explain why kids turn out the way they do.

In science, the gold standard of research is to randomly assign groups of subjects to undergo different treatments or experiences and watch what happens to them. But it would be unethical to expose pregnant mothers to stress. So, researchers examine the effects of stress on pregnant animals, or they try to look backwards to find women who were stressed while pregnant and examine how it may have affected their offspring.

In this study, researchers looked at the genes of women and their children that are thought to be connected to stress.

They found that genetically, mothers stressed by domestic violence appear to "program their offspring to respond in a more costly way when exposed to stressors," Meyer said. The genes in the women themselves weren't affected by exposure to domestic violence.

Meyer said the ongoing stress of the domestic relationships may have been the key problem for the women. "Data from many studies suggest that stressors need not be physical," he said. "Emotional neglect, ongoing familial conflict, and other severe forms of adversity may also take their toll."

Could something in the women that makes them more likely to become victims of domestic violence be passed down to their children? Probably not. The researchers linked domestic violence during pregnancy to genetic differences in their children, but they didn't find a link to mothers who experienced domestic violence before pregnancy.

How is the research helpful? "If it really were the case that stress in pregnancy did have persistent effects, then we should invest a great deal more effort and resources in trying to improve well-being in pregnancy," said O'Connor. "It would presumably be cost-effective because you're preventing something from happening."

The study appears in the July 19, 2011, issue of *Translational Psychiatry*.

Chapter 18

Family Violence against Women with Disabilities

Why It Matters

Women with developmental disabilities have among the highest rates of physical, sexual, and emotional violence perpetrated by intimate partners and family members.[1] Disabled individuals are at greater risk of severe physical and sexual violence than nondisabled persons, and many disabled victims of violence experience multiple assaults.[2,3] Domestic abuse victims with disabilities are often more dependent on their caretakers than victims without disabilities, and face many barriers to reporting abuse and seeking services.[4] Victims who do report abuse or seek services often do not find adequate help, since many programs that serve domestic violence victims are not equipped or trained to offer proper care to disabled victims.[4]

Did You Know?

- Women with disabilities had a 40 percent greater risk of violence than women without disabilities.[5]

- Women with disabilities are at particular risk for severe violence.[5]

- The most common perpetrators of violence against women with disabilities are their male partners.[5]

- Studies estimate that 80 percent of disabled women have been sexually assaulted.[6]

- Women with disabilities are three times more likely to be sexually assaulted than women without disabilities.[7]

- One study showed that 47 percent of sexually abused women with disabilities reported assaults on more than ten occasions.[8]

- Approximately 48 percent of substantiated cases of abuse involve elder adults who are not physically able to care for themselves.[9]

- Disabled children are more than twice as likely as children without disabilities to be physically abused, and almost twice as likely to be sexually abused.[10]

- Virtually all women with disabilities who were sexually assaulted also reported social, emotional, and behavioral harm.[11]

Reporting Abuse

- Studies estimate that between 70 and 85 percent of cases of abuse against disabled adults go unreported.[12]

- One study found that only 5 percent of reported crimes against people with disabilities were prosecuted, compared to 70 percent for serious crimes committed against people with no disabilities.[12]

- Disabled victims are more vulnerable to threats by their abusers if they report the abuse.[13]

Barriers to Seeking Services

- People with disabilities often lack accessible services due to limited resources, lack of transportation (especially in rural communities), or structural limitations of service facilities.[14]

- Some disabled victims lack the skills or abilities necessary to act independently to seek help.[13]

- Many disabled victims lack knowledge about services. Public information and awareness education are generally not distributed in Braille, large print, or audiotape and do not define domestic violence in ways that people with disabilities can relate to.[13]

- Disabled victims of violence are heavily dependent on their abusive primary caretakers and run the risk of losing their caretaker if they report abuse.[13]

- Victims may experience an increased risk of being institutionalized or losing their basic decision-making rights if they are viewed as unable to take care of themselves without the help of their abuser.[13]

- Disabled victims may be at greater risk for losing child custody if they are viewed as being unable to care for children independently from an abusive primary caretaker.[13]

Disability Training

- Only 35 percent of shelters surveyed have disability awareness training for their staff and only 16percent have a dedicated staff person to deliver services to women with disabilities.[15]

- Service providers often lack the training and sensitivity necessary to serve victims with disabilities.[14]

- Some people see people with disabilities as less credible than nondisabled victims.[16]

- Some people think abusive treatment is necessary to manage people with disabilities or blame disabled victims for the abuse they suffer, and because they hold these beliefs they consider domestic violence against people with disabilities to be justified.[13]

Protections for Disabled Victims of Violence[16]

The Violence Against Women Act and Victims with Disabilities

The Violence Against Women Act (VAWA) provides support to victims with disabilities. Although the original version of VAWA did not provide funding for victims with disabilities, the 2000 reauthorization authorized a grant program to provide education and technical assistance to service providers to better meet the needs of disabled victims of violence.

The 2005 reauthorization of VAWA further expanded coverage for disabled victims. The 2005 reauthorization:

- expanded education, training, and services grant programs;

- Included added construction and personnel costs for shelters that serve disabled victims of domestic violence to the purpose areas that can receive VAWA funding;

- focused on the development of collaborative relationships between victim service organizations and organizations that serve individuals with disabilities;

- provided funding for the development of model programs that implement advocacy and intervention services within organizations servicing disabled individuals.

Protection and Services for Disabled Victims

Although the Department of Justice authorized $10 million per year for fiscal year (FY) 2007 through FY 2011, only $7.1 million was allocated for protections and services for disabled victims in FY 2007. The Campaign for Funding to End Domestic and Sexual Violence requests $10 million for FY 2008 and subsequent years to be allocated to serve victims with disabilities.

Sources

1.   Abramson, W., et al. (Ed). "Violence Against Women with Developmental or Other Disabilities." *Impact* 13(3).

2.   Brownridge, Douglas. (2006) "Partner Violence Against Women With Disabilities: Prevalence, Risk, and Explanations." *Violence Against Women* (12)9.

3.   Abramson, W., et al. (Ed). "Violence Against Women with Developmental or Other Disabilities." *Impact* 13(3).

4.   West Virginia Coalition Against Domestic Violence. "People With Disabilities." Resources. Accessed online at http://www .wvcadv.org/people_with_disabilities.htm, July 2007.

5.   Brownridge, Douglas. (2006) "Partner Violence Against Women With Disabilities: Prevalence, Risk, and Explanations." *Violence Against Women* (12)9.

6.   Protection and Advocacy, Inc. (2003) "Abuse and Neglect of Adults with Developmental Disabilities: A Public Health Priority for the State of California."

7.   Brownridge, Douglas. (2006) "Partner Violence Against Women With Disabilities: Prevalence, Risk, and Explanations." *Violence Against Women* (12)9.

8. Abramson, W., et al. (Ed). "Violence Against Women with Developmental or Other Disabilities." *Impact* 13(3).

9. Metropolitan Life Insurance Company. (2004) "Preventing Elder Abuse." *Since You Care Guide*. New York.

10. Abramson, W., et al. (Ed). "Violence Against Women with Developmental or Other Disabilities." *Impact* 13(3).

11. Abramson, W., et al. (Ed). "Violence Against Women with Developmental or Other Disabilities." *Impact* 13(3).

12. Protection and Advocacy, Inc. (2003) "Abuse and Neglect of Adults with Developmental Disabilities: A Public Health Priority for the State of California."

13. West Virginia Coalition Against Domestic Violence. "People With Disabilities." Resources. Accessed online at http://www .wvcadv.org/people_with_disabilities.htm, July 2007.

14. Chang, J. C., et al. (2003). "Helping women with disabilities and domestic violence: Strategies, limitations, and challenges of domestic violence programs and services." *Journal of Women's Health* 12(7): 699–708.

15. Nosek, Ph.D. Margaret A. et al. "Violence Against Women with Disabilities—Fact Sheet #1: Findings from Studies 1992–2002." Baylor College of Medicine.

16. National Coalition Against Domestic Violence. (2006) "Comparison of VAWA 1994, VAWA 2000 and VAWA 2005 Reauthorization Bill." Accessed online at http://www.ncadv.org/files/ VAWA_94_00_05.pdf, July 2007.

Chapter 19

Abuse of Men

Chapter Contents

Section 19.1

About Domestic Violence against Men

"Information For and About Male Victims of Domestic Abuse," © 2008 Domestic Abuse Helpline for Men and Women. Reprinted with permission. The Domestic Abuse Helpline for Men and Women offers a National twenty-four-hour helpline for information and support, and referrals to other programs and resources. For additional information, call the Helpline at 888-7HELPLINE (888-743-5754) or visit http://dahmw.org.

Have You Been Abused?

- Does your partner block an exit to keep you from leaving during an argument? Open personal mail? Keep you from seeing friends or family? Use name-calling?

- Does your partner denigrate you in the presence of others? Say no one else would want you? Threaten suicide if you were to leave?

- Do you feel like you're "walking on eggshells" around your partner? Does she act like two different people (e.g., Dr. Jekyll/ Mr. Hyde)?

- Does she threaten that if you leave you will never see the children again? Destroy or threaten to destroy your property?

- Have you been shoved, slapped, punched, bitten, or kicked? Even once?

- Does your partner anger easily, especially when drinking or on drugs?

If any number of these factors are true in your relationship, there is a problem. Victims of intimate partner violence come from all walks of life—all cultures, incomes, professions, ages, and religions. Intimate partner violence is not always defined by who's the stronger and/or bigger person in the relationship. However, it is about one person having and maintaining power and control over another person through physical, psychological, and/or verbally abusive means.

Why Men Don't Tell

Men typically face disbelief and ridicule when reporting abuse. As a result, male victims of domestic abuse tend to make excuses for injuries—"It was an accident"—when questioned by friends or medical personnel, which only allows perpetrators to continue the abuse.

Abusers are experts at making their victims feel like no one is on their side. Feeling like no one cares can create a spiral of isolation—the more you withdraw from friends and family, the less those who care about you will be able to help.

Though you may have been injured far worse on an athletic field, it is not the same thing as being physically attacked by your intimate partner, which hurts emotionally as well as physically. Allowing this pattern to continue can result in depression, substance abuse, loss of confidence, and even suicide.

For over thirty years, domestic violence has been defined as "the chronic abuse of power that men use to control women." Public awareness campaigns have focused solely on men as the perpetrators, never as victims. And yet, a Department of Justice study indicates that over 834,000 men report being domestically assaulted annually.

The general public has been desensitized by sit-coms and commercials depicting men being hit over the head with frying pans, kicked in the groin, and slapped in the face by their intimate female partners. What message does this give society? A woman hitting a man is humorous and acceptable behavior. But it's not. No one deserves to be abused whether man, woman or child.

What You Can Do

- Keep a record of incidents of abuse.
- Take photographs.
- Always seek medical attention for your injuries, and be truthful about what caused them.
- Tell family and friends what is happening.
- Avoid being provoked into physical retaliation. When it is safe for you to do so, leave.

Document! Document! Document!

Reasons Why Men Stay in Abusive Relationships

- **Shame:** What will people think? OR I don't want to be laughed at OR No one will believe me.

- **Self-worth:** I probably deserved it.

- **Denial:** I can handle it, it's not that bad OR All I have to do is leave the house until she cools down OR It's premenstrual syndrome (PMS); the kids are giving her a hard time.

- **Reluctance to give up the good:** She is a really creative, or loving, or wonderful person most of the time OR She didn't mean it.

- **Inertia:** It's too hard to do anything about it OR I'm not ready to change my life OR I'll deal with it later.

Help for Victims of Domestic Abuse

Academic studies indicate that both men and women are victims as well as perpetrators of domestic violence. Historically, men are more likely to inflict injury. However, domestic violence, by definition, is not limited to physical abuse. It is a pattern of behavior in any relationship that is used to gain or maintain power and control over an intimate partner. Abuse is physical, sexual, emotional, economic, or psychological actions or threats of actions that manipulate, intimidate, paralyze, hurt, humiliate, blame, or put fear in another person. Domestic violence can happen to anyone of any race, age, gender, religion, or sexual orientation. It can happen to couples who are married, living together, or who are dating. Domestic violence affects people of all socioeconomic backgrounds and educational levels.

Section 19.2

Sexual Assault of Men

Rape is a men's issue for many reasons. For one, we don't often talk about the fact that men are sexually assaulted. We need to start recognizing the presence of male survivors and acknowledging their unique experience.

The following questions and answers can help us all learn about male survivors so that we stop treating them as invisible and start helping them heal.

How often are men sexually assaulted?

While the numbers vary from study to study, most research suggests that 10 to 20 percent of males will be sexually violated at some point in their lifetimes. That translates into tens of thousands of boys and men assaulted each year alongside hundreds of thousands of girls and women.

If there are so many male survivors, why don't I know any?

Like female survivors, most male survivors never report being assaulted. Perhaps worst of all, men fear being blamed for the assault because they were not "man enough" to protect themselves in the face of an attack.

Can a woman sexually assault a man?

Yes, but it's not nearly as common as male-on-male assault. A recent study shows that more than 86 percent of male survivors are sexually abused by another male. That is not to say, however, that we should overlook boys or men who are victimized by females. It may be tempting to dismiss such experiences as wanted sexual initiation (especially in the case of an older female assaulting a younger male),

257

but the reality is that the impact of female-on-male assault can be just as damaging.

Don't only men in prison get raped?

While prison rape is a serious problem and a serious crime, many male survivors are assaulted in everyday environments, often by people they know—friends, teammates, relatives, teachers, clergy, bosses, partners. As with female survivors, men are also sometimes raped by strangers. These situations tend to be more violent and more often involve a group of attackers rather than a single attacker.

How does rape affect men differently from women?

Rape affects men in many ways similar to women. Anxiety, anger, sadness, confusion, fear, numbness, self-blame, helplessness, hopelessness, suicidal feelings and shame are common reactions of both male and female survivors.

In some ways, though, men react uniquely to being sexually assaulted. Immediately after an assault, men may show more hostility and aggression rather than tearfulness and fear. Over time, they may also question their sexual identity, act out in a sexually aggressive manner, and even downplay the impact of the assault.

Don't men who get raped become rapists?

No! This is a destructive myth that often adds to the anxiety a male survivor feels afterwards. Because of this myth, it is common for a male survivor to fear that he is now destined to do to others what was done to him.

While many convicted sex offenders have a history of being sexually abused, most male survivors do not become offenders. The truth is that the great majority of male survivors have never sexually assaulted and will never sexually assault anyone.

If a man is raped by another man, does it mean he's gay?

No! A man getting raped by another man says nothing about his sexual orientation before the assault, nor does it change his sexual orientation afterwards.

Rape is prompted by anger or a desire to intimidate or dominate, not by sexual attraction or a rapist's assumption about his intended victim's sexual preference.

Because of society's confusion about (1) the role that attraction plays in sexual assault and (2) whether victims are responsible for provoking an assault, even heterosexual male survivors may worry that they somehow gave off "gay vibes" that the rapist picked up and acted upon. This is hardly the case.

How should I respond if a man tells me he has been assaulted?

The basics of supporting female survivors are the same for males. Believe him. Don't push and don't blame. Be cautious about physical contact until he's ready. Ask him if he wants to report it to the authorities and if he wants to talk to a counselor. If you need to, get counseling for yourself as well.

Where can male survivors go for help?

Most community resources—local or campus-based rape crisis centers—have on-site counselors trained in working with male survivors. Or they can refer survivors to professionals who can help. Know the resources in your area to help male survivors heal.

Chapter 20

Elder Abuse

Chapter Contents

Section 20.1

Facts about Elder Abuse and Neglect

"Elder Abuse and Neglect," by Lawrence Robinson, Tina de Benedictis, Ph.D., and Jeanne Segal, Ph.D., updated April 2012. © 2012 Helpguide.org. All rights reserved. Reprinted with permission. Helpguide provides a detailed list of references and resources for this article, with links to related Helpguide topics and information from other websites. For a complete list of these resources, go to http://helpguide.org/mental/elder_abuse_physical_emotional_sexual_neglect.htm

Many elderly adults are abused in their own homes, in relatives' homes, and even in facilities responsible for their care. If you suspect that an elderly person is at risk from a neglectful or overwhelmed caregiver, or being preyed upon financially, it's important to recognize the warning signs.

Your Elderly Neighbor

There's an elderly neighbor you've chatted with at civic meetings and block parties for years. When you see her coming to get her mail as you walk up the street, you slow down and greet her at the mailbox. She says hello but seems wary, as if she doesn't quite recognize you. You ask her about a nasty bruise on her forearm. Oh, just an accident, she explains; the car door closed on it. She says goodbye quickly and returns to the house. Something isn't quite right about her. You think about the bruise, her skittish behavior. Well, she's getting pretty old, you think; maybe her mind is getting fuzzy. But there's something else—something isn't right.

What Is Elder Abuse?

As elders become more physically frail, they're less able to stand up to bullying or fight back if attacked. They may not see or hear as well or think as clearly as they used to, leaving openings for unscrupulous people to take advantage of them. Mental or physical ailments may make them more trying companions for the people who live with them.

Tens of thousands of seniors across the United States are being abused: harmed in some substantial way, often by people who are directly responsible for their care.

More than half a million reports of abuse against elderly Americans reach authorities every year, and millions more cases go unreported.

Where Does Elder Abuse Take Place?

Elder abuse tends to take place where the senior lives: most often in the home, where abusers are apt to be adult children, other family members such as grandchildren, or spouses/partners of elders. Institutional settings, especially long-term care facilities, can also be sources of elder abuse.

The Different Types of Elder Abuse

Abuse of elders takes many different forms, some involving intimidation or threats against the elderly, some involving neglect, and others involving financial chicanery. The most common are defined below.

Physical Abuse

Physical elder abuse is nonaccidental use of force against an elderly person that results in physical pain, injury, or impairment. Such abuse includes not only physical assaults such as hitting or shoving but the inappropriate use of drugs, restraints, or confinement.

Emotional Abuse

In emotional or psychological senior abuse, people speak to or treat elderly persons in ways that cause emotional pain or distress.

Verbal forms of emotional elder abuse include:

- intimidation through yelling or threats;
- humiliation and ridicule;
- habitual blaming or scapegoating.

Nonverbal psychological elder abuse can take the form of:

- ignoring the elderly person;
- isolating an elder from friends or activities;
- terrorizing or menacing the elderly person.

Sexual Abuse

Sexual elder abuse is contact with an elderly person without the elder's consent. Such contact can involve physical sex acts, but activities such as showing an elderly person pornographic material, forcing the person to watch sex acts, or forcing the elder to undress are also considered sexual elder abuse.

Neglect or Abandonment by Caregivers

Elder neglect, failure to fulfill a caretaking obligation, constitutes more than half of all reported cases of elder abuse. It can be active (intentional) or passive (unintentional, based on factors such as ignorance or denial that an elderly charge needs as much care as he or she does).

Financial Exploitation

This involves unauthorized use of an elderly person's funds or property, either by a caregiver or an outside scam artist.

An unscrupulous caregiver might:

- misuse an elder's personal checks, credit cards, or accounts;
- steal cash, income checks, or household goods;
- forge the elder's signature;
- engage in identity theft.

Typical rackets that target elders include:

- announcements of a "prize" that the elderly person has won but must pay money to claim;
- phony charities;
- investment fraud.

Healthcare Fraud and Abuse

Carried out by unethical doctors, nurses, hospital personnel, and other professional care providers, examples of healthcare fraud and abuse regarding elders include:

- not providing healthcare, but charging for it;
- overcharging or double-billing for medical care or services;

- getting kickbacks for referrals to other providers or for prescribing certain drugs;

- overmedicating or undermedicating;

- recommending fraudulent remedies for illnesses or other medical conditions;

- Medicaid fraud.

Signs and Symptoms of Elder Abuse

At first, you might not recognize or take seriously signs of elder abuse. They may appear to be symptoms of dementia or signs of the elderly person's frailty—or caregivers may explain them to you that way. In fact, many of the signs and symptoms of elder abuse do overlap with symptoms of mental deterioration, but that doesn't mean you should dismiss them on the caregiver's say-so.

General Signs of Abuse

The following are warning signs of some kind of elder abuse:

- Frequent arguments or tension between the caregiver and the elderly person

- Changes in personality or behavior in the elder

If you suspect elderly abuse, but aren't sure, look for clusters of the following physical and behavioral signs.

Signs and Symptoms of Specific Types of Abuse

Physical abuse:

- Unexplained signs of injury such as bruises, welts, or scars, especially if they appear symmetrically on two side of the body

- Broken bones, sprains, or dislocations

- Report of drug overdose or apparent failure to take medication regularly (a prescription has more remaining than it should)

- Broken eyeglasses or frames

- Signs of being restrained, such as rope marks on wrists

- Caregiver's refusal to allow you to see the elder alone

Emotional abuse:

- Threatening, belittling, or controlling caregiver behavior that you witness

- Behavior from the elder that mimics dementia, such as rocking, sucking, or mumbling to oneself

Sexual abuse:

- Bruises around breasts or genitals

- Unexplained venereal disease or genital infections

- Unexplained vaginal or anal bleeding

- Torn, stained, or bloody underclothing

Neglect by caregivers or self-neglect:

- Unusual weight loss, malnutrition, dehydration

- Untreated physical problems, such as bed sores

- Unsanitary living conditions: dirt, bugs, soiled bedding and clothes

- Being left dirty or unbathed

- Unsuitable clothing or covering for the weather

- Unsafe living conditions (no heat or running water; faulty electrical wiring, other fire hazards)

- Desertion of the elder at a public place

Financial exploitation:

- Significant withdrawals from the elder's accounts

- Sudden changes in the elder's financial condition

- Items or cash missing from the senior's household

- Suspicious changes in wills, power of attorney, titles, and policies

- Addition of names to the senior's signature card

- Unpaid bills or lack of medical care, although the elder has enough money to pay for them

- Financial activity the senior couldn't have done, such as an ATM withdrawal when the account holder is bedridden

- Unnecessary services, goods, or subscriptions

Healthcare fraud and abuse:

- Duplicate billings for the same medical service or device
- Evidence of overmedication or undermedication
- Evidence of inadequate care when bills are paid in full
- Problems with the care facility:
  - poorly trained, poorly paid, or insufficient staff
  - crowding
  - inadequate responses to questions about care

Risk Factors for Elder Abuse

It's difficult to take care of a senior when he or she has many different needs, and it's difficult to be elderly when age brings with it infirmities and dependence. Both the demands of caregiving and the needs of the elder can create situations in which abuse is more likely to occur.

Risk Factors among Caregivers

Many nonprofessional caregivers—spouses, adult children, other relatives and friends—find taking care of an elder to be satisfying and enriching. But the responsibilities and demands of elder caregiving, which escalate as the elder's condition deteriorates, can also be extremely stressful. The stress of elder care can lead to mental and physical health problems that make caregivers burned out, impatient, and unable to keep from lashing out against elders in their care.

Among caregivers, significant risk factors for elder abuse are:

- inability to cope with stress (lack of resilience);
- depression, which is common among caregivers;
- lack of support from other potential caregivers;
- the caregiver's perception that taking care of the elder is burdensome and without psychological reward;
- substance abuse.

Even caregivers in institutional settings can experience stress at levels that lead to elder abuse. Nursing home staff may be prone to elder abuse if they lack training, have too many responsibilities, are unsuited to caregiving, or work under poor conditions.

The Elder's Condition and History

Several factors concerning elders themselves, while they don't excuse abuse, influence whether they are at greater risk for abuse:

- The intensity of an elderly person's illness or dementia

- Social isolation (i.e., the elder and caregiver are alone together almost all the time)

- The elder's role, at an earlier time, as an abusive parent or spouse

- A history of domestic violence in the home

- The elder's own tendency toward verbal or physical aggression

In many cases, elder abuse, though real, is unintentional. Caregivers pushed beyond their capabilities or psychological resources may not mean to yell at, strike, or ignore the needs of the elders in their care.

Reporting Elder Abuse

If you are an elder who is being abused, neglected, or exploited, tell at least one person. Tell your doctor, a friend, or a family member whom you trust. Other people care and can help you.

And if you see an older adult being abused or neglected, don't hesitate to report the situation. Don't assume that someone else will take care of it or that the person being abused is capable of getting help if he or she really needs it.

Many seniors don't report the abuse they face even if they're able. Some fear retaliation from the abuser, while others believe that if they turn in their abusers, no one else will take care of them. When the caregivers are their children, they may be ashamed that their children are behaving abusively or blame themselves: "If I'd been a better parent when they were younger, this wouldn't be happening." Or they just may not want children they love to get into trouble with the law.

How Do I Report Elder Abuse?

Every state in the United States has at least one toll-free elder abuse hotline or helpline for reporting elder abuse in the home, in the community, or in nursing homes and other long-term care facilities.

For help in your area, talk to your local hospital or a trusted doctor or therapist.

The first agency to respond to a report of elderly abuse, in most states, is Adult Protective Services (APS). Its role is to investigate abuse cases, intervene, and offer services and advice. Again, the power and scope of APS varies from state to state.

Preventing Elder Abuse and Neglect

We can help reduce the incidence of elder abuse, but it'll take more effort than we're making now. Preventing elder abuse means doing three things:

- Listening to seniors and their caregivers
- Intervening when you suspect elder abuse
- Educating others about how to recognize and report elder abuse

What You Can Do As a Caregiver to Prevent Elder Abuse

If you're overwhelmed by the demands of caring for an elder, do the following:

- Request help, from friends, relatives, or local respite care agencies, so you can take a break, if only for a couple of hours.
- Find an adult day care program.
- Stay healthy and get medical care for yourself when necessary.
- Adopt stress reduction practices.
- Seek counseling for depression, which can lead to elder abuse.
- Find a support group for caregivers of the elderly.
- If you're having problems with drug or alcohol abuse, get help.

And remember, elder abuse helplines offer help for caregivers as well. Call a helpline if you think there's a possibility you might cross the line into elder abuse.

What You Can Do As a Concerned Friend or Family Member

- Watch for warning signs that might indicate elder abuse. If you suspect abuse, report it.
- Take a look at the elder's medications. Does the amount in the vial jive with the date of the prescription?

269

- Watch for possible financial abuse. Ask the elder if you may scan bank accounts and credit card statements for unauthorized transactions.

- Call and visit as often as you can. Help the elder consider you a trusted confidante.

- Offer to stay with the elder so the caregiver can have a break— on a regular basis, if you can.

How You Can Protect Yourself, As an Elder, Against Elder Abuse

- Make sure your financial and legal affairs are in order. If they aren't, enlist professional help to get them in order, with the assistance of a trusted friend or relative, if necessary.

- Keep in touch with family and friends and avoid becoming isolated, which increases your vulnerability to elder abuse.

- If you are unhappy with the care you're receiving, whether it's in your own home or in a care facility, speak up. Tell someone you trust and ask that person to report the abuse, neglect, or substandard care to your state's elder abuse helpline or long-term-care ombudsman, or make the call yourself.

Finally, if you aren't in a position to help an elder personally, you can volunteer or donate money to the cause of educating people about elder abuse, and you can lobby to strengthen state laws and policing so that elder abuse can be investigated and prosecuted more readily. The life you save down the line may be your own.

Reporting Elder Abuse

As difficult as reporting elder abuse can be, it's important for you to stand up for an older adult in need. Learn how to communicate effectively in different situations and put a stop to elder abuse and neglect.

Section 20.2

Elder Abuse and Substance Abuse

Substance abuse has been identified as the most frequently cited risk factor associated with elder abuse and neglect. It may be the victim and/or the perpetrator who has the substance abuse problem. Substance abuse is believed to be a factor in all types of elder abuse, including physical mistreatment, emotional abuse, financial exploitation, and neglect. It is also a significant factor in self-neglect.

Researchers and practitioners have observed the following patterns with respect to perpetrators of elder abuse who abuse drugs or alcohol:

- Persons with alcohol or substance abuse problems may view older family members, acquaintances, or strangers as easy targets for financial exploitation. The perpetrator may be seeking money to support a drug habit or because they are unable to hold a job and have no source of income.

- Perpetrators may move into an older person's home and use it as a base of operation for drug use or trafficking.

- The research on domestic violence shows that abusive partners are more likely to be violent while they're under the influence of drugs or alcohol. The relationship between domestic violence and substance abuse, however, is not fully understood. Although it has been assumed that alcohol and drugs reduce users' inhibitions, it has also been observed that perpetrators of domestic violence use drugs and alcohol to rationalize their behavior.

- Caregivers who are having difficulty coping with the demands of providing care may use drugs as a misguided coping mechanism.

They have observed the following patterns with respect to victims who abuse drugs or alcohol:

- Alcoholic or substance-abusing older persons are at risk for several reasons. They may have substance-abuse-related impairments, such as cognitive loss, that reduces their ability to resist or detect coercion or fraud. Physical disabilities associated with substance abuse increase risk by rendering the older person dependant on others for assistance or care, and giving caregivers physical access to the older person and their home. Caregivers are also likely to have access to an older person's financial resources and to wield significant influence.

- Seniors may be encouraged to take drugs or drink excessively, or even forced to do so. A perpetrator's motive may be to make the older person easier to exploit financially or, in the case of illegal drug use, less likely to report. Abusive caregivers may encourage older people to drink excessively or use drugs to make them more compliant or easier to care for.

- Some victims use drugs or alcohol as a coping mechanism to relieve their anxiety and fear.

- Seniors who have longstanding alcohol or substance abuse problems are likely to have poor relationships with their families or to be estranged entirely. If the older person needs care, their family members may be unwilling to help or may harbor resentments that impede their ability to provide good care.

- Older persons who self-neglect are likely to have substance abuse or alcohol problems.

Resources for learning more about the relationship between substance abuse and elder abuse:

Elder Abuse and Substance Abuse: Making the Connection. An interview with Charmaine Spencer and Jeff Smith. In *Nexus, a Publication for NCPEA Affiliates*. April 2000.

Bradshaw, D., and Spencer, C. (1999). The role of alcohol in elder abuse cases. In J. Pritchard (Ed.). *Elder abuse work: Best practices in Britain and Canada*. London: Jessica Kingsley Press.

Section 20.3

Prevalence and Consequences of Elder Maltreatment

"Elder Maltreatment Consequences," U.S. Centers for Disease
Control and Prevention, June 9, 2010.

Prevalence of Elder Maltreatment

The true incidence of elder maltreatment is difficult to determine.
Findings from the National Elder Abuse Incidence Study (NEAIS)—
a seminal study conducted in 1996—indicate that roughly 551,000
persons age sixty and older experienced elder abuse, neglect, or self-
neglect in domestic settings (National Center on Elder Abuse 1998).

Of these cases, only 21 percent (about 115,000) were reported to and
substantiated by Adult Protective Service (APS) agencies; the remaining 79 percent were either not reported to APS or not substantiated.

The best available estimate of prevalence suggests that between one
and two million residents of the United States age sixty-five or older
have been abused, neglected, or exploited by persons on whom they
depended for care or protection (National Research Council 2003).

Consequences of Elder Maltreatment

The possible physical and psychosocial consequences of elder maltreatment are numerous and varied. Few studies have examined the
consequences of elder maltreatment and distinguished them from
those linked to normal aging (National Research Council 2003; Wolf
1997; Wolf et al 2002).

Physical Effects

The most immediate probable physical effects include:

- welts, wounds, and injuries (e.g., bruises, lacerations, dental
  problems, head injuries, broken bones, pressure sores);

- persistent physical pain and soreness;

273

- nutrition and hydration issues;

- sleep disturbances;

- increased susceptibility to new illnesses (including sexually transmitted diseases);

- exacerbation of preexisting health conditions; and

- increased risks for premature death.

(Anetzberger 2004; American Medical Association 1990; Lachs et al 1998; Lindbloom et al. 2007)

Psychological Effects

Established psychological effects of elder maltreatment include higher levels of distress and depression (Comijs et al 1999; Pillemer & Prescott 1989).

Other potential psychological consequences that need further scientific study are:

- increased risks for developing fear/anxiety reactions;

- learned helplessness; and

- post-traumatic stress syndrome.

References

American Medical Association. 1990. American Medical Association white paper on elderly health. Report of the Council on Scientific Affairs. *Arch Intern Med*;150:2459–72.

Anetzberger G. 2004. *The clinical management of elder abuse*. New York: Hawthorne Press.

Lachs MS, Williams CS, O'Brien S, et. al. 1998. The mortality of elder mistreatment. *JAMA*;280:42832.

Lindbloom EJ, Brandt J, Hough, L., Meadows SE. 2007. Elder mistreatment in the nursing home: A systematic review. *J Am Med Dir Assoc*;8(9):610–16.

National Center on Elder Abuse. 1998. *National elder abuse incidence study: final report*. Washington DC: American Public Human Services Association.

National Research Council. 2003. Elder mistreatment: abuse, neglect, and exploitation in an aging America. In: Bonnie RJ. and Wallace RB, editors. *Panel to Review Risk and Prevalence of Elder Abuse and Neglect*. Washington DC: The National Academies Press.

Wolf R, Daichman L, Bennett G. 2002. Abuse of the elderly. In: Krug E, Dahlberg L, Mercy J, Zwi A, Lozano R, editors. *World Report on Violence and Health*. Geneva: World Health Organization. p.123–46.

Wolf RS. 1997. Elder abuse and neglect: an update. *Rev Clin Gerontol*;7:177–82.

Chapter 21

Abuse in the Lesbian, Gay, Bisexual, and Transgender Community

Chapter Contents

Section 21.1

Domestic Violence and Lesbian, Gay, Bisexual, and Transgender Relationships

Why It Matters

Domestic violence is defined as a pattern of behaviors utilized by one partner (the batterer or abuser) to exert and maintain control over another person (the survivor or victim) where there exists an intimate and/or dependent relationship. Experts believe that domestic violence occurs in the lesbian, gay, bisexual, and transgender (LGBT) community with the same amount of frequency and severity as in the heterosexual community. Society's long history of entrenched racism, sexism, homophobia, and transphobia prevents LGBT victims of domestic violence from seeking help from the police, legal and court systems for fear of discrimination or bias.[1]

Did You Know?

- In ten cities and two states alone, there were 3,524 incidents of domestic violence affecting LGBT individuals, according to the National Coalition of Anti-Violence Programs 2006 Report on Lesbian, Gay, Bi-Sexual and Transgender Domestic Violence.[1]

- LGBT domestic violence is vastly underreported, unacknowledged, and often reported as something other than domestic violence.[1]

- Delaware, Montana, and South Carolina explicitly exclude same-sex survivors of domestic violence from protection under criminal laws. Eighteen states have domestic violence laws that are gender neutral but apply to household members only.[2]

- Thirty states and the District of Columbia have domestic violence laws that are gender neutral and include household members as well as dating partners.[2]

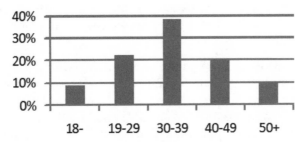

Figure 21.1. *Reported cases of lesbian, gay, bisexual, and transgender violence, by age of victim.*

Survivors

- Gay and bisexual men experience abuse in intimate partner relationships at a rate of two in five, which is comparable to the amount of domestic violence experienced by heterosexual women.[3]

- Approximately 50 percent of the lesbian population has experienced or will experience domestic violence in their lifetimes.[1]

- In one year, 44 percent of victims in LGBT domestic violence cases identified as men, while 36 percent identified as women.[1]

- Seventy-eight percent of lesbians report that they have either defended themselves or fought back against an abusive partner. Eighteen percent of this group described their behavior as self-defense or "trading blow for blow or insult for insult."[4]

Types of Abuse[5]

- **Physical:** The threat of harm or any forceful physical behavior that intentionally or accidentally causes bodily harm or property destruction.

- **Sexual:** Any forced or coerced sexual act or behavior motivated to acquire power and control over the partner. It is not only forced sexual contact but also contact that demeans or humiliates the partner and instigates feelings of shame or vulnerability—particularly in regards to the body, sexual performance, or sexuality.

- **Emotional/Verbal:** Any use of words, voice, action, or lack of action meant to control, hurt, or demean another person. Emotional abuse typically includes ridicule, intimidation, or coercion.

- **Financial:** The use or misuse, without the victim's consent, of the financial or other monetary resources of the partner or of the relationship.

- **Identity abuse:** Using personal characteristics to demean, manipulate, and control the partner. Some of these tactics overlap with other forms of abuse, particularly emotional abuse. This category is comprised of the social "isms," including racism, sexism, ageism, able-ism, beauty-ism, as well as homophobia. Includes threats to "out" victim.

Transgender Abuse[1]

Specific forms of abuse occur in relationships where one partner is transgender, including:

- using offensive pronouns such as "it" to refer to the transgender partner;

- ridiculing the transgender partner's body and/or appearance;

- telling the transgender partner that he or she is not a real man or woman;

- ridiculing the transgender partner's identity as "bisexual," "trans," "femme," "butch," "gender queer," etc.;

- denying the transgender partner's access to medical treatment or hormones or coercing him or her to not pursue medical treatment.

Human Immunodeficiency Virus (HIV)/Acquired Immune Deficiency Syndrome (AIDS)–Related Abuse[1]

The presence of HIV/AIDS in an abusive relationship may lead to specific forms of abuse, which include:

- "outing" or threatening to tell others that the victim has HIV/AIDS;

- an HIV-positive abuser suggesting that she or he will sicken or die if the partner ends the relationship;

- preventing the HIV-positive partner from receiving needed medical care or medications;

- taking advantage of an HIV-positive partner's poor health status, assuming sole power over a partner's economic affairs, creating the partner's utter dependency on the abuser;

- an HIV-positive abuser infecting or threatening to infect a partner.

Barriers to Seeking Services[1]

Barriers to addressing LGBT intimate partner violence (both for service providers and survivors) include:

- the belief that domestic violence does not occur in LGBT relationships and/or is a gender-based issue;

- societal anti-LGBT bias (homophobia, biphobia, and transphobia);

- Lack of appropriate training regarding LGBT domestic violence for service providers;

- A fear that airing of the problems among the LGBT population will take away from progress toward equality or fuel anti-LGBT bias.

- Domestic violence shelters are typically female only, thus transgender people may not be allowed entrance into shelters or emergency facilities due to their gender/genital/legal status.

Sources

1. National Coalition of Anti-Violence Programs. (2006) "Anti-Lesbian, Gay, Bisexual and Transgender Violence in 2006." www.ncavp.org.

2. National Gay and Lesbian Task Force. (2005) "Domestic Violence Laws in the U.S." www.thetaskforce.org.

3. Greenwood, Gregory, et. al. (2002) "Battering and Victimization Among a Probability-Based Sample of Men Who Have Sex With Men." *American Journal of Public Health*. 92 (12).

4. Renzetti, C.M. (1992). "Violent Betrayal: Partner Abuse in Lesbian Relationships." *Violence Against Women*. Sage Publications.

5. Gay Men's Domestic Violence Project. "Types of Abuse." www.gmdvp.org.

Section 21.2

Unique Concerns in Lesbian, Gay, Bisexual, and Transgender Violence

"Lesbian/Gay/Bisexual/Transgender/Queer Domestic Violence Information Guide," reprinted with permission from the New York State Office for the Prevention of Domestic Violence (www.opdv.ny.gov), © 2012. The complete text of this document is available at http://www.opdv.ny.gov/whatisdv/lgbtqdvinfo.html.

What Does Domestic Violence in the LGBTQ Community Look Like?

LGBTQ abusers use many of the same tactics as non-LGBTQ abusers, such as social isolation, emotional and psychological abuse, economic control, and physical and sexual violence, to perpetrate domestic violence against their intimate partners. However, domestic violence within same-sex relationships is comprised of some unique characteristics requiring specific responses and resources that aren't typically necessary or available when responding to domestic violence perpetrated in heterosexual relationships, usually by a male abuser against his female intimate partner.

Specific Issues/Concerns Unique to LGBTQ Victims of Domestic Violence

- LGBTQ domestic violence abusers may "out" (or threaten to "out") their victims, thereby exposing victims' sexual orientation, gender identity, and/or human immunodeficiency virus (HIV) status to family, employers, police, religious institutions, the community, or child protective workers.

- LGBTQ domestic violence perpetrators often control their partners' expressions of sexual identity and connections to and within the larger LGBTQ community.

- LGBTQ domestic violence perpetrators may sabotage or disallow a transgendered partner access to his/her prescribed hormones, often medically required during the transition process.

- LGBTQ domestic violence perpetrators may use children in common to manipulate and control the victim around issues of custody and visitation, particularly in cases where the child(ren) are biologically related to the perpetrator and may or may not be legally adopted by the victim.

- Leaving an abusive LGBTQ relationship is not easy despite a common false assumption that because LGBTQ relationships are not legally recognized in the same way that heterosexual relationships are, that the abuse is not serious and the victim should easily be able to leave the relationship.

- Service providers and/or first responders often make assumptions and perpetuate the myth that same-sex intimate partners cannot perpetuate (or be victims of) domestic violence, as both partners are assumed to share equal social standing, earning potential, and physical strength, and are therefore unable to exert power and control over, or be controlled by, an intimate partner.

- Dual Arrests are common within the LGBTQ community, as the lack of gender disparity often makes primary aggressor determinations more challenging than the statistically established norm of male perpetrator/ female victim within heterosexual domestic violence.

Barriers to Addressing LGBTQ Domestic Violence

- LGBTQ individuals may be overlooked by mandatory domestic violence victim notification at hospitals.

- Service availability and appropriately trained staff are often limited or nonexistent.

- Many domestic violence shelters prohibit male victims from entering their facilities.

- Most domestic violence victim support groups are designed for female victims of male partners.

- Individuals who have not publicly disclosed their LGBTQ status, who have that information exposed by an abusive partner, become more visible, putting them at risk for becoming vulnerable targets for general criminal behavior even outside of their intimate relationships.

Section 21.3

What Rights Do I Have as a Lesbian, Gay, Bisexual, or Transgender Victim of Domestic Violence?

Reprinted with permission from "What Rights Do I Have as an LGBT Victim of Domestic Violence?" published by the American Bar Association Section of Individual Rights and Responsibilities. Copyright © 2011 by the American Bar Association. This information or any portion thereof may not be copied or disseminated in any form or by any means or stored in an electronic database or retrieval system without the express written consent of the American Bar Association.

How do I know if I am in an abusive relationship?

If you believe you might be in an abusive relationship, here are some questions to ask yourself:[1]

When you are with your partner, do you sometimes feel as if:

- you are not safe?
- you have to watch what you do and say?
- things are either really great, or there are problems—but things are never just okay?

Has your partner ever:

- told you where to go or what not to say?
- told you what to wear?
- told you how you could spend money?
- gotten in the way of you receiving medical care?
- told you not to hang out with certain people?

Has your partner ever:

- threatened you physically?
- pushed, hit, or held you down?

- threatened to "out" you to anyone?

- threatened to report you to an authority, such as immigration?

- refused to have safer sex or forced you to have sex against your will?

If you answer yes to some or all of these questions, you may be experiencing domestic violence. You are not alone and help is available.

How is domestic violence in lesbian, gay, bisexual, or transgender (LGBT) relationships different from domestic violence in heterosexual relationships?

Between one-third and one-fourth of lesbian, gay, bisexual, and transgender (LGBT) people in relationships experience domestic violence—the same as women in heterosexual relationships.

Although the abuse is often similar in LGBT and heterosexual relationships, perpetrators of domestic violence in LGBT relationships may also use society's bias against their partner's sexual orientation or gender identity to abuse and isolate their partner. These tactics may include:[2]

- threatening to "out" or outing the partner's sexual orientation and/or gender identity to their family, employer, or community;

- threatening to tell or telling others the partner's human immunodeficiency virus (HIV)/acquired immune deficiency syndrome (AIDS) status;

- reinforcing fears that no one will help because she or he is lesbian, gay, bisexual, and/or transgender; or

- telling the partner that abusive behavior is a normal part of lesbian, gay, bisexual, and/or transgender relationships.

What legal options do I have if I am afraid of my partner?

As an LGBT person who may be a victim of domestic violence, you have legal rights, regardless of whether you are married or in a recognized domestic partnership with your partner. Access to legal assistance will depend on the laws in your state.

A person can request protection from an abuser under both civil and criminal law. In almost all states, an LGBT victim can request a civil protection order, an order available to victims of domestic violence that requires your partner to stay away from you. In most states, victims of stalking, repeated violence, or harassment can request a protection order which prevents the person from harming or contacting them.

What is a civil protection order?

A civil protection order is a civil court order, requested by a victim (petitioner) and signed by a judge. A civil protection order can, for example:

- order the abuser to stop threatening, abusing or harassing you;

- order the abuser to stay a certain distance from you (also known as a "stay-away order");

- order the abuser not to come to your home (sometimes even if you share the home);

- order the abuser to stop contacting you;

- say who your children will live with temporarily and whether the abuser can visit them; or

- in some states, order the abuser to get treatment or counseling (often a condition of child visitation).

A victim does not have to press criminal charges against a partner in order to get a civil protection order. The choice to get the police and criminal justice system involved is completely separate from filing a civil protection order.

A civil protection order goes by different names in different states. It is also referred to as a protection order, a protective order, a restraining order, a protection from abuse order, a domestic protection order, or a no contact order, among others.

Do I qualify for a civil protection order as an LGBT victim of domestic violence?

A survivor in an LGBT relationship can qualify for a civil protection order in almost every state. Civil protection orders can only be filed between people with specific types of relationships, as defined by state statutes. Most state statutes include individuals in romantic or dating relationships while others limit the relationships to categories such as "spouses," "family members," or "roommates."

It is important to know your state's laws so that you can know whether you qualify for a civil protection order.

What are my options if I live in a state where I do not qualify for a civil protection order?

There are options for LGBT victims who are denied or prevented from obtaining civil protection orders. Each state has its own individual laws which allow victims of violence or harassment not considered to be "domestic violence" to get protection. These options might also be useful in situations where survivors do not want to be "out" about the nature of their relationship to their abuser.

In most states, victims of stalking can file protection orders against their stalker. In many states, a victim of repeated violence or harassment can request a protection order against the person who has assaulted or harassed them.

These protection orders, in most states, can order the respondent to not harm or contact the petitioner. However in most states a person cannot request other relief such as custody. Like in a civil protection order, these orders are civil in nature, and do not require that criminal charges be filed.

How can I get a civil protection order?

The process for requesting a domestic violence civil protection order and other protection orders are the same in most states. First, go to the state courthouse (municipal, superior, or district court) in the district where you live. There, you will fill out a request (petition) where you explain in writing why you want the order and describe recent incidences of abuse. The more details you can provide the better. Once you fill out the petition and submit it to the clerk of the court, you will be given a court date to appear before a judge, who will decide whether or not to grant the petition.

In many states, when you file for a civil protection order you may be awarded a temporary (or emergency) order. In states where they do not automatically grant a temporary protection order, you can request it in your petition. A judge will decide on the spot whether to grant the temporary protection order. If the temporary protection order is granted, the abuser (usually called the respondent in court documents) must be notified.

The order will begin once the respondent is notified. The temporary order will last until your court date, when a judge will decide whether to grant you a permanent order, extend the temporary order, or terminate the order.

In many states, the police will deliver the temporary order, your petition for civil protection, and a notice about the court date to the

287

respondent. In other states or if the police are unable to serve the respondent, you may be responsible for finding a third party to serve the notice.

The time between when you file your petition and the court date varies from state to state. In general, courts try to schedule the hearings as quickly as possible; typically, not more than a month away.

At your court date, if both you and the respondent are present, you will be given a chance to present to a judge why you believe that a protection order is necessary to protect you. You should be prepared to provide evidence such as other witnesses, photographs, voicemails, or emails. The respondent, if she or he decides to participate, will be given the opportunity present evidence as to why the order should not be granted. The judge will make a decision and either grant a civil protection order or deny the order and terminate the temporary protection order.

A protection order lasts different amounts of times in different states. In some states, they last for only six months. In others, they can last up to two years, or even permanently. You will need to go back to court to extend a protection order once it expires.

An abuser who violates either a temporary or long-term civil protection order may be subject to civil or criminal contempt charges. If you have an order that an abuser violates, you can call the police to report the violation. The government may then decide to prosecute the abuser for violating the order. In some states, you can also file a motion for criminal or civil contempt yourself.

What further legal protections are available to me if my abuser is charged with a crime related to the abuse?

When an abuser is charged with a violence-related crime, the victim can get access to special criminal orders of protection. In most states, when a person is charged with committing such crimes as harassment, battery, or assault, the court has the right to place a no-contact (or restraining) order against the person. Under a no-contact order, the defendant cannot contact the victim or come near the victim. If the defendant does contact the victim, the defendant will be breaking the law and could face criminal penalties.

What if I am afraid to get help because I believe that I will be harassed by the police for being LGBT?

Some victims may be hesitant to call the police or seek other assistance because they are afraid that they or their partner will be mistreated because of their sexual orientation and/or gender identity.

Legally, neither the courts nor the police can discriminate against victims and abusers because of their sexual orientation and/or gender identity.

Many states are working to improve their interactions with LGBT people. Numerous states now provide training to their police officers regarding same-sex domestic violence.[4] Some jurisdictions have begun to adopt policies that allow them to better serve the LGBT community. Some examples of policies are those requiring police to treat same-sex instances of domestic violence the same as heterosexual instances,[5] creating a gay and lesbian unit of the police,[6] and attempting to forge a workplace where LGBT police officers do not feel that they have to hide their sexual orientation.[7]

Even with increasing efforts to eradicate homophobia and transphobia in police and court systems, many LGBT survivors still reasonably fear mistreatment by police and court systems. If you want to get help and do not want to contact the police or courts first, contact your local antiviolence program. These are groups that work specifically with LGBT survivors of domestic violence, sexual violence, and hate violence, and who can help you navigate the legal system.

Will my abuser automatically be charged with a crime if I call the police?

If you call the police, your partner will not automatically be charged with a crime, even if she or he is arrested. The state prosecutor's office, with the assistance of the police, decides whether to file criminal charges against an abuser. A victim does not decide whether a criminal case is brought against an abuser once the police are involved.

Once a criminal investigation is underway, a victim does not have the ability to "drop" criminal charges against their abuser. A victim is a witness in the case, and not a party to it. While a victim's cooperation is very helpful in prosecuting a criminal case, it is not always necessary. Victims who do not want charges to be brought can talk with the police or prosecutor, but this does not assure the case will be "dropped" and may not excuse the victim from having to testify for the government in the case. Even if the victim does not testify, an abuser can be prosecuted based on other evidence, such as the police report.

Where can I find more information about my rights as an LGBT victim of domestic violence?

Remember that only a legal professional who is knowledgeable in this area of law can advise you on the availability of rights and protections. For information on attorneys in your area, contact your state or local bar association.

Notes

1. These questions have been developed by the National Coalition of Anti-Violence Programs (http://www.ncavp.org/issues/DomesticViolence.aspx).

2. National Coalition of Anti-Violence Programs, available at http://www.ncavp.org/issues/DomesticViolence.aspx.

3. Whether a transgender person can get a civil protection order under a state's definition of relationship may depend on whether that person identifies or is legally categorized as the same sex as their partner. For example, a transgender woman who is legally female should have the same rights as a non-transgender woman to file against her abusive male partner.

4. Eighty-three percent of police departments report providing training on issues around same-sex domestic violence. Amnesty International, Stonewalled: Police Abuse and Misconduct Against Lesbian, Gay and Transgender People in the U.S.

5. For example, both Arlington, Virginia, and New York City recently enacted such a policy.

6. Washington, D.C. has created such a unit.

7. Philadelphia, Pennsylvania, has made such an effort to become more LGBT friendly.

Chapter 22

Abuse within the Military

Chapter Contents

Section 22.1

Domestic Violence
and the Military: Basic Facts

Statistics

- Between 1998 and 2004, there were on average 11,372 reports of spousal abuse reported to the Family Advocacy Program. This includes physical, sexual, and emotional abuse. (Lloyd, Davis, Family Advocacy Program, http://www.ncdsv.org/images/Spouse AbuseReportedFAP1998-2004.pdf)

- In one study, 30 percent of active duty military women reported intimate partner abuse in their lifetime and 21.6 percent reported such violence during service. (Campbell et al, Violence against Women 9(9), 2003.)

- In 2001, more than eighteen thousand incidents of spousal abuse were reported to the military services. More than ten thousand were substantiated. Of these, 62 percent of perpetrators were an active duty military member, and 38 percent civilian spouses of active duty members. Sixty-six percent of victims were female and 34 percent male. (Family Advocacy Program [FAP] Data, Department of Defense [DOD], 2002.)

- Domestic violence homicides in military communities from 1995 to 2001 included 54 in the Navy and Marine Corps, 131 in the Army and 32 in the Air Force. (Initial Report of Defense Task Force on Domestic Violence, 2001.)

Overview of the Issue

- If the abuser is a military member, domestic violence situations are handled on two separate tracks: The military justice system and the Family Advocacy System. These are two separate systems, not connected. Family advocacy is an identification, intervention, and treatment program, not a punishment system. It does not enjoy the right of confidentiality under military law (such as chaplains and attorneys), and evidence gathered and statements made during Family Advocacy investigations may be used in military justice proceedings, which will determine the punishment under provisions of military justice.

- Additional factors include limited or lacking victim services and training, and victims who are unaware of their options, such as transitional compensation that provides financial support, healthcare, and housing benefits to victims of military family violence.

- Many victims fear retaliation from the abuser. Those with children fear the loss of pay and benefits if prosecution leads to discharge. Active duty victims fear adverse career consequences if they are seen by Command as weak.

- Disciplinary actions, punishment, sanctions, or prosecution of an active duty offender is the responsibility of and at the discretion of his Command, who will often base their decision on the service's financial investment and the offenders' military record. Misdemeanor assaults rarely result in prosecution, and felony assaults often result in nonjudicial punishment like demotion, loss of pay, and extra duty.

What You Can Do

- Civilian advocates can educate themselves about military practices and procedures by getting to know their local military installation and how it operates. Find out what memoranda of understanding (MOUs) exist between military and civilian support systems in your community. Family Advocacy Programs and civilian advocates who cross-train are better able to provide effective responses to victims and batterers.

- Geography and mobility can create many barriers. Friends and family who stay in touch with military loved ones can reduce the risk of isolation.

Impact on Victims

- Military protective orders are not judicial but administrative, subject to review, short term, and not enforceable off base. Conversely, civilian protective orders are not enforceable on base; victims must file for both.

- The military does not recognize domestic violence unless it is occurring between legally married spouses, so many dating, engaged, and LGBT victims will not be assisted. Immigrant wives are also vulnerable.

- Under the Soldiers and Sailors Relief Act, service members may avoid responding to criminal charges, civil lawsuits, or restraining orders for up to a year if they are deployed.

Quotable

The military environment includes domestic violence situations and can deter reporting efforts and options for victims. Basic rights of safety and health for spouses and children should not be ignored and need the protection of both civilian and military support.

Section 22.2

Frequently Asked Questions about Dealing with Domestic Abuse among Military Personnel

"General Military Information," reprinted from WomensLaw.org and last updated in April 2011. It does not reflect any changes to the policies, procedures, and laws cited since that time. Please continue to check WomensLaw.org for updated information to this section. © 2011 National Network to End Domestic Violence. All rights reserved. Citations in the original WomensLaw.org content were omitted for this reprinting. For additional information and resources, visit http://www.womenslaw.org or http://nnedv.org.

What are the differences between the military and the civilian justice systems?

One of the main differences is that in the military, the commanding officer has the authority to decide what behavior to address and whether to use judicial, administrative, or other means to deal with domestic abuse or domestic violence. There are some general guidelines, but the important point is that the commander can use his/her full discretion to decide what to do.

The civilian justice system deals with domestic violence/abuse in a different way than the military system does. The civilian justice system makes decisions based on the state's laws. Courts will decide what punishment or other action to take, based on testimony and evidence from both sides.

In both the military and civilian justice systems, you can seek a protective order requiring the abuser to stay away from you and your children, your home, your workplace, or school and not engage in any violent conduct. Protective orders have different names in the various states, but the MPO or military protective order is consistently called that among all the services. You can have both an MPO and a civil protective order at the same time. However, the procedure for getting an MPO and a civilian protective order and the duration of the orders are quite different in both systems.

I have heard the terms "domestic abuse" and "domestic violence" used by military personnel. Is there a difference?

Yes. In the military, "domestic abuse" and "domestic violence" mean two different things. In both cases, you must be in a heterosexual relationship with the abuser and the abuser must be:

- your current or former spouse; or

- a person who you have a child in common with; or

- a current or former "intimate partner" who you live/lived with.

Domestic abuse is defined as a pattern of behavior resulting in emotional/psychological abuse, economic control, and/or interference with personal liberty. There does not have to be any physical violence involved.

Domestic violence in the military is a crime (under the United States Code, the Uniform Code of Military Justice, or state law) that involves the use, attempted use, or threatened use of force or violence *or* a violation of an order of protection.

If your relationship with the abuser does not meet any of these requirements, you could still qualify for a civilian protective order (CPO) in the state you live in.

I am being abused. How do I go get help in the military system?

Anyone who is a victim of domestic abuse or domestic violence by someone who is serving in the military can seek assistance from a victim advocate at the Family Advocacy Program on the installation. The victim advocate may be able to work with you to get a military protective order and provide other services *and* also help you with any civilian resources that may be helpful too.

However, even if you are not married to the offender, have no child in common, or never lived together (and therefore, do not meet the military's definition of domestic abuse or violence), the victim advocate is still required to provide basic information about how the military system works and to help you access services offered in the civilian community. Every installation is required to have at least one victim advocate, and the larger ones will have several.

If I tell someone in the military that I am being abused, will it be kept confidential?

Whether or not what you say will be kept confidential depends on who you report it to. If you want the information to be confidential, this is known as making a "restricted report" (a nonconfidential report is an "unrestricted report"). There are just three groups of professionals who've been granted the ability to keep information about domestic abuse or violence confidential. They are victim advocates, chaplains, and medical professionals (healthcare providers). However, even those three groups of professionals would have to reveal the abuse if they believe that it is necessary to prevent or lessen a serious and immediate threat to the health or safety of you or another person. In that case, it will likely be reported to the FAP, the commander, and/or law enforcement.

If you report the abuse to other staff at the FAP (aside from a victim advocate or supervisor of a victim advocate) it will not be confidential. FAP works with military command and law enforcement personnel. The abuser will also be interviewed to have the chance to respond to the complaint.

All others are required to make an immediate report of the abuse or violence to FAP. Even if you, personally, do not report the abuse, all military personnel and civilians employed by the military (with the exception of the three groups of professionals mentioned above) are required to report suspected domestic violence to other parts of the system. What this means is that, regardless of how information about suspected domestic violence comes into the system (i.e., emergency room report, routine medical screening, police response, or victim disclosure), the command and others will be notified, whether or not you want this to occur.

While there are others who can offer assistance, such as the military police or the Staff Judge Advocate or Judge Advocate General, contacting them may result in a formal report. If you are concerned about the abuser being aware that you've asked for assistance, then begin with the victim advocate, the chaplain, or a medical professional. They can then assist you to consider when and how to make a more formal report of the abuse/violence and to access other needed information and support from the professionals who do not have the ability to keep it confidential.

You may also decide to seek help outside of the military, where stricter confidentiality rules apply. Shelters and agencies in your area can help you think through your options. Shelters near military installations are typically familiar with the policies, practices, and people and can also help you access a victim advocate.

Can victims in homosexual relationships receive help?

Currently, only victims in heterosexual relationships can get help from the Family Advocacy Program (FAP) and/or receive a military protective order ("MPO"). However, with President Obama's repeal of the "Don't Ask, Don't Tell" policy, effective in September 2011, it is expected that soon, victims in homosexual relationships will be entitled to benefits and services that were only available to married heterosexual couples.

Section 22.3

Military Sexual Trauma and Harassment

Excerpted from "Military Sexual Trauma," U.S. Department of Veterans Affairs, February 2010.

What is military sexual trauma (MST)?

In both civilian and military settings, women and men can experience a range of unwanted sexual behaviors that they may find distressing. Within the Department of Veterans Affairs (VA), Veterans are likely to hear these sorts of experiences described as "military sexual trauma," the overarching term the VA uses to refer to experiences of sexual assault or repeated, threatening acts of sexual harassment. The definition used by the VA is given by U.S. Code (1720D of Title 38) and is "psychological trauma, which in the judgment of a VA mental health professional, resulted from a physical assault of a sexual nature, battery of a sexual nature, or sexual harassment which occurred while the Veteran was serving on active duty or active duty for training." Sexual harassment is further defined as "repeated, unsolicited verbal or physical contact of a sexual nature which is threatening in character."

More concretely, MST includes any sexual activity where someone is involved against his or her will—he or she may have been pressured into sexual activities (for example, with threats of negative consequences for refusing to be sexually cooperative or with implied faster promotions or better treatment in exchange for sex), may have been unable to consent to sexual activities (for example, when intoxicated), or may have been physically forced into sexual activities. Other experiences that fall into the category of MST included unwanted sexual touching or grabbing; threatening, offensive remarks about a person's body or sexual activities; and/or threatening and unwelcome sexual advances. If these experiences occurred while an individual was on active duty or active duty for training, they are considered to be MST.

How common is MST?

Information about how commonly MST occurs comes from VA's universal screening program. Under this program, all veterans seen at Veterans Health Administration (VHA) facilities are asked whether they experienced sexual trauma during their military service; veterans who respond "yes" are asked if they are interested in learning about MST-related services available. Not every veteran who responds "yes" needs or is necessarily interested in treatment. It's important to note that rates obtained from VA screening cannot be used to make any estimate of the rate of MST among all those serving in the U.S. Military, as they are drawn only from Veterans who have chosen to seek VA healthcare. Also, a positive response does not indicate that the perpetrator was a member of the military.

About one in five women and one in one hundred men seen in VHA respond "yes" when screened for MST. Though rates of MST are higher among women, because of the disproportionate ratio of men to women in the military there are actually only slightly fewer men seen in VA that have experienced MST than there are women.

How can MST affect veterans?

It's important to remember that MST is an experience, not a diagnosis or a mental health condition in and of itself. Given the range of distressing sexually related experiences that veterans report, it is not surprising that there are a wide range of emotional reactions that veterans have in response to these events. Even after severely distressing experiences, there is no one way that everyone will respond—the type, severity, and duration of a veteran's difficulties will all vary based on factors like whether he or she has a prior history of abuse, the types of responses from others he or she received at the time of the experiences, and whether the experience happened once or was repeated over time. For some veterans, experiences of MST may continue to affect their mental and physical health, even many years later.

Some of the difficulties both female and male survivors of MST may have include the following:

- **Strong emotions:** Feeling depressed; having intense, sudden emotional reactions to things; feeling angry or irritable all the time

- **Feelings of numbness:** Feeling emotionally "flat"; difficulty experiencing emotions like love or happiness

- **Trouble sleeping:** Trouble falling or staying asleep; disturbing nightmares

- **Difficulties with attention, concentration, and memory:** Trouble staying focused; frequently finding their mind wandering; having a hard time remembering things

- **Problems with alcohol or other drugs:** Drinking to excess or using drugs daily; getting intoxicated or "high" to cope with memories or emotional reactions; drinking to fall asleep

- **Difficulty with things that remind them of their experiences of sexual trauma:** Feeling on edge or "jumpy" all the time; difficulty feeling safe; going out of their way to avoid reminders of their experiences; difficulty trusting others

- **Difficulties in relationships:** Feeling isolated or disconnected from others; abusive relationships; trouble with employers or authority figures

- **Physical health problems:** Sexual difficulties; chronic pain; weight or eating problems; gastrointestinal problems

Among users of VA healthcare, medical record data indicates that diagnoses of posttraumatic stress disorder (PTSD) and other anxiety disorders, depression and other mood disorders, and substance use disorders are most frequently associated with MST.

Fortunately, people can recover from experiences of trauma, and VA has services to help veterans do this.

Section 22.4

Military Protective Orders

What is a military protective order (MPO)?

Unit commanders may issue military protective orders (MPOs) to an active duty service member to protect a victim of domestic abuse/violence or child abuse (the victim could be a service member or a civilian). To qualify, you must be in a heterosexual relationship with the abuser and be the spouse/ex-spouse, current or former intimate partner, or have a child in common. A victim, victim advocate, installation law enforcement agency, or Family Advocacy Program (FAP) clinician may request a commander to issue an MPO.

MPOs may order the abuser (referred to as "the subject") to:

- have no contact or communication (including face to face, by telephone, in writing, or through a third party) with you or members of the your family or household;
- stay away from the family home (whether it is on or off the installation);
- stay away from the children's schools, child development centers, youth programs, and your place of employment;
- move into government quarters (barracks);
- leave any public place if the victim is in the same location or facility;
- do certain activities or stop doing certain activities;
- attend counseling; and
- surrender his or her government weapons custody card.

Commanders may tailor the order to meet your specific needs.

An MPO is only enforceable while the service member is attached to the command that issued the order. When the service member is transferred to a new command, the order will no longer be valid. If the victim still believes that the MPO is necessary to keep him or her safe, the victim, a victim advocate, or an FAP staff member may ask the commander who issued the MPO to contact the new commander to advise him or her of the MPO and to request the issuance of a new one. The commander who issued the MPO is supposed to recommend to the new command that a new MPO is issued when the service member is transferred to a new command and an MPO is still necessary to protect the victim.

Civilian abusers cannot be subject to MPOs. They may only be subject to a civil protection order issued by a state or tribal court. However, a commanding officer may order that the civilian abuser stay away from the installation.

Make sure that you get the MPO in writing from the commanding officer so that you can have it with you at all times.

Am I eligible to get a military protective order (MPO)?

You are eligible to file for a MPO against an active duty member of the military who has abused you or your children and who is your spouse/ex-spouse, intimate partner you live(d) with (but not a same-sex partner), or someone you have a child in common with. An MPO will be ordered if the commander agrees to it.

Can victims in homosexual relationships receive help?

Currently, only victims in heterosexual relationships can get help from the Family Advocacy Program and/or receive a military protective order. However, with President Obama's repeal of the "Don't Ask, Don't Tell" policy, effective in September 2011, it is expected that soon, victims in homosexual relationships will be entitled to benefits and services that were only available to married heterosexual couples.

For how long is an MPO valid?

MPOs are generally short term and can last as little at ten days. An MPO is generally issued for the period of time that it will take the FAP to investigate your claims and to provide the commander additional information. The victim advocate at your installation will know how long it generally takes for the FAP's Case Review Committee (CRC) to provide the commander with the results of their investigation, so you may want to ask the commander to take that time frame into account when issuing the MPO. Your MPO may or may not have an expiration date. However, whether it has an expiration date or not, the commanding officer may review the MPO at any time to change it or dissolve (end) it.

Also, an MPO is only enforceable while the service member is attached to the command that issued the order. When the service member is transferred to a new command, the order will no longer be valid. If you still need the protection of an MPO, the commander who issued the MPO should contact the new commander to advise him or her of the MPO and recommend that a new one be issued.

What will the process be like for getting an MPO? Will I have to be in the same room as the abuser?

Unlike civilian court, there is no trial or hearing. You will not have to appear in front of a judge. You will not have to testify in front of the abuser or even be in the same room as he or she.

The commander is the one who decides whether or not to issue an MPO. The commander may or may not meet with you before issuing the MPO. Oftentimes, the victim advocate at the FAP may call the commander on your behalf to ask for the MPO. If the commander does want to meet with you before granting the MPO, you might go to his or her office or meet him or her at the FAP or the local precinct. If the commander has a reasonable belief that an MPO is necessary to protect you, one will be issued.

What can I do if I am not granted an MPO?

Most likely the commander will issue an MPO if recommended by FAP as part of its review of the case. However, if you are not granted a MPO, you might still be eligible for a civil protective or restraining order issued by your home state, or the state you are currently living in. Unlike civil protective order proceedings, there is no real appeal process in the military if you are denied an MPO or if you disagree with the decision of the commanding officer. You can seek assistance in a variety of ways if the MPO is denied, and you can continue to inform the commander of further abuse, but you cannot "appeal" the decision. Please note that even though there is a law requiring military bases to enforce protective orders and civil restraining orders, this law may not be fully enforced.

Chapter 23

Police-Involved Abuse

When Your Batterer Is a Police Officer
Your Situation Is Different

Thirty years ago, there was no such thing as a battered women's shelter, a domestic violence agency, or an order of protection. Battered women and their advocates have worked hard to raise public awareness and lower society's tolerance of this crime. As a result of their work, today there are hundreds of shelters and domestic violence agencies across the country and every state has laws against domestic violence. The federal government spends millions of dollars annually to combat this crime against women.

There is a wealth of information and resources available to help victims of domestic violence recognize and escape the violence in their lives, except if your batterer happens to be a police officer.

Extraordinary Obstacles

If your batterer is a police officer, most of the progress that has been made in developing resources and assistance for battered women is of

This chapter includes the following information: "When Your Batterer Is a Police Officer," from *Police Domestic Violence: A Handbook for Victims* by Diane Wetendorf, © 2000, 2006; "Calling 911," © 2012 Diane Wetendorf, Inc.; "Police Power and Control Wheel," © 1998, 2007 Diane Wetendorf, Inc., adapted from Domestic Abuse Intervention Project, Duluth, MN; and "Safety and Technology," and "Domestic Violence Shelters," © 2012 Diane Wetendorf, Inc. All rights reserved. Reprinted with permission. For additional information and resources about officer-involved domestic violence, visit www.abuseofpower.info.

little benefit to you. Victims of police officers are still as isolated and invisible as all the victims of this crime were thirty years ago. Work now needs to be done to raise the public's awareness of domestic violence in the police home. Society must hold police officers accountable to not only enforce the law, but live by it.

As the victim of a police officer, your situation is very different than that of other victims. If you have ever tried to get help, you may have become discouraged because no one seemed to understand your plight. Even domestic violence counselors probably offered you the same options they offer other battered women, such as calling the police for intervention, seeking refuge in a shelter, or obtaining an order of protection.

Few people fully realize how extremely complex common remedies become when the perpetrator is a police officer.

Because of the extraordinary obstacles you face on your journey to safety, you will need to make extraordinarily creative plans to overcome those obstacles.

Focus On Your Survival

You may or may not be thinking about ending your relationship right now. But the fact that you are reading this means that you're at the point of wanting to change your life. You may still be in love with your partner and desperately want things to work out between you. You and your children may be financially dependent on him. You may be terrified of what he'll do to you if you ever try to leave him. You will probably do everything you can think of to make him change his behavior.

Most women try several avenues to change. The most common attempts include asking the abuser's colleagues or supervisors to talk to him, persuading him to go to counseling, offering to go to counseling with him, getting an order of protection, separating from him, even filing for divorce. Though it is possible that any of these strategies could work, often no matter what you or others do, the abuser continues to be manipulating, controlling, and/or violent. After you have exhausted all of your options to get him to change, you may be left with no choice but to focus on your own emotional and/or physical survival.

You Can Get Your Life Back

Focusing on your own survival means that you have decided to take back control of your own life. To do that, you must regain trust in your own thought processes, intuition, and your own gut feelings. It is very hard to rebuild confidence in yourself after your abuser has destroyed it, so you might want to talk to a domestic violence counselor or therapist who can give you support and encouragement. It helps to have someone with whom you can discuss all of your options for safety and learn how to minimize the involved risks. You will want to thoroughly consider the personal, financial, and legal ramifications of every option available to you as you make your decisions. This may seem overwhelming at times, especially if you are in the middle of a crisis while having to make important decisions.

There are no easy answers. The fact that many, many women have survived domestic violence at the hands of a police officer attests to the fact that your escape and your survival are possible.

Calling 9-1-1

It doesn't matter who calls 911—you, a child, neighbor, or stranger. A call to 911 starts a process that often goes far beyond your immediate need for help. It draws the complexity of the criminal justice system into your life.

He's One of Us

When police respond to a domestic violence call, officers are to use all reasonable means to prevent further abuse. Their actions can differ depending on whether the responding officers are from your abuser's department or another jurisdiction.

When co-workers are the responders, personal relationships, his rank, and department policies influence how they handle the situation. Responding officers may know him even if they are from another department. Even if they don't know him, once he identifies himself as a cop or firefighter, they usually treat him differently than they do a civilian abuser.

They may be reluctant to believe that a fellow officer or friend is a batterer. They may be less likely to believe and be sympathetic to you. They may feel conflicted between upholding the law and protecting another officer's job.

Officer Discretion

Responding officers may use their discretion on how to handle the call despite department policy. They may extend "professional courtesy" by not filing an official report, by not collecting evidence at the scene, by not making an arrest, or by not notifying supervisors about the incident.

They may pressure you not to pursue charges. There may be a blatant or a subtle threat to your safety if you decide to cooperate with an investigation or prosecution.

Your abuser may be able to manipulate responding officers into arresting you by claiming that you assaulted him. They may not listen to your story or believe that you were acting in self-defense.

Police Report

The police report is a key factor in the prosecutor's decision to pursue charges. A well-prepared report clearly identifies all parties present at the time of the incident, provides an account of events from everyone present, details the responding officers' observations of the scene, and summarizes the responding officers' actions.

It is important that you read the report to verify that it is accurate. This guards against any discrepancies between the batterer's account of events and yours, plus any tendency the responding officers may have to describe the incident in a way that is favorable to their colleague. If the report is inaccurate, you should request that the department amend the report to include your account of the incident.

Access to the police report will vary across jurisdictions. Some police agencies or prosecutors readily provide a copy of the report to you. Other departments and prosecutors may only provide a copy of the criminal complaint, not the report.

What You Can Do

Many departments have policies for responding to general domestic violence calls. Fewer have policy specific to officer-involved domestics. Your local domestic violence advocate may be able to help you determine whether proper procedures were followed.

To help ensure appropriate response, you can:

- Try to get the police report number, the names and badge numbers of responding officers.

- Insist that a supervisor is called to the scene. (Many departments require this by policy.)

- Give an honest account of what happened. Include if you have been drinking, if you used physical force against the abuser in response or because you felt threatened. If you do not provide a complete account of events at this point, any inconsistencies that emerge later will hurt your credibility or could lead to your arrest.

308

- Write down everything you can remember about the incident as soon as possible. Your account should include who was present (including children and other witnesses); what everyone said and did; any threats, physical attacks, and property damage; the cause and severity of any injuries; and what the police said and did when they were there. Don't forget to include the date and time.

- Take pictures of the scene and ask someone to photograph any bruises or other injuries, even if photos were taken by responding officers and/or at the emergency room. (Pictures should also be taken two to five days later because bruises darken with time.) Take pictures of any damaged furniture, broken doors, damage to your car, or other property damage. The photographer should not be a family member or friend that the defense could portray as biased. The pictures should be processed with a date and time stamp and signed by the photographer.

- Keep notes, photos, and other documentation in a secure location that the abuser can't easily access. For example, a locked cabinet in an advocate's office, a safe deposit box, or with your attorney.

Safety and Technology

Police Have Access to Information

Police officers have access to an immense amount of private and public information. This includes information from the Department of Motor Vehicles, criminal records, telephone and utility companies, credit bureaus, banks, landlords, mortgage companies, school personnel, hospital staff, insurance companies, government agencies, and other sources.

Communication, banking, and transportation services use interconnected networks and databases. A batterer who is in law enforcement has the investigative skills and knowledge to obtain and use personal information against you, your family, and friends.

Sophisticated and affordable surveillance products are readily available to anyone who wants to track or stalk another person. Standard telephones, cell phones, computers, e-mail, credit cards, automated teller machines (ATMs), automobiles, and public transportation leave a trail of information about where you are and what you are doing. Your abuser is trained to find people using these trails.

Note: If you are still in the relationship with your abuser, some of the following safety points (such as changing passwords on accounts or voice mail) could increase his suspicion.

309

Police Power and Control Wheel

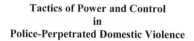

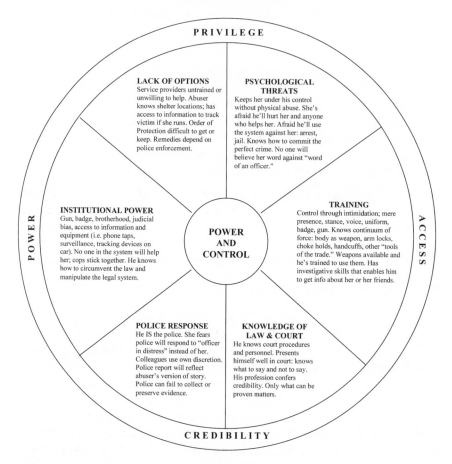

Figure 23.1. Police Power and Control Wheel: Tactics of Power and Control in Police-Perpetrated Domestic Violence (© 1998, 2007 Diane Wetendorf, Inc. Adapted from Domestic Abuse Intervention Project, Duluth MN).

Internet Safety

It doesn't matter whether your abuser has physical access to your computer. If you think your computer usage is being monitored, it probably is.

He doesn't have to be a computer programmer or have special skills to monitor your computer and internet activities. There are many programs he can use to track all your computer usage—websites you visit, documents you create or edit, and all your e-mail activity. It doesn't matter if you try to delete files or hide your work behind passwords. He can also discover internet-based phone calls, online purchases and banking, and many other activities.

If you are looking for information on abuse or planning your escape, don't use your home computer. If you can, use a "safer" computer such as a friend's computer or a public computer in a library, hotel, or other free public access. Avoid using public access that requires identifying information such as your driver's license or credit card information.

There is no way you can completely erase what you have done on any computer. If you think your computer usage is being monitored, it probably is. Remember that as a police officer, your abuser is trained to notice anything out of the ordinary, so it may be dangerous to delete cookies, change passwords, or erase your internet history if you usually don't do so.

E-mail and Electronic Posting

- E-mail, instant messaging (IM), and text messaging are never confidential means of communication. They are equivalent to sending a postcard.

- Use a safer computer and an account that your abuser does not know about.

- Create difficult passwords for your e-mail, voice mail, and home security access. Even though your abuser can break a password, one that combines numbers, letters, and symbols will make it more difficult.

- Be aware that employers have access to all your computer and e-mail activity.

- Avoid posting any personal information or abuse history on a blog, public or private forum, or social networking site. It does not matter if you create an alias. Whatever you post is ultimately traceable.

Telephones

- Avoid using cellular or cordless phones. Your calls can be picked up on a police scanner or other eavesdropping equipment.

- Use someone else's phone or a pay phone to make confidential calls. Your abuser may have tapped or put a bug on your line.

- Remember that cell phones transmit signals that give your relatively specific location at any given time. There is also a record of every call you make and receive.

- Guard your cell phone! It contains a wealth of information about you.

Save Evidence

- Save all correspondence from your abuser even if it is not threatening. If your order of protection prohibits your abuser from contacting you, this violates the order. These records are your evidence.

- Save all threatening e-mail or voice mail messages. Set up your e-mail and voice mail to automatically record the date and time of messages.

- Make copies of all correspondence and important documents and keep them in a safe place that your abuser does not know. If you can, keep a diary of everything that has been happening. Consider asking your domestic violence counselor to keep your papers, mail them to yourself at a rented mailbox, or put them in a safe deposit box.

Domestic Violence Shelters

No Guarantee

While going to a battered women's shelter can be a life-saving option for many victims, there are serious limitations to what any shelter can offer.

If you succeed in leaving your abuser, he may become obsessed with tracking you down. The established domestic violence shelter system may or may not work for you.

Using the shelter network may be possible, but it will be more complicated for you because your abuser is in law enforcement.

Police officers have access to information, including the locations of local shelters and the ability to discover the location of any shelter. Your batterer may remind you that he works closely with shelter staff. His message is clear: "Don't bother going to them, they know me; they won't believe you."

Valid Fears

You may be very reluctant to confide in any advocate. Your fears are well grounded about using any established system:

- Advocates work closely with the criminal justice system and can inadvertently or intentionally share information that will get back to the batterer.

- The abuser can discover the location of any shelter.

- The batterer may have been inside the shelter.

- Other women in the shelter may know your abuser as the officer who rescued them.

- The abuser may retaliate when you let others in the community know that he is a batterer.

- Shelter staff and other residents may be put in danger.

- The shelter is too isolated to feel safe.

- The shelter's only source of protection is the local police, who may not be of any help to you.

- Shelter staff may blame you for hurting their good relationship with the local police.

Shelter Advantages

- Shelter staff are trained in domestic violence issues. They can give you information on domestic violence laws and assist you in obtaining an order of protection.

- Staying in a domestic violence shelter can protect you from child abduction charges.

- If your abuser does track you to the shelter, the staff are trained to deal with this situation. It may be harder for him to manipulate the staff or the police if you are not in a local shelter.

- Women staying at the shelter are in situations similar to yours. They understand what you're going through and can give you emotional support.

- If you decide not to return home, the staff can help you apply for public benefits.

- Some shelter programs have transitional housing, which is longer-term housing than emergency shelter.

Shelter Disadvantages

- Life in a shelter is not home. You and your children are away from everything that is familiar to you.

- Some shelters are overcrowded and afford you little, if any, privacy.

- Some of the other residents may be difficult to live with because they, too, are in the midst of a crisis.

- Shelters have house rules, curfews, and requirements that you help with chores and participate in group counseling.

- You will have to agree to keep the shelter's address secret, to not have any contact with your abuser, and to send your children to a school near the shelter.

- You may not be able to go to work.

- Use of alcohol or drugs is reason for eviction from the shelter.

Shelter Intake Procedures

As you may already have learned, you can't just call a shelter and "reserve" a room. Shelters are often filled to capacity. Shelter intake policies vary, but most shelters only take women who are in immediate danger.

Shelter staff are required to interview you on the phone to make sure that you are eligible for shelter services. The way you tell your story and how you answer their questions will determine whether you are accepted into the shelter. They usually ask you if there has been recent physical abuse and if you are in immediate danger. They may require you to have or to get an order of protection.

They will ask questions regarding your physical and mental health. Some shelters hesitate to accept women who have a history of mental illness. They will also ask if you have any special needs and if you are on any medications. They will ask if you have any alcohol or drug problems. They may ask questions about your abuser, including what his occupation is. They may hesitate accepting you because your abuser is a firefighter or police officer. They may consider you a security risk, or they may not want to threaten their relationship with local law enforcement.

Staff will ask you if you have children with you. Many shelters do not take boys who are over twelve years old. If you have several children it might be harder to find a shelter that has enough space to accommodate you.

The shelter may not accept you if your abuser has filed criminal charges against you. You may be prevented from receiving victim services if he has an order of protection naming you as the perpetrator. Talk to an attorney or legal advocate about counter-petitioning for your own order of protection or vacating the abuser's order.

If You Go

If you do go to a shelter, you and shelter staff must review the pros and cons of notifying local police. If there is reason to believe that they will extend "professional courtesy" to another officer and respond to his inquiries about your whereabouts, then the police should not be notified. If you both trust the local department to respond appropriately, then they should alert the police about your batterer's likely attempts to locate and harm you.

Chapter 24

Abuse within Immigrant Communities

Chapter Contents

Section 24.1

Violence against Immigrant and Refugee Women: What You Need to Know

"Violence against Immigrant and Refugee Women," U.S. Department of Health and Human Services Office on Women's Health, May 18, 2011.

No one deserves to be hit or mistreated. You can get help, even if you do not have legal papers giving you permission to be in the United States. Keep reading to learn more about getting help.

An immigrant or refugee woman may face many of the same challenges as any other abused woman. In addition, she may face some unique challenges, such as being:

- made to "lose face" in her community;

- taught by her culture that family duty comes first;

- accused of leaving or failing her culture and background;

- lied to about her partner's ability to have her deported and keep their children;

- told that in the United States the law says she must have sex with her partner;

- told that her abuser is allowed to hit her or use other forms of physical punishment.

Although immigrant and refugee women may face such challenges, they also often have strong family ties and other sources of support. If you think you are being abused, reach out to someone who cares about you.

Remember, violence is against the law. If your partner abuses you, the police can make an arrest and help you leave safely. If you have been abused, the police usually will not report you to immigration authorities. If the police officers do not speak your language, find someone other than your abuser to translate for you.

318

Leaving Your Partner

If you decide to leave an abusive partner, go to a safe place such as the home of a trusted friend or relative or a local domestic violence shelter. Try to choose a place where your partner will not be able to find you. Keep in mind that shelters will help you no matter what your immigration status.

If you are leaving someone who is an immigrant, it can be helpful to have important information, so try to copy down the number on his resident card or naturalization papers. Take your children with you when you leave.

Court Order of Protection (Restraining Order)

If you are being abused, you can get a court order of protection to protect yourself and your children. You don't have to be a U.S. citizen or legal resident to get a court order of protection.

A court order of protection can do the following:

- Order the abuser not to have any contact with you and your children

- Order the abuser to move out of your home and give you use of the car

- Order the abuser to give you money for you and your children or to continue your insurance coverage

You can get an application for a court order of protection at courthouses, women's shelters, lawyers' offices, and some police stations.

You do not need a lawyer to get a protection order. Still, you may want to get help from a lawyer if you are not legal or if you do not understand your rights. Often, a local domestic violence agency can help you find a lawyer. Some lawyers will help you at no charge.

If an order is issued and the abuser does anything that the order forbids, call the police right away. The police can arrest the abuser for not following the order.

Protecting Your Children

Your partner may threaten to take your children if you leave him. Here are some ways you can work to protect your children:

- Apply for a court order of protection that says your partner has to stay away from you and your children.

319

- Apply for a custody order that says your children have to live with you. You can also ask for the order to say that your partner is not allowed to take your children out of the United States.

- If you have a court order of protection or custody order, give a copy to your children's school. Ask the school not to release the children to the abuser.

- Try to prevent your abuser from leaving the country with your child using a U.S. passport. Usually, if your child is under sixteen, your partner cannot get a U.S. passport for your child without your permission. Also, the U.S. Department of State has an alert program that may let you object to a passport being given to children up to the age of eighteen.

- Try to prevent your child from leaving the United States using a passport from another country. Your child may have citizenship from another country (either instead of U.S. citizenship or in addition to it). If so, contact that country's embassy in the United States, and ask that your child not be given a passport. Include a copy of a custody order or a court order that prevents your child from leaving the country. This may help convince the embassy to grant your request.

- Keep important items handy. Make sure you have recent pictures of your children and their passports and birth certificates. The police can help you better if you have these items.

- Compile contact information. Make a list of your partner's family and friends, including their addresses and phone numbers. This can help if your partner takes your children.

You may be able to get child support from your partner. A lawyer can help you with this. Ask your local domestic violence shelter for help finding a lawyer.

Deportation Concerns

If you are a U.S. citizen or a legal resident or have a valid visa, you cannot be deported unless you used fake documents to enter the country, broke the rules of your visa, or committed certain crimes.

If you are undocumented (don't have legal papers to be in the United States) or are not sure about your immigration status, you should talk to an immigration lawyer. Your local domestic violence shelter can help you find an immigration lawyer. There are lawyers who will help you at no charge.

If you report domestic violence to the police, they usually will not report you to immigration authorities. Still, you should carry the name of an immigration lawyer in case you need it.

Becoming Legal

You should talk to an immigration lawyer before taking steps to become legal. Your local domestic violence shelter can help you find a lawyer. Some lawyers will help you at no charge if you don't have much money. Remember that your lawyer will not tell anyone what you say without your permission.

If you are married to a U.S. citizen or a lawful permanent resident, usually your spouse has to apply for legal permanent residency for you. But in cases of domestic abuse you can apply for residency for you and your children by yourself, and your partner doesn't have to know. This is called self-petitioning, and there are specific rules about who can apply for residency this way.

If you are already in deportation hearings and are a victim of domestic abuse, you may be able to have your deportation cancelled and become a permanent resident. This is called a cancellation of removal and also has specific rules about who can apply for it.

Talk to an immigration lawyer to find out more about these and other options. Also keep in mind that you should not say you are a U.S. citizen if you are not. You also should not use false papers to work in the United States.

Section 24.2

Basic Questions and Answers about Residency Laws for Victims of Domestic Violence

"Questions and Answers about U-Visas" is excerpted from "Questions and Answers: Victims of Criminal Activity, U Nonimmigrant Status," U.S. Department of Homeland Security, November 2010; and "Questions and Answers about VAWA" is excerpted from "Battered Spouse, Children and Parents," U.S. Department of Homeland Security, April 2011.

Questions and Answers about U-Visas

The U nonimmigrant status (U visa) is set aside for victims of crimes who have suffered substantial mental or physical abuse and are willing to assist law enforcement and government officials in the investigation or prosecution of the criminal activity. Below are questions and answers pertaining to U nonimmigrant visas.

How does one become eligible for U nonimmigrant status?

There are four statutory eligibility requirements:

- The individual must have suffered substantial physical or mental abuse as a result of having been a victim of a qualifying criminal activity.

- The individual must have information concerning that criminal activity.

- The individual must have been helpful, is being helpful, or is likely to be helpful in the investigation or prosecution of the crime.

- The criminal activity must have violated U.S. laws

What qualifies as "criminal activity"?

Qualifying criminal activity is defined as being an activity involving one or more activities that violate U.S. criminal law, including abduction, abusive sexual contact, blackmail, domestic violence, extortion, false imprisonment, genital female mutilation, felonious assault, incest, involuntary servitude, kidnapping, murder, obstruction of justice, peonage, perjury, prostitution, rape, sexual assault, sexual exploitation, slave trader, torture, trafficking, witness tampering, unlawful criminal restraint, and other related crimes.

What are the Procedures to Request U Nonimmigrant Status?

Foreign national victims of crime must file a Form I-918, Petition for U Nonimmigrant Status. The form requests information regarding the petitioner's eligibility for such status, as well as admissibility to the United States.

How long can one maintain the U nonimmigrant classification?

U nonimmigrant status cannot exceed four years. However, extensions are available upon certification by a certifying agency that the foreign national's presence in the United States is required to assist in the investigation or prosecution of the qualifying criminal activity.

Can a foreign national petition for U nonimmigrant status from outside the United States?

Yes. The United States Citizenship and Immigration Services (US-CIS) has determined that the legal framework for U nonimmigrant status permits foreign national victims of criminal activity to petition for such status either inside or outside the United States.

If not admissible to enter the United States as a foreign national, an applicant for a U visa must obtain a waiver of inadmissibility through submission of a Form I-192, Application for Advance Permission to Enter as a Non-Immigrant. This waiver is adjudicated by the Vermont Service Center of USCIS on a discretionary basis, allowing the petitioner to continue with the U nonimmigrant visa process.

Can family members of the petitioner receive U nonimmigrant status?

Family members who accompany the petitioner can, under certain circumstances, obtain a U nonimmigrant derivative visa. The U nonimmigrant visa principal must petition on behalf of qualifying family members.

If the principle petitioner is under twenty-one years of age, then they may petition on behalf of spouse, children, parents, and unmarried siblings under age eighteen.

If the principle petitioner is twenty-one years of age or older, they may petition on behalf of spouse and children.

The principal petitioner needs to file a Form I-918, Supplement A, Petition for Qualifying Family Member of U-1 Recipient, on behalf of their qualifying family members.

Can an individual who has held U nonimmigrant status eventually apply for a green card (permanent residence)?

Yes. The individual must have been physically present in the United for a continuous period of at least three years since the date of admission as a U nonimmigrant; the individual must not have unreasonably refused to provide assistance to law enforcement since receiving a U nonimmigrant visa; and the certifying agency must determine that the individual's continued presence in the country is justified on humanitarian grounds to ensure continuation of a cohesive family, or is otherwise in the national or public interest.

Can qualifying family members apply for permanent residence (a green card)?

Yes. There are two ways family members of a U nonimmigrant visa holder can apply for a green card. First, family members who hold a derivative U nonimmigrant visa themselves may be eligible for a green card. Second, certain family members who have never held a derivative U nonimmigrant visa may be eligible for a green card.

Questions and Answers about VAWA

As a battered spouse, child or parent, you may file an immigrant visa petition under the Violence against Women Act (VAWA). VAWA allows certain spouses, children, and parents of U.S. citizens and permanent residents (green card holders) to file a petition for themselves without the abuser's knowledge. This will allow you to seek both safety and independence from the abuser. The provisions of VAWA apply equally to women and men. Your abuser will not be notified that you have filed for immigration benefits under VAWA.

Who is eligible to file?

Spouse: You may file for yourself if you are, or were, the abused spouse of a U.S. citizen or permanent resident. You may also include on your petition your unmarried children who are under twenty-one if they have not filed for themselves.

Parent: You may file for yourself if you are the parent of a child who has been abused by your U.S. citizen or permanent resident spouse. You may include on your petition your children, including those who have not been abused, if they have not filed for themselves. You may also file if you are the parent of a U.S. citizen, and you have been abused by your U.S. citizen son or daughter.

Child: You may file for yourself if you are an abused child under twenty-one, unmarried, and have been abused by your U.S. citizen or permanent resident parent. Your children may also be included on your petition. You may file for yourself as a child after age twenty-one but before age twenty-five if you can demonstrate that the abuse was the main reason for the delay in filing.

What are the eligibility requirements for a spouse?

- You are married to a U.S. citizen or permanent resident abuser; or your marriage to the abuser was terminated by death or a divorce (related to the abuse) within the two years prior to filing; or your spouse lost or renounced citizenship or permanent resident status within the two years prior to filing due to an incident of domestic violence; or you believed that you were legally married to your abusive U.S. citizen or permanent resident spouse but the marriage was not legitimate solely because of the bigamy of your abusive spouse.

- You have been abused in the United States by your U.S. citizen or permanent resident spouse; or you have been abused by your U.S. citizen or permanent resident spouse abroad while your spouse was employed by the U.S. government or a member of the U.S. uniformed services; or you are the parent of a child who has been subjected to abuse by your U.S. citizen or permanent spouse.

- You entered into the marriage in good faith, not solely for immigration benefits.

- You have resided with your spouse.

- You are a person of good moral character.

What are the eligibility requirements for a child?

You:

- are the child of a U.S. citizen or permanent resident abuser;

- were the child of a U.S. citizen or permanent resident abuser who lost citizenship or lawful permanent resident status due to an incident of domestic violence;

- have been abused in the United States by your U.S. citizen or permanent resident parent;

- have been abused by your U.S. citizen or permanent resident parent abroad while your parent was employed by the U.S. government or a member of the U.S. uniformed services;

- have resided with the abusive parent;

- have evidence to prove your relationship to your parent;

- must provide evidence of good moral character if you are over the age of fourteen.

What are the eligibility requirements for a parent?

- You are the parent of a U.S. citizen son or daughter or were the parent of a U.S. citizen son or daughter who lost or renounced citizenship status related to an incident of domestic violence or died within two years prior of filing.

- You have been abused by your U.S. citizen son or daughter.

- You have resided with the abusive son or daughter.

- You are a person of good moral character.

Chapter 25

Human Trafficking

Chapter Contents

Section 25.1

What Is Human Trafficking?

"Human Trafficking," U.S. Department of Health and
Human Services Office on Women's Health, May 18, 2011.

Human trafficking is when a person is forced or tricked into working in terrible conditions. Victims of human trafficking may be kidnapped, for example. They also may be lured with false promises of a better life in a new country. A person who is trafficked may be drugged, locked up, beaten, starved, or made to work for many hours a day. Types of work a trafficked person may be forced to do include prostitution, farm work, cleaning, childcare, or sweatshop work.

Ways traffickers control a woman may include the following:

- Making her work to pay back money they say she owes them

- Threatening to hurt her or her family

- Threatening to have her deported

- Taking away her passport, birth certificate, or identification card

- Preventing her from having contact with friends, family, or the outside world

Sometimes, a woman may end up trafficked after being forced to marry someone against her will. In a forced marriage, a woman's husband and his family can have great control over her life. They may then place her in domestic or sexual slavery against her will.

Help for Victims of Human Trafficking

If you think you have come in contact with a victim of human trafficking, call the National Human Trafficking Resource Center hotline at 888-373-7888. Hotline staff can help you figure out if you have seen a victim of human trafficking and can suggest local resources.

Anyone who is brought into the United States for forced labor may be able to get a special visa and other help rebuilding his or her life.

Section 25.2

Sex Trafficking

Excerpted from "Fact Sheet: Sex Trafficking," U.S.
Department of Health and Human Services, June 28, 2011.

Sex trafficking is a modern-day form of slavery in which a commercial sex act is induced by force, fraud, or coercion, or in which the person induced to perform such an act is under the age of eighteen years. Enactment of the Trafficking Victims Protection Act of 2000 (TVPA) made sex trafficking a serious violation of federal law.

Victims of Sex Trafficking and What They Face

Victims of sex trafficking can be women or men, girls or boys, but the majority are women and girls. There are a number of common patterns for luring victims into situations of sex trafficking, including the following:

- A promise of a good job in another country

- A false marriage proposal turned into a bondage situation

- Being sold into the sex trade by parents, husbands, or boyfriends

- Being kidnapped by traffickers

Sex traffickers frequently subject their victims to debt-bondage, an illegal practice in which the traffickers tell their victims that they owe money (often relating to the victims' living expenses and transport into the country) and that they must pledge their personal services to repay the debt.

Sex traffickers use a variety of methods to "condition" their victims, including starvation, confinement, beatings, physical abuse, rape, gang rape, threats of violence to the victims and the victims' families, forced drug use, and the threat of shaming their victims by revealing their activities to their family and their families' friends.

Victims face numerous health risks. Physical risks include drug and alcohol addiction; physical injuries (broken bones, concussions, burns, vaginal/anal tearings); traumatic brain injury (TBI) resulting in memory loss, dizziness, headaches, numbness; sexually transmitted diseases (e.g., human immunodeficiency virus [HIV]/ acquired immune deficiency syndrome [AIDS], gonorrhea, syphilis, urinary tract infections, pubic lice); sterility, miscarriages, menstrual problems; other diseases (e.g., tuberculosis, hepatitis, malaria, pneumonia); and forced or coerced abortions.

Psychological harms include mind/body separation/disassociated ego states, shame, grief, fear, distrust, hatred of men, self-hatred, suicide, and suicidal thoughts. Victims are at risk for posttraumatic stress disorder (PTSD)—acute anxiety, depression, insomnia, physical hyperalertness, and self-loathing that is long-lasting and resistant to change (complex-PTSD).

Victims may also suffer from traumatic bonding—a form of coercive control in which the perpetrator instills in the victim fear as well as gratitude for being allowed to live.

Types of Sex Trafficking

Victims of trafficking are forced into various forms of commercial sexual exploitation, including prostitution, pornography, stripping, live-sex shows, mail-order marriages, military prostitution, and sex tourism.

Victims trafficked into prostitution and pornography are usually involved in the most exploitive forms of commercial sex operations. Sex trafficking operations can be found in highly visible venues, such as street prostitution, as well as more underground systems, such as closed brothels that operate out of residential homes. Sex trafficking also takes place in a variety of public and private locations, such as massage parlors, spas, strip clubs, and other fronts for prostitution. Victims may start off dancing or stripping in clubs and then be coerced into situations of prostitution and pornography.

Assistance for Victims of Sex Trafficking

When victims of trafficking are identified, the U.S. government can help them adjust their immigration status and obtain support and assistance in rebuilding their lives in the United States through various programs. By certifying victims of trafficking, the U.S. Department of Health and Human Services (HHS) enables trafficking victims who are non–U.S. citizens to receive federally funded benefits and services to the same extent as a refugee. Victims of trafficking who are U.S.

citizens do not need to be certified to receive benefits. As U.S. citizens, they may already be eligible for many benefits.

Through HHS, victims can access benefits and services including food, health care, and employment assistance. Certified victims of trafficking can obtain access to services that provide English language instruction and skills training for job placement. Since many victims are reluctant to come forward for fear of being deported, one of HHS's most important roles is to connect victims with nonprofit organizations prepared to assist them and address their specific needs. These organizations can provide counseling, case management, and benefit coordination.

If you think you have come in contact with a victim of human trafficking, call the National Human Trafficking Resource Center at 888-373-7888. This hotline will help you determine if you have encountered victims of human trafficking, will identify local resources available in your community to help victims, and will help you coordinate with local social service organizations to help protect and serve victims so they can begin the process of restoring their lives.

Section 25.3

Victim Assistance

Excerpted from "Fact Sheet: Victim Assistance," U.S. Department of Health and Human Services, May 31, 2012.

Benefits and Services Available to Victims of Human Trafficking

Certified and eligible victims of human trafficking can receive benefits and services necessary for their safety, protection, and basic well-being. These include:

- Housing assistance
- Food assistance
- Income assistance
- Employment assistance

- English language training

- Health care

- Mental health services

- Foster care

Temporary Immigration Status and Relief

The TVPA created the T visa, a nonimmigrant status that allows a foreign victim of human trafficking to remain in the United States for up to four years. The law also allows certain members of a T visa holder's family to apply for derivative T visa status.

There are several benefits to a T visa, including the following:

- Employment authorization (EAD);

- Possibility of adjusting status to lawful permanent resident; and

- Ability of certain family members to obtain nonimmigrant status as T visa derivatives.

Eligible family members of trafficking victims who have received T nonimmigrant status can apply for a special T visa for derivatives. These family members include the spouse, child, parent, or an unmarried minor sibling of a victim of trafficking victim who is under twenty-one years of age, or the spouse or child of a victim of trafficking who is twenty-one years of age or older. Like certified trafficking victims, T visa derivatives are eligible for federal and state benefits and services to the same extent as refugees. Also, derivatives can apply for EADs.

The following are some of the specific benefit programs for which trafficking victims with a certification or eligibility letter can apply:

- **Temporary Assistance for Needy Families (TANF):** A federally subsidized, state-run cash-benefit and work-opportunities program for needy families with children when the parents or other caretaker relatives are unable to provide for the family's basic needs, and for pregnant women.

- **Supplemental Security Income (SSI):** A monthly benefit for persons who are blind or disabled, or are at least sixty-five years old and have limited income and resources.

- **Refugee Cash Assistance (RCA):** HHS/ORR program available to victims who are ineligible for TANF and SSI. RCA benefits are available for up to eight months from the date of ORR certification. RCA recipients must register for employment services and participate in employability service programs unless specifically exempted by state criteria. Minors who cannot comply with the employability service requirements cannot receive RCA.

- **Supplemental Nutrition Assistance Program (SNAP), formerly Food Stamps:** Federal benefits to buy food that is provided to low-income individuals and families through an electronic card that is used like an ATM card at participating grocery stores.

- **Women, Infants and Children (WIC):** Provides supplemental food packages for nutritionally at-risk, low-income pregnant, breastfeeding, and postpartum women; infants; and children up to five years of age.

- **Medicaid:** The federally subsidized, state-run program that provides health coverage for low-income pregnant women, children, parents, adults, and those with disabilities who may have no insurance or inadequate medical insurance.

- **Children's Health Insurance Program (CHIP):** The public health insurance program for low-income, uninsured children eighteen years of age or younger who do not qualify for Medicaid.

- **Refugee Medical Assistance (RMA):** HHS/ORR program available to victims who are ineligible for Medicaid or CHIP. RMA benefits are available for up to eight months from the date of ORR certification, or the date of eligibility if the victim is a minor.

- **Medical screening:** Conducted by state or local health departments or their proxies for the diagnosis, treatment, and prevention of communicable diseases and other conditions of public health importance. This usually includes screening for tuberculosis (TB), parasites, and hepatitis B, as well as school vaccinations.

- **One-Stop Career Center System:** Department of Labor (DOL)–funded nationwide network of employment centers that provide information and assistance for people who are looking for jobs, or who need education and training to get a job. Services include training referrals, career counseling, job listings, and other employment services.

- **Job Corps:** DOL-funded centers to help eligible youth aged sixteen to twenty-four achieve employment, earn a high school diploma or general equivalency degree (GED) and/or learn a vocational trade.

- **Matching Grant:** HHS/ORR self-sufficiency program administered by private agencies as an alternative to public assistance and designed to enable clients to become self-sufficient within four to six months from the date of certification or eligibility. Provides case management; cash assistance and housing, when needed; and employment services. Clients must complete enrollment in Matching Grant within thirty-one days of the date of certification or eligibility.

- **Housing:** Eligibility for affordable rental housing for low-income families, the elderly, and persons with disabilities, and Housing Choice Vouchers issued by low-income housing agencies to very-low-income individuals and families so that they can lease privately owned rental housing.

- **Unaccompanied Refugee Minors (URM) Program:** Provides specialized, culturally appropriate foster care or other licensed care settings according to children's individual needs. Provides family reunification assistance when appropriate.

Part Four

Preventing and Intervening in Domestic Violence

Chapter 26

Healthy Relationships Are Key to Preventing Domestic Violence

Chapter Contents

Section 26.1

What Should I Look for in a Boy- or Girlfriend?

Relationships require respect, trust, and open communication. Whether you're looking for a relationship or are already in one, make sure you and your partner agree on what makes a relationship healthy. It's not always easy, but you can build a healthy relationship. Look for someone who:

- treats you with respect;
- doesn't make fun of things you like or want to do;
- never puts you down;
- doesn't get angry if you spend time with your friends or family;
- listens to your ideas and compromises sometimes;
- isn't excessively negative;
- shares some of your interests such as movies, sports, reading, dancing, or music;
- isn't afraid to share their thoughts and feelings;
- is comfortable around your friends and family;
- is proud of your accomplishments and successes;
- respects your boundaries and does not abuse technology;
- doesn't require you to "check in" or need to know where you are all the time;
- is caring and honest;
- doesn't pressure you to do things that you don't want to do;
- doesn't constantly accuse you of cheating or being unfaithful;
- encourages you to do well in school or at work;

- doesn't threaten you or make you feel scared;

- understands the importance of healthy relationships.

Remember that a relationship consists of two people. Both you and your partner should have equal say and should never be afraid to express how you feel. It's not just about speaking up for yourself—you should also listen and seriously consider what your partner says.

Every relationship has arguments and disagreements sometimes—this is normal. How you choose to deal with your disagreements is what really counts. Both people should work hard to communicate effectively.

Section 26.2

Building Healthy Relationships

"Healthy Relationships," by Joyce Woodford, resources updated by Dorinda Lambert. © 2002, 2012 Counseling Services, Kansas State University (www .k-state.edu/counseling). All rights reserved. Reprinted with permission.

Healthy relationships:

- make people happier and ease stress;

- are realistic and flexible;

- mean sharing and talking;

- include self-care;

- use fair fighting techniques.

Ten Tips for Healthy Relationships

Healthy relationships bring happiness and health to our lives. Studies show that people with healthy relationships really do have more happiness and less stress. There are basic ways to make relationships healthy, even though each one is different ... parents, siblings, friends, boyfriends, girlfriends, professors, roommates, and classmates. Here are ten tips for healthy relationships!

1. Keep expectations realistic. No one can be everything we might want him or her to be. Sometimes people disappoint us. It's not all-or-nothing, though. Healthy relationships mean accepting people as they are and not trying to change them!

2. Talk with each other. It can't be said enough: communication is essential in healthy relationships! It means: take the time. Really be there. Genuinely listen. Don't plan what to say next while you're trying to listen. Don't interrupt. Listen with your ears and your heart. Sometimes people have emotional messages to share and weave it into their words. Ask questions. Ask if you think you may have missed the point. Ask friendly (and appropriate!) questions. Ask for opinions. Show your interest. Open the communication door. Share information. Studies show that sharing information especially helps relationships begin. Be generous in sharing yourself, but don't overwhelm others with too much too soon.

3. Be flexible. Most of us try to keep people and situations just the way we like them to be. It's natural to feel apprehensive, even sad or angry, when people or things change and we're not ready for it. Healthy relationships mean change and growth are allowed!

4. Take care of you. You probably hope those around you like you, so you may try to please them. Don't forget to please yourself. Healthy relationships are mutual!

5. Be dependable. If you make plans with someone, follow through. If you have an assignment deadline, meet it. If you take on a responsibility, complete it. Healthy relationships are trustworthy!

6. Fight fair. Most relationships have some conflict. It only means you disagree about something, it doesn't have to mean you don't like each other! When you have a problem:

    *   **Negotiate a time to talk about it:** Don't have difficult conversations when you are very angry or tired. Ask, "When is a good time to talk about something that is bothering me?" Healthy relationships are based on respect and have room for both.

    *   **Don't criticize:** Attack the problem, not the other person. Open sensitive conversations with "I" statements; talk about how you struggle with the problem. Don't open with

"you" statements; avoid blaming the other person for your thoughts and feelings. Healthy relationships don't blame.

- **Let others speak for themselves:** Healthy relationships recognize each person's right to explain themselves.

- **Stay with the topic:** Don't use a current concern as a reason to jump into everything that bothers you. Healthy relationships don't use ammunition from the past to fuel the present. Say, "I'm sorry" when you're wrong. It goes a long way in making things right again. Healthy relationships can admit mistakes.

- **Don't assume things:** When we feel close to someone it's easy to think we know how he or she thinks and feels. We can be very wrong! Healthy relationships check things out.

- **Ask for help if you need it:** Talk with someone who can help you find resolution—like a counselor, a teacher, a minister, or even parents. Healthy relationships aren't afraid to ask for help. There may not be a resolved ending. Be prepared to compromise or to disagree about some things. Healthy relationships don't demand conformity or perfect agreement.

- **Don't hold grudges:** You don't have to accept anything and everything, but don't hold grudges—they just drain your energy. Studies show that the more we see the best in others, the better healthy relationships get. Healthy relationships don't hold on to past hurts and misunderstandings.

- **The goal is for everyone to be a winner:** Relationships with winners and losers don't last. Healthy relationships are between winners who seek answers to problems together.

- **You can leave a relationship:** You can choose to move out of a relationship. Studies tell us that loyalty is very important in good relationships, but healthy relationships are now, not some hoped-for future development.

7. Show your warmth. Studies tell us warmth is highly valued by most people in their relationships. Healthy relationships show emotional warmth!

8. Keep your life balanced. Other people help make our lives satisfying but they can't create that satisfaction for us. Only you can fill your life. Don't overload on activities, but do use your time at

college to try new things—clubs, volunteering, lectures, projects. You'll have more opportunities to meet people and more to share with them. Healthy relationships aren't dependent!

9. It's a process. Sometimes it looks like everyone else on campus is confident and connected. Actually, most people feel just like you feel, wondering how to fit in and have good relationships. It takes time to meet people and get to know them ... so, make "small talk" ... respond to others ... smile ... keep trying. Healthy relationships can be learned and practiced and keep getting better!

10. Be yourself! It's much easier and much more fun to be you than to pretend to be something or someone else. Sooner or later, it catches up anyway. Healthy relationships are made of real people, not images!

Section 26.3

Traits of a Healthy Family

"Traits of a Healthy Family," reprinted with permission from the Corporate Alliance to End Partner Violence, © 2012. All rights reserved. For additional information, visit www.caepv.org.

1. The healthy family communicates and listens.

2. The healthy family affirms and supports one another.

3. The healthy family teaches respect for others.

4. The healthy family develops a sense of trust.

5. The healthy family has a sense of play and humor.

6. The healthy family exhibits a sense of shared responsibility.

7. The healthy family teaches a sense of right and wrong.

8. The healthy family has a strong sense of family in which rituals and traditions abound.

9. The healthy family has a balance of interaction among members.

10. The healthy family has a shared sense of values.

11. The healthy family respects the privacy of one another.

12. The healthy family values service to others.

13. The healthy family fosters honest conversation.

14. The healthy family shares leisure time.

15. The healthy family admits and seeks help with problems.

Section 26.4

Tips for Being a Nurturing Parent

Reprinted from the U.S. Health and Human Services Department, 2006.
Reviewed by David A. Cooke, M.D., FACP, May 2012.

A healthy, nurturing relationship with your child is built through countless interactions over the course of time. It requires a lot of energy and work, but the rewards are well worth it. When it comes to parenting, there are few absolutes (one, of course, being that every child needs to be loved) and there is no one "right way." Different parenting techniques work for different children under different circumstances. These tips provide suggestions as you discover what works best in your family. Do not expect to be perfect; parenting is a difficult job.

Help Your Children Feel Loved and Secure

We can all take steps to strengthen our relationships with our children, including the following:

- Make sure your children know you love them, even when they do something wrong.

- Encourage your children. Praise their achievements and talents. Recognize the skills they are developing.

- Spend time with your children. Do things together that you both enjoy. Listen to your children.

- Learn how to use nonphysical options for discipline. Many alternatives exist. Depending on your child's age and level of development, these may include simply redirecting your child's attention, offering choices, or using "time out."

Realize that Community Resources Add Value

Children need direct and continuing access to people with whom they can develop healthy, supportive relationships. To assist this, parents may do the following things:

- Take children to libraries, museums, movies, and sporting events.

- Enroll children in youth enrichment programs, such as sports or music.

- Use community services for family needs, such as parent education classes or respite care.

- Communicate regularly with childcare or school staff.

- Participate in religious or youth groups.

Seek Help If You Need It

Being a parent is difficult. No one expects you to know how to do it all. Challenges such as unemployment or a child with special needs can add to family tension. If you think stress may be affecting the way you treat your child, or if you just want the extra support that most parents need at some point, try the following:

- **Talk to someone:** Tell a friend, healthcare provider, or a leader in your faith community about what you are experiencing. Or, join a support group for parents.

- **Seek respite care when you need a break:** Everyone needs time for themselves. Respite care or crisis care provides a safe place for your children so you can take care of yourself.

- **Call a help line:** Most states have help lines for parents. Childhelp USA® offers a national twenty-four-hour hotline (800-4-A-CHILD) for parents who need help or parenting advice.

- **Seek counseling:** Individual, couple, or family counseling can identify and reinforce healthy ways to communicate and parent.

- **Take a parenting class:** No one is born knowing how to be a good parent. It is an acquired skill. Parenting classes can give you the skills you need to raise a happy, healthy child.

- **Accept help:** You do not have to do it all. Accept offers of help from trusted family, friends, and neighbors. Do not be afraid to ask for help if you feel that you need it.

Chapter 27

Men's Role in Domestic Violence Prevention

Chapter Contents

Section 27.1

Teaching Boys about Relationship Abuse

Excerpted from "Ways You Can Coach Boys into Men," © 2012 Futures
Without Violence. All rights reserved. Reprinted with permission. For additional information, visit www.futureswithoutviolence.org.

Teach early: It's never too soon to talk to a child about violence.
Let him know how you think he should express his anger and frustration—and what is out of bounds. Talk with him about what it means
to be fair, share, and treat others with respect.

Be there: If it comes down to one thing you can do, this is it. Just
being with boys is crucial. The time doesn't have to be spent in activities. Boys will probably not say this directly—but they want a male
presence around them, even if few words are exchanged.

Listen: Hear what he has to say. Listen to how he and his friends
talk about girls. Ask him if he's ever seen abusive behavior in his
friends. Is he worried about any of his friends who are being hurt in
their relationships? Are any of his friends hurting anyone else?

Tell him how: Teach him ways to express his anger without using
violence. When he gets mad, tell him he can walk it out, talk it out, or
take a time out. Let him know he can always come to you if he feels
like things are getting out of hand. Try to give him examples of what
you might say or do in situations that could turn violent.

Bring it up: A kid will never approach you and ask for guidance
on how to treat women. But that doesn't mean he doesn't need it. Try
watching TV with him or listening to his music. If you see or hear
things that depict violence against women, tell him what you think
about it. Never hesitate to let him know you don't approve of sports
figures that demean women, or jokes, video games, and song lyrics that
do the same. And when it comes time for dating, be sure he knows that
treating girls with respect is important.

Be a role model: Fathers, coaches, and any man who spends time
with boys or teens will have the greatest impact when they "walk
the walk." They will learn what respect means by observing how you

treat other people. So make respect a permanent way of dealing with people—when you're driving in traffic, talking with customer service reps, in restaurants with waiters, and with your family around the dinner table. He's watching what you say and do and takes his cues from you, both good and bad. Be aware of how you express your anger. Let him know how you define a healthy relationship and always treat women and girls in a way that your son can admire.

Teach often: Your job isn't done once you get the first talk out of the way. Help him work through problems in relationships as they arise. Let him know he can come back and talk to you again anytime. Use every opportunity to reinforce the message that violence has no place in a relationship.

Section 27.2

What Men Can Do to End Violence against Women

"Ten Things Men Can Do to Prevent Domestic and Sexual Violence," © 2007 A Call to Men, Inc. (www.acalltomen.org). Reviewed for currency by copyright holder April 2012. All rights reserved. Reprinted with permission.

1. Acknowledge and understand how male dominance and aspects of unhealthy manhood are at the foundation of domestic and sexual violence.

2. Examine and challenge our individual beliefs and the role that we play in supporting men who are abusive.

3. Recognize and stop colluding with other men by getting out of our socially defined roles, and take a stance to prevent domestic and sexual violence.

4. Remember that our silence is affirming. When we choose not to speak out against domestic and sexual violence, we are supporting it.

5. Educate and re-educate our sons and other young men about our responsibility in preventing domestic and sexual violence.

6. "Break out of the man box"—Challenge traditional images of manhood that stop us from actively taking a stand in domestic and sexual violence prevention.

7. Accept and own our responsibility that domestic and sexual violence will not end until men become part of the solution to end it. We must take an active role in creating a cultural and social shift that no longer tolerates violence and discrimination against women and girls.

8. Stop supporting the notion that domestic and sexual violence is due to mental illness, lack of anger management skills, chemical dependency, stress, etc. Domestic and sexual violence is rooted in male dominance and the socialization of men.

9. Take responsibility for creating appropriate and effective ways to educate and raise awareness about domestic and sexual violence prevention.

10. Create responsible and accountable men's initiatives in your community to support domestic and sexual violence prevention.

Chapter 28

Parents' Role in Preventing Dating Violence

Chapter Contents

Section 28.1

Talking to Your Teen about Dating Violence

Excerpted from "Talk with Your Teen about Healthy Relationships,"
National Health Information Center, 2012.

When Do I Start Talking with My Child about Relationships?

It's never too early to teach your child about healthy relationships. In fact, you've probably been doing it all along. When you taught your son to say "please" and "thank you" as a toddler, you were teaching him about respect and kindness.

Your own relationships also teach your kids how to treat others. When you treat your kids, partner, and friends in healthy, supportive ways, your kids learn from your choices.

Kids learn from unhealthy experiences, too. If your child is experiencing violence at home or in the community, he may be more likely to be in an unhealthy relationship later on.

When Do I Start Talking about Dating Relationships?

The best time to start talking about healthy dating relationships is before your child starts dating. Start conversations about what to look for in a romantic partner. For example, you could ask your child:

- How do you want to be treated?

- How do you want to feel about yourself when you are with that person?

What Makes a Relationship Healthy?

In a healthy relationship:

- both people feel respected, supported, and valued;

- decisions are made together;

- both people have friends and interests outside of the relationship;

- disagreements are settled with open and honest communication;
- there are more good times than bad.

What Makes a Relationship Unhealthy?

In an unhealthy relationship:

- one person tries to change the other;
- one person makes most or all of the decisions;
- one or both people drop friends and interests outside of the relationship;
- one person yells, threatens, hits, or throws things during arguments;
- one person makes fun of the other's opinions or interests;
- one person keeps track of the other all the time by calling, texting, or checking in with other friends;
- there are more bad times than good.

What Is Dating Violence?

Dating violence is when one person in a romantic relationship is abusive to the other person. Dating violence includes emotional, physical, and sexual abuse. It can happen in same-sex and opposite-sex relationships.

Both boys and girls can be unhealthy or unsafe in a relationship. That's why it's so important to talk to all kids and teens about how to be in respectful, healthy relationships.

Who Is at Risk for Dating Violence?

While dating violence can happen to anyone, teens may be more at risk of unhealthy relationships if they:

- use alcohol or drugs;
- are depressed;
- hang out with friends who are violent;
- have trouble controlling their anger;
- struggle with learning in school;
- have sex with more than one person.

What Are the Warning Signs of Dating Violence?

It's common for teens to have mood swings and to try out different behaviors. However, sudden changes in your teen's attitude or behavior could be a sign that something more serious is going on.

If you think this may be the case, talk to your teen to find out more.

Watch for signs that your teen may have a partner who is violent. Here are some changes you might see in a teen whose partner uses violence:

- Avoiding friends, family, and school activities
- Making excuses for a partner's behavior
- Looking uncomfortable or fearful around a partner
- Losing interest in favorite activities
- Getting bad grades
- Having unexplained injuries, like bruises or scratches

Watch for signs that your teen may be violent. People who use physical, emotional, or sexual violence to control their partners also need help to stop. If you see these signs in your child, your teen might need help with violent behaviors:

- Jealousy and possessiveness
- Blaming other people for anything that goes wrong
- Damaging or ruining a partner's things
- Wanting to control someone else's decisions
- Constantly texting or calling a partner
- Posting embarrassing information about a partner on websites like Facebook (including sexual information or pictures)

People in unhealthy relationships may have many excuses to try to explain away the hurtful parts of the relationship. If you see these signs, talk to your teen.

Take Action!

Set Rules for Dating

As kids get older, they gain more independence and freedom. However, teens still need parents to set boundaries and expectations for their behavior.

Here are some things you may want to talk about with your teen ahead of time:

- Can friends come over when you aren't home?
- Can your son go on a date with someone you haven't met?
- How can your daughter reach you if she ever needs a ride home?

Be a Role Model

You can teach your kids a lot by treating them and others with respect. As you have conversations with your teen about healthy relationships, think about your own behavior. Does it match the values you are talking about?

Treating your kids with respect also helps you build healthy relationships with them. This can make it easier to communicate with your teen about important issues like staying safe.

Section 28.2

How You Can Help If Your Child Is in an Abusive Relationship

Knowing that your son or daughter is in an unhealthy relationship can be both frustrating and frightening. But as a parent, you're critical in helping your child develop healthy relationships and can provide life-saving support if they're in an abusive relationship. Remember, dating violence occurs in both same-sex and opposite-sex couples and either gender can be abusive.

What Do I Need to Know?

You can look for some early warning signs of abuse that can help you identify if your child is in an abusive relationship before it's too late. Some of these signs include:

- Your child's partner is extremely jealous or possessive.

- You notice unexplained marks or bruises.

- Your child's partner emails or texts excessively.

- You notice that your son or daughter is depressed or anxious.

- Your son or daughter stops participating in extracurricular activities or other interests.

- Your child stops spending time with other friends and family.

- Your child's partner abuses other people or animals.

- Your child begins to dress differently.

What Can I Do?

- **Tell your child you're concerned for their safety:** Point out that what's happening isn't "normal." Everyone deserves a safe and healthy relationship. Offer to connect your son or daughter with a professional, like a counselor or attorney, who they can talk to confidentially.

- **Be supportive and understanding:** Stress that you're on their side. Provide information and nonjudgmental support. Let your son or daughter know that it's not their fault and no one "deserves" to be abused. Make it clear that you don't blame them and you respect their choices.

- **Believe them and take them seriously:** Your child may be reluctant to share their experiences in fear of no one believing what they say. As you validate their feelings and show your support, they can become more comfortable and trust you with more information. Be careful not to minimize your child's situation due to age, inexperience, or the length of their relationship.

- **Help develop a safety plan:** One of the most dangerous times in an abusive relationship is when the victim decides to leave. Be especially supportive during this time and try to connect your child to support groups or professionals that can help keep them safe.

- **Remember that ultimately your child must be the one who decides to leave the relationship:** There are many complex reasons why victims stay in unhealthy relationships. Your support can make a critical difference in helping your son or daughter find their own way to end their unhealthy relationship.

But My Child Isn't in an Unhealthy Relationship

It's never too early to talk to your child about healthy relationships and dating violence. Starting conversations—even if you don't think your child is dating—is one of the most important steps you can take to help prevent dating violence. Here are some sample questions to start the conversation:

- Are any of your friends dating? What are their relationships like? What would you want in a partner?

- Have you witnessed unhealthy relationships or dating abuse at school? How does it make you feel? Were you scared?

- Do you know what you would do if you witnessed or experienced abuse?

- Has anyone you know posted anything bad about a friend online? What happened afterwards?

- Would it be weird if someone you were dating texted you all day to ask you what you're doing?

Need more tips to get started? Here are some other ways you can prepare to talk to your child about healthy and unhealthy relationships:

- Do your own research on dating abuse to get the facts before talking to your teen or twenty-something.

- Provide your child with examples of healthy relationships, pointing out unhealthy behavior. Use examples from your own life, television, movies, or music.

- Ask questions and encourage open discussion. Make sure you listen to your son or daughter, giving them a chance to speak. Avoid analyzing, interrupting, lecturing, or accusing.

- Keep it low key. Don't push it if your child is not ready to talk. Try again another time.

- Be supportive and nonjudgmental so they know they can come to you for help if their relationship becomes unhealthy in the future.

- Admit to not knowing the answer to a particular question. This response builds trust.

- Reinforce that dating should be fun! Stress that violence is never acceptable.

- Discuss the options your child has if they witness dating abuse or experience it themselves.

- Remind your son or daughter they have the right to say no to anything they're not comfortable with or ready for. They also must respect the rights of others.

- If your child is in a relationship that feels uncomfortable, awkward, or frightening, assure them they can come to you. And remember—any decisions they make about the relationship should be their own.

- Contact Break the Cycle to find out if there are dating violence prevention programs in your community. If not, work with Break the Cycle to bring abuse prevention to your local school or community group.

Chapter 29

Preventing and Intervening in Child Abuse

Chapter Contents

Section 29.1

Responding to a Disclosure of Child Abuse

Reprinted with permission from "Responding to a Disclosure of Abuse," by Jackie Reilly, M.S., Extension Youth Development Specialist/Associate Professor, University of Nevada Cooperative Extension, and Sally S. Martin, Ph.D., Family Life Specialist/Associate Professor, Human Development and Family Studies, University of Nevada Cooperative Extension. © 2001, reviewed 2011. All rights reserved. For additional information and related publications, visit the website of the University of Nevada Cooperative Extension at www.unce.unr.edu.

When a Child Discloses

Hearing a disclosure—a child telling you that someone has abused or hurt him— can be scary. How you respond can be critical. A lot of thoughts may run through your mind:

- You may be worried about the child and yourself.
- You may be unsure of how to respond or what to say.
- You may be unsure of the child's comments and information.
- You may not be sure if the child has been abused.
- You may be angry with the parent or alleged abuser.
- You may be worried about retaliation from the alleged abuser. If so, ask that your report remain confidential.

You may even want to take the child home with you. How you respond is very important. Responding to a disclosure of abuse or neglect is a big responsibility. This section has suggestions about how to respond in ways that help the child, her parents, and yourself.

Children Often Are Reluctant to Tell about Abuse

In over 80 percent of the cases of physical abuse, emotional abuse, or neglect, the birth parents are the abusers. The majority of perpetrators in sexual abuse cases are nonrelated caregivers, that is, baby-sitters, step-parents, boyfriends, girlfriends, or adoptive parents.

Children often love the person who is abusing them and simply want the abusive behavior to stop. Because they love and care about the person, they may be reluctant to get the person in trouble. Many perpetrators tell children to keep the abuse a secret and frighten them with unpleasant consequences.

Children may start to tell someone about the abuse. If the person reacts with disgust or doesn't believe them, they may stop disclosing the events. Then they may not tell anyone about it until they feel brave enough or have established a sense of trust with someone else. This may delay them from seeking help. If a child begins to tell you about possible abuse, please listen carefully.

He or She?

We give equal time and space to both sexes! That's why we take turns referring to children as "he" or "she." So keep in mind that even if we say "he" or "she" we are talking about all children.

Ideas That Can Help

- Be on the same eye level as the child; be tactful and have no physical barriers between you and the child.

- Assess the child's safety needs and the urgency of the situation.

- Don't interrogate or interview the child.

- Listen to the child.

- Don't comment on the child's situation as being bad or good; let the child tell her own story; leave out your own assumptions and value judgments.

- Be calm and in control of your responses and emotions.

- Find out what the child wants from you.

- Validate the child's feelings.

- Believe the child and be supportive.

- Assure the child that you care, you are still her friend, and she is not to blame.

- Don't react with disgust.

- Let the child know what you will do.

- Tell the child you're glad she told you.

- Tell the child you will try to get him some help.

- Tell the child you will have to tell someone whose job it is to help kids with these kinds of situations.

- Do not talk about the disclosure to other children or adults, other than to report suspicions.

Section 29.2

How to Report Suspected Child Maltreatment

Excerpted from the U.S. Department of Health
and Human Services, 2012.

Anyone can report suspected child abuse or neglect. Reporting abuse or neglect can protect a child and get help for a family—it may even save a child's life. In some states, any person who suspects child abuse or neglect is required to report.

Childhelp® is a national organization that provides crisis assistance and other counseling and referral services. The Childhelp National Child Abuse Hotline is staffed twenty-four hours a day, seven days a week, with professional crisis counselors who have access to a database of fifty-five thousand emergency, social service, and support resources. All calls are anonymous. Contact them at 800-4-A-CHILD (800-422-4453).

If you suspect a child is being abused or neglected, or if you are a child who is being maltreated, contact your local child protective services office or law enforcement agency so professionals can assess the situation. Many states have a toll-free number to call to report suspected child abuse or neglect.

Chapter 30

How the Legal System Can Help

Chapter Contents

Section 30.1

Common Legal Intervention Strategies and Their Effectiveness

Reprinted from the following documents from the U.S. Department of Justice: "Arrests Can Be an Effective Intervention for Intimate Partner (Domestic) Violence," May 18, 2009; "Protections Orders May Reduce Intimate Partner (Domestic) Violence," June 30, 2011; "The Threat of Prosecution May Reduce Further Intimate Partner (Domestic) Violence," May 19, 2009; and excerpted from "Batterer Intervention Programs Often Do Not Change Offender Behavior," July 6, 2011.

Arrests Can Be an Effective Intervention for Intimate Partner (Domestic) Violence

Police executives and lawmakers can do several things to lower dual arrest rates and make arrest more effective:

- **Police can arrest offenders who have left the crime scene:** Officers should canvass the area more thoroughly to find and arrest offenders who have left the crime scene.

- **Police can make fewer dual arrests in incidents involving same-sex couples:** High rates of dual arrest in these incidents indicate a need to train officers to recognize patterns of abuse in same-sex relationships and identify the primary aggressor. Policies and training should address potential gender-role stereotyping and the significance of victimization for same-sex couples.

- **Police executives and lawmakers can institute primary aggressor laws and policies:** States and police departments that wish to lower dual arrest rates may want to institute primary aggressor laws and policies, and enhance officer training on how to identify the primary offender in an incident. Officers should, for example, be able to distinguish between injuries inflicted in attacking someone and injuries inflicted in self-defense, such as biting an offender to make him or her let go of a stranglehold.

Background: Research Tackles the Problem, Offers Recommendations

Police have been making more arrests in domestic violence incidents. In 2000, about 50 percent of intimate partner violence cases[1] resulted in arrests, compared to 7 to 15 percent in the 1970s and 1980s. Research has revealed that some aspects of the change cause problems: too many victims are arrested and too few cases are accepted by prosecutors.

The problem appears to arise in part from the practice of dual arrests—situations in which police arrest both parties involved in the altercation rather than trying to identify the primary aggressor. About 2 percent of domestic violence incidents result in dual arrests.

The research comes from a study that examined data from National Incident-Based Reporting System, and involved a multistate survey of incident records kept by police.

Findings pointed to the practice recommendations that could improve the effectiveness of arrests, conserve police resources, and raise conviction rates:

- Contrary to previous beliefs, arrests do not appear to be gender biased. The research showed that police arrested men and women with equal frequency when other factors, such as seriousness of offense, were taken into account. Additionally, police were equally likely to make arrests in same-sex and heterosexual incidents.

- Officers were four times more likely to make an arrest if an offender stayed at the scene of the crime. If the offender left, the officers were unlikely to follow up and obtain an arrest warrant. Even if a warrant was obtained, it might not be served.

- Police were more likely to make dual arrests when responding to an incident that involved a same-sex couple. For example, if the domestic incident involved two males, officers apparently assumed that, as in a barroom fight, both men were equally responsible and thus both should be arrested.

- Police made the highest number of dual arrests in jurisdictions with mandatory arrest laws, particularly if state laws or department policies did not instruct officers to arrest only the main offender at a domestic violence incident. Jurisdictions with such primary aggressor laws reported one-fourth the dual arrest rate observed in jurisdictions without such policies or laws.

Protections Orders May Reduce Intimate Partner (Domestic) Violence

When domestic violence cases first come to court, most domestic violence courts (88 percent) issue a temporary protection order or restraining order (unless one has already been issued). At sentencing, almost as many domestic violence courts impose a final protection order prohibiting or limiting contact with the victim.[2]

The National Institute of Justice (NIJ) funded a study of protection orders, consequences for violating them, and costs in rural and urban jurisdictions in Kentucky. This study found that:[3]

- Protection orders deter further violence and increase victim safety:

- In 50 percent of the cases studied, victims experienced considerably less abuse and fear of abuse in the months after obtaining a protection order, even when the offender violated the terms of the order.

- Protection orders save justice and social service systems money and improve victims' quality of life:

  - The Kentucky study measured a wide range of costs for each participant, including medical, mental health, criminal justice, legal, lost earnings, property losses, and time lost for family and civic responsibilities. The study also produced a quality of life index six months before the protection order and six months after the protective order was issued. Overall, protection orders saved the state $85 million in a single year and improved victim safety at very little cost.

- Rural and urban communities may differ in the processing and enforcement of protection orders, but victims in both the country and city benefit from protection orders:

  - Rural victims encountered more barriers to obtaining protective orders, more negativity and blame from administering agencies, weaker enforcement of protection orders, and ultimately less relief from fear and abuse over time after obtaining a protection order.

  - Urban victims reported more difficulty navigating the justice system. Rural victims reported protection order violations less frequently.

- Both rural and urban victims experienced similar reductions in abuse after obtaining a protection order, and overall a large majority felt that protection orders were effective.

The Threat of Prosecution May Reduce Further Intimate Partner (Domestic) Violence

The threat of, or offer to drop, prosecution may provide leverage for abused women. For victim-initiated complaints, permitting victims to drop charges following an arrest significantly lowered the chance of new violence during and six months following the court appearance. These women also experienced less violence, less severe violence, and a longer delay before the onset of new violence.[4]

Batterer Intervention Programs Often Do Not Change Offender Behavior

Courts often mandate that convicted abusive partners attend batterer intervention programs in addition to serving a probation term. NIJ researchers have evaluated the most common batterer intervention programs. Most findings show that these programs do not change batterers' attitudes toward women or domestic violence, and that they have little to no impact on reoffending.

One study did find that men who were married and had a stake in the community (such as owning a home) and men who completed the full program were slightly less likely to reoffend.[5]

Other batterer program evaluations have been conducted, but with inconsistent results. One approach that researchers may use to integrate the results from various evaluations is known as meta-analysis. Two separate meta-analyses carried out on the more rigorous batterer intervention studies found that these programs have, at best, a modest or minimal benefit.[6, 7]

Notes

1. These are cases of aggravated assault, simple assault, and intimidation that involve spouses, ex-spouses, same-sex couples, and boyfriends and girlfriends.

2. Labriola, M., S. Bradley, C. S. O'Sullivan, M. Rempel, S. Moore, *A National Portrait of Domestic Violence Courts*, Final report to the National Institute of Justice, 2010, NCJ 229659.

3. Logan, T. K., R. Walker, W. Hoyt, T. Faragher, The Kentucky Civil Protective Order Study: A Rural and Urban Multiple Perspective Study of Protective Order Violation Consequences, Responses, and Costs, Final report to the National Institute of Justice, 2009, NCJ 228350.

4. Ford, D. A., and S. Breall. "Violence Against Women: Synthesis of Research for Prosecutors." Final report to the National Institute of Justice, 2000, NCJ 199660.

5. Jackson, S., L. Feder, D. R. Forde, R. C. Davis, C. D. Maxwell, and B. G. Taylor. Batterer Intervention Programs: Where Do We Go From Here? Research Report, Washington, DC: U.S. Department of Justice, National Institute of Justice, June 2003, NCJ 195079.

6. Feder, L., and D. B. Wilson. "A Meta-Analytic Review of Court-Mandated Batterer Intervention Programs: Can Courts Affect Abusers' Behavior?" *Journal of Experimental Criminology* 1 (2005): 239–62.

7. Babcock, J. C., C. E. Green, and C. Robie. "Does Batterers' Treatment Work? A Meta-Analytic Review of Domestic Violence Treatment." *Clinical Psychology Review* 23 (2004): 1023–53.

Section 30.2

Laws on Violence against Women

U.S. Department of Health and Human Services
Office on Women's Health, May 18, 2011.

The U.S. Congress has passed two main laws related to violence against women, the Violence Against Women Act and the Family Violence Prevention and Services Act.

The Violence Against Women Act

The Violence Against Women Act (VAWA) was the first major law to help government agencies and victim advocates work together to fight domestic violence, sexual assault, and other types of violence against women. It created new punishments for certain crimes and started programs to prevent violence and help victims. Over the years, the law has been expanded to provide more programs and services. Currently, some included items are as follows:

- Violence prevention programs in communities

- Protections for victims who are evicted from their homes because of events related to domestic violence or stalking

- Funding for victim assistance services like rape crisis centers and hotlines

- Programs to meet the needs of immigrant women and women of different races or ethnicities

- Programs and services for victims with disabilities

- Legal aid for survivors of violence

- Services for children and teens

The National Advisory Committee on Violence Against Women works to help promote the goals and vision of VAWA. The committee is a joint effort between the U.S. Department of Justice and the U.S. Department of Health and Human Services. Examples of the committee's

369

efforts include the Community Checklist initiative to make sure each community has domestic violence programs and the Toolkit to End Violence Against Women, which has chapters for specific audiences.

The Family Violence Prevention and Services Act

The Family Violence Prevention and Services Act (FVPSA) provides the main federal funding to help victims of domestic violence and their dependents (such as children). Programs funded through FVPSA provide shelter and related help. They also offer violence prevention activities and try to improve how service agencies work together in communities. FVPSA works through a few main ways:

- **Formula grants:** This money helps states, territories, and tribes create and support programs that work to help victims and prevent family violence. The amount of money is determined by a formula based partly on population. The states, territories, and tribes distribute the money to thousands of domestic violence shelters and programs.

- **The National Domestic Violence Hotline:** This is a twenty-four-hour, confidential, toll-free hotline. Hotline staff connect the caller to a local service provider. Trained advocates provide support, information, referrals, safety planning, and crisis intervention in more than 170 languages to hundreds of thousands of domestic violence victims each year.

- **The Domestic Violence Prevention Enhancements and Leadership Through Alliances (DELTA) Program:** Like many public health problems, intimate partner violence is not simply an individual problem—it is a community problem. DELTA supports local programs that teach people ways to prevent violence.

Section 30.3

Mandatory Reporters of Child Abuse and Neglect

"Mandatory Reporters of Child Abuse and Neglect: Summary of State Laws," U.S. Department of Health and Human Services, 2010.

All states, the District of Columbia, American Samoa, Guam, the Northern Mariana Islands, Puerto Rico, and the U.S. Virgin Islands have statutes identifying persons who are required to report child maltreatment under specific circumstances.

Professionals Required to Report

Approximately forty-eight states, the District of Columbia, American Samoa, Guam, the Northern Mariana Islands, Puerto Rico, and the Virgin Islands designate professions whose members are mandated by law to report child maltreatment.[1] Individuals designated as mandatory reporters typically have frequent contact with children. Such individuals may include the following:

- Social workers

- Teachers and other school personnel

- Physicians and other healthcare workers

- Mental health professionals

- Child care providers

- Medical examiners or coroners

- Law enforcement officers

Some other professions frequently mandated across the states include commercial film or photograph processors (in eleven states, Guam, and Puerto Rico), substance abuse counselors (in fourteen states), and probation or parole officers (in seventeen states).[2] Seven states and the District of Columbia include domestic violence workers on the list of mandated reporters, while seven states and the District of Columbia include animal control or humane officers.[3] Court-appointed special advocates are mandatory reporters in nine states.[4] Members of the clergy now are required to report in twenty-six states.[5]

Reporting by Other Persons

In approximately eighteen states and Puerto Rico, any person who suspects child abuse or neglect is required to report. Of these eighteen states, sixteen states and Puerto Rico specify certain professionals who must report but also require all persons to report suspected abuse or neglect, regardless of profession.[6] New Jersey and Wyoming require all persons to report without specifying any professions. In all other states, territories, and the District of Columbia, any person is permitted to report. These voluntary reporters of abuse are often referred to as "permissive reporters."

Standards for Making a Report

The circumstances under which a mandatory reporter must make a report vary from state to state. Typically, a report must be made when the reporter, in his or her official capacity, suspects or has reasons to believe that a child has been abused or neglected. Another standard frequently used is when the reporter has knowledge of, or observes a child being subjected to, conditions that would reasonably result in harm to the child. Permissive reporters follow the same standards when electing to make a report.

Privileged Communications

Mandatory reporting statutes also may specify when a communication is privileged. "Privileged communications" is the statutory recognition of the right to maintain confidential communications between professionals and their clients, patients, or congregants. To enable states to provide protection to maltreated children, the reporting laws in most states and territories restrict this privilege for mandated reporters. All but three states and Puerto Rico currently address the issue of privileged communications within their reporting laws, either affirming the privilege or denying it (i.e., not allowing privilege to be grounds for failing to report).[7] For instance:

- The physician-patient and husband-wife privileges are the most common to be denied by states.

- The attorney-client privilege is most commonly affirmed.

- The clergy-penitent privilege is also widely affirmed, although that privilege usually is limited to confessional communications and, in some states, denied altogether.[8]

Inclusion of the Reporter's Name in the Report

Most states maintain toll-free telephone numbers for receiving reports of abuse or neglect.[9] Reports may be made anonymously to most of these reporting numbers, but states find it helpful to their investigations to know the identity of reporters. Approximately eighteen states, the District of Columbia, American Samoa, Guam, and the Virgin Islands currently require mandatory reporters to provide their names and contact information, either at the time of the initial oral report or as part of a written report.[10] The laws in Connecticut, Delaware, and Washington allow child protection workers to request the name of the reporter. In Wyoming, the reporter does not have to provide his or her identity as part of the written report, but if the person takes and submits photographs or X-rays of the child, his or her name must be provided.

Disclosure of the Reporter's Identity

All jurisdictions have provisions in statute to maintain the confidentiality of abuse and neglect records. The identity of the reporter is specifically protected from disclosure to the alleged perpetrator in thirty-nine states, the District of Columbia, Puerto Rico, American Samoa, Guam, Puerto Rico, and the Northern Mariana Islands.[11] This protection is maintained even when other information from the report may be disclosed.

Release of the reporter's identity is allowed in some jurisdictions under specific circumstances or to specific departments or officials. For example, disclosure of the reporter's identity can be ordered by the court when there is a compelling reason to disclose (in California, Mississippi, Tennessee, Texas, and Guam) or upon a finding that the reporter knowingly made a false report (in Alabama, Arkansas, Connecticut, Kentucky, Louisiana, Minnesota, South Dakota, Vermont, and Virginia). In some jurisdictions (California, Florida, Minnesota, Tennessee, Texas, Vermont, the District of Columbia, and Guam), the reporter can waive confidentiality and give consent to the release of his or her name.

Notes

1. The word "approximately" is used to stress the fact that states frequently amend their laws. This information is current only through April 2010. At that time, New Jersey and Wyoming were the only two states that did not enumerate specific professional groups as mandated reporters but required all persons to report.

2. Film processors are mandated reporters in Alaska, California, Colorado, Georgia, Illinois, Iowa, Louisiana, Maine, Missouri, Oklahoma, and South Carolina. Substance abuse counselors are required to report in Alaska, California, Connecticut, Illinois, Iowa, Kansas, Massachusetts, Nevada, New York, North Dakota, Oregon, South Carolina, South Dakota, and Wisconsin. Probation or parole officers are mandated reporters in Arkansas, California, Colorado, Connecticut, Hawaii, Illinois, Louisiana, Massachusetts, Minnesota, Missouri, Nevada, North Dakota, South Dakota, Texas, Vermont, Virginia, and Washington.

3. Domestic violence workers are mandated reporters in Alaska, Arizona, Arkansas, Connecticut, Illinois, Maine, and South Dakota. Humane officers are mandated reporters in California, Colorado, Illinois, Maine, Ohio, Virginia, and West Virginia.

4. Arkansas, California, Louisiana, Maine, Montana, Oregon, Virginia, Washington, and Wisconsin.

5. Alabama, Arizona, Arkansas, California, Colorado, Connecticut, Illinois, Louisiana, Maine, Massachusetts, Michigan, Minnesota, Mississippi, Missouri, Montana, Nevada, New Hampshire, New Mexico, North Dakota, Ohio, Oregon, Pennsylvania, South Carolina, Vermont, West Virginia, and Wisconsin. For more information, see Child Welfare Information Gateway's Clergy as Mandatory Reporters of Child Abuse and Neglect at www.childwelfare.gov/systemwide/laws_policies/statutes/clergymandated.cfm.

6. Delaware, Florida, Idaho, Indiana, Kentucky, Maryland, Mississippi, Nebraska, New Hampshire, New Mexico, North Carolina, Oklahoma, Rhode Island, Tennessee, Texas, and Utah.

7. Connecticut, Mississippi, and New Jersey do not currently address the issue of privileged communications within their reporting laws. The issue of privilege may be addressed elsewhere in the statutes of these states, such as rules of evidence.

8. New Hampshire, North Carolina, Oklahoma, Rhode Island, Texas, and West Virginia disallow the use of the clergy-penitent privilege as grounds for failing to report suspected child abuse or neglect. For a more complete discussion of the requirement for clergy to report child abuse and neglect, see the Information Gateway's Clergy as Mandatory Reporters of Child Abuse and Neglect at www.childwelfare.gov/systemwide/laws_policies/statutes/clergymandated.cfm.

9. For state-specific information about these hotlines, see Information Gateway's State Child Abuse Reporting Numbers at www.childwelfare.gov/pubs/reslist/rl_dsp.cfm?rs_id=5&rate_chno=W-00082.

10. California, Colorado, Florida, Illinois, Indiana, Iowa, Louisiana, Maine, Massachusetts, Minnesota, Mississippi, Missouri, Nebraska, New Mexico, New York, North Carolina, Pennsylvania, and Vermont have this requirement.

11. The statutes in Alaska, Arizona, Delaware, Idaho, Maryland, Massachusetts, New Hampshire, Oklahoma, Rhode Island, West Virginia, Wyoming, and the Virgin Islands do not specifically protect reporter identity but do provide for confidentiality of records in general.

Chapter 31

How You Can Help Someone Who Is in an Abusive Situation

Chapter Contents

Section 31.1

How to Help a Friend Who Is Being Abused

U.S. Department of Health and Human Services
Office on Women's Health, May 18, 2011.

Here are some ways to help a friend who is being abused:

- **Set up a time to talk:** Try to make sure you have privacy and won't be distracted or interrupted.

- **Let your friend know you're concerned about her safety:** Be honest. Tell her about times when you were worried about her. Help her see that what she's going through is not right. Let her know you want to help.

- **Be supportive:** Listen to your friend. Keep in mind that it may be very hard for her to talk about the abuse. Tell her that she is not alone, and that people want to help.

- **Offer specific help:** You might say you are willing to just listen, to help her with child care, or to provide transportation, for example.

- **Don't place shame, blame, or guilt on your friend:** Don't say, "You just need to leave." Instead, say something like, "I get scared thinking about what might happen to you." Tell her you understand that her situation is very difficult.

- **Help her make a safety plan:** Safety planning includes picking a place to go and packing important items.

- **Encourage your friend to talk to someone who can help:** Offer to help her find a local domestic violence agency. Offer to go with her to the agency, the police, or court.

- **If your friend decides to stay, continue to be supportive:** Your friend may decide to stay in the relationship, or she may leave and then go back many times. It may be hard for you to understand, but people stay in abusive relationships for many reasons. Be supportive, no matter what your friend decides to do.

- **Encourage your friend to do things outside of the relationship:** It's important for her to see friends and family.

- **If your friend decides to leave, continue to offer support:** Even though the relationship was abusive, she may feel sad and lonely once it is over. She also may need help getting services from agencies or community groups.

- **Keep in mind that you can't "rescue" your friend:** She has to be the one to decide it's time to get help. Support her no matter what her decision.

- **Let your friend know that you will always be there, no matter what.**

Section 31.2

Helping a Friend through the Criminal Justice System

"Helping a Friend Through the Criminal Justice System,"
copyright © 2010 Marie De Santis, Women's Justice Center,
www.justicewomen.com. Reprinted with permission.

The following tips can be adapted for helping victims with work, schools, social services, churches, or any other institution victims may turn to for help. We highlight the criminal justice system because in crimes of violence against women and children the responses of police, prosecutors, and courts are most important of all. Only the criminal justice system has the power and authority to control the violent offender.

Accompany your friend to law enforcement and courts whenever possible. Just being physically present with your friend during court hearings and police and prosecutor interviews keeps the process from becoming overwhelming. In fact, your presence can turn the criminal case into the empowerment for your friend that it should be; her turn for her truth to be heard and vindicated. Another good reason to accompany your friend is to help keep track of information.

While answering questions about the crime, it's hard for victims to remember new information and questions they wanted to ask. If you carry a notebook and jot things down, you're a friend indeed. Another important reason for accompanying friends to law enforcement is that, despite improvements, there are still too many police and prosecutors who don't take crimes of violence against women seriously. Your presence alone tells officials that someone else cares very much about the victim and is watching out that the system cares too.

Help your friend start and keep a notebook. Once a criminal case gets rolling, there's a flood of vital information coming at the victim and much of it's packaged in the unfamiliar language of law enforcement. Criminal charges, hearing dates, bail conditions, case numbers, pleadings, official's names and titles, protective orders, all quickly become frightening to someone who is already worried. A small notebook collects it all in one place for her so she can focus on other things. If the victim isn't getting this information, you and she should ask, and keep asking, until you do get it. It's also a good idea for a victim to take notes on telephone conversations with officials, to write down questions she wants to remember to ask, comments she wants to make, and additional information she may remember about the crime. Sometimes just helping your friend get started on a notebook is all she needs to get going. Sometimes she may need you or someone else to keep notes updated.

Insist on good translations. In crimes of rape, domestic violence, and child abuse, language translations must be accurate, and the translator must be someone who won't cause the victim to withhold parts of her story. A non-English-speaking victim should never have to tell her story through neighbors or family members. (Would you tell a neighbor all the details of a beating by your husband?) Statements given by victims to officials are too important to be translated carelessly or unprofessionally. Prosecutors and police always have access to professional translators. Even at the scene, police can call AT&T interpreters by phone. They should use them!

Don't ignore yours or the victim's intuition that things may not be going the way they should. If you and your friend feel that she's getting treated badly, or that the case isn't being properly investigated, you may very well be right. Remember, it's only very recently that women's groups have pressed law enforcement to treat violence against women as serious violent crime. The response of some law enforcement officials has been excellent, but there are still too many who would like to make the women and their cases go away. Some officials try to wash their hands of these cases. They may lead the victim to believe the case isn't workable, may misinform her about her rights or about the law, or carry out halfhearted investigations. They may minimize the offense, imply the victim had responsibility in the attack, or allow long delays in taking action or responding to the victim's calls. Or they may just make things so uncomfortable for the victim that she simply doesn't want to continue. Pay attention to your gut feelings about how things are going. Ask questions! Don't let things slide by that you don't understand or that don't make sense.

Try to get good information. This can be the hard part. You may be getting your questions answered but you may not always be getting straight answers. If things don't sound right, try to get answers from other sources such as victim advocates, your county law librarian, a trusted official not involved in the case, or the district attorney's office in another county. Probation officers are also well informed and often very helpful.

If you still feel things aren't going right, don't hesitate a moment to go to supervisors, to call other officials, to write letters, and in general make noise. It's easy to feel intimidated about making complaints, especially when you're not one hundred percent certain how the process should work, and even more so when an official is trying to bully you into thinking that there's nothing that can be done. It's also true that not every case has enough evidence to bring a conviction. But when women sense these cases are not being handled properly, they are usually right. Your friend has a right to be treated with respect, no matter what the circumstances of the crime, she has the right to a full investigation, and to accurate and honest answers. Many attacks and serious injuries to women occur because the system has failed to take action. So make that call to the officer's or prosecutor's supervisor. Or ask for a meeting. Tell them why you aren't happy. Ask all your questions. Tell them what you want. Why weren't all the witnesses interviewed? Why didn't the officer issue an emergency protective order? Why wasn't the suspect arrested? Why was his bail reduced? Why can't this case be charged as a felony? Go to the chief, the city council, or the press if necessary. Put your complaint in writing. Too many times the only real problem is that one official or another didn't want to be bothered. Your willingness to complain is often enough to get your friend the protection and justice she deserves and needs.

Bring evidence into the case yourself. It's always better if you can persuade a police officer or a district attorney to gather all the evidence and witness statements. But if they don't respond to your requests, you can do it yourself. Witnesses can write out complete statements, or they can write out something that was previously left out. The same is true for the victim. For example, officers sometimes don't ask victims about the history of abuse that occurred before this incident. The victim can simply write it down and enter it into the case. Photographs, medical records, and other forms of physical evidence can also be entered by you into the case. To enter evidence into the case, simply go to the police department or district attorney's office and ask that the items be made part of the case file. It's always best if you can sit down with an officer or deputy district attorney so they can ask you questions about the origin of the items. Always make and keep copies of all written statements.

Get more help! The only thing better than your help is more help. A criminal case takes a long time and a lot of attention. Make a list with your friend of all the people who might be able to help: friends, teachers, neighbors, classmates, coworkers, church members, etc. Don't be shy about asking. Most people want to do something to help stop the violence. And everyone wants to make a difference.

Section 31.3

How to Help a Child Who Is Witnessing Domestic Violence: Tips for Caregivers

Reprinted from "How to Intervene," "When and Where to Seek Help," and "How to Support the Child," © 2012 Child Witness to Violence Project, Boston Medical Center. All rights reserved. Reprinted with permission. For additional information, visit www.childwitnesstoviolence.org.

How to Intervene

There is no age at which a child is immune to the effects of violence. As health professionals, concerned parents, caregivers, and citizens, we must work tirelessly to reduce, if not eliminate violence in the lives of children. Interventions with children who are affected by violence require multiple disciplines and careful collaboration. No one profession can succeed alone. Families are best helped when health providers, mental health providers, educators, police, and the courts work together.

What Parents and Caregivers Can Do

Remember: Children are not little adults. They have different and unique ways of understanding violence. Listen carefully to how they make sense of what happened:

- Use reassurance and a calm voice when talking to a child, especially in the aftermath of violence. Give children permission to tell their stories. Sometimes it is difficult to listen to the child's distress, but talking helps children heal.

- Remind children that the violence is not their fault, and it is not their job to solve adult problems.

- Remember, you can get specific help from professionals in planning how to talk to children about the violence they may have witnessed.

- Work to create a stable, safe environment for the child.

What Neighbors Can Do

- If you know of a child who is witnessing violence, you can help the child by helping his or her parents. In the case of domestic violence, you can help by supporting and helping the battered partner.

- Be supportive of your neighbor or friend and express your concern. Simple statements like, "I am concerned about you. How have you been doing?" can make a lasting difference.

- Share the telephone numbers of support services with the person you think is in need of the information. If the violence is domestic violence, share those numbers privately.

- Be willing to make a phone call for your friend or neighbor.

- If needed, help them get to a safe place. Perhaps give them a ride or call a taxi for them.

- If possible, help them find a safe place to stay.

- If necessary, support them in getting legal or housing assistance.

- Remember that if the violence you are concerned about is domestic violence, you don't help the victim by confronting the batterer yourself. Have trained professionals respond.

What Professionals Can Do

There are many counseling treatments for children who are exposed to violence that have been carefully evaluated for their effectiveness. A list of evidence-based trauma-focused counseling interventions can be found at www.nctsn.org.

While there are differences in how these interventions are delivered, they share the same core components of focus. They:

- Stabilize the environment for the child and the family.

- Give family members support and information about how children respond to witnessing violence. Caregivers may be unaware of how affected young children are from exposure to violent behavior.

- Work with caregivers to create strategies for reducing symptoms and managing challenging behaviors.

- Help the child and the caregiver understand the child's perspective of the violent event(s).

- Help the child to tell the story of the traumatic event in play or words.

- Correct cognitive distortions or misunderstandings about the event.

- Provide activities that promote a child's competence and self-esteem.

- Collaborate with all agencies and care providers that are part of a child's life.

When and Where to Seek Help

When Do Children Need Professional Help?

Many children exposed to violence can resolve their feelings and concerns with the help of their family and community. However, there are instances when professional help is needed. Consider seeking professional help in the following situations:

- The child is vulnerable because of other stressful events or losses they have experienced.

- The child was related to or is a close friend of the victim.

- Parents are highly upset and less able to respond to the child's needs.

- A child is physically hurting him- or herself or others.

- A child's parent has been the victim of violence.

- A child's problems have gone on for three to four months with no improvement.

If you are a parent worried about your child, remember that you know your child best. Don't hesitate to consult a professional.

If you are worried about a child you know well, remember that you play a very important role!

Where Can You Seek Professional Help?

There are a number of institutions and agencies that provide help. Typically, all offer a specific set of services. For example, courts provide services around legal matters. Below is a partial list of helping agencies:

- Schools

- Courts

- Mental health providers

- Religious institutions

- Shelters for battered women

- Police departments

- District attorney's office

Who Can You Contact for Help or a Referral?

Talk to someone who knows your child well. He or she may be able to provide counseling or a referral. Consider contacting the following professionals:

- **Healthcare providers (the child's pediatrician):** Pediatricians are committed to keeping their patients' bodies and minds healthy. They can help parents to understand their child's symptoms and behaviors, address medical and emotional concerns, and offer appropriate referrals. Many providers have a list of counselors, advocates, or other resources to help children and families. They can also help the parent navigate the managed care system.

- **School counselors and administrators:** School counselors are trained to recognize problems that may affect a child's developmental growth and learning. Administrators include school principals, department heads, and head teachers. They may refer the family to experts in the field of children exposed to violence as well as set up teaching, learning, and counseling programs that take into account the educational needs of children exposed to violence.

- **Teachers:** Most teachers see children every day of the week. Children learn best when teachers can collaborate with parents and other service providers. Since their goal is to help children be successful in school, they can make classroom adjustments that help stressed children learn the material with which they are presented. They often are aware of local services that are available and can tell you how to access them.

- **Clergy and the religious community:** Of course, clergy look out for our spiritual well-being. They can help us keep our faith in the face of difficult times, and that faith can serve as an important resource when we are worried about our children. Sometimes faith communities join hands in an attempt to end violence. For example, a model interfaith nonprofit organization, Safe Havens, exists in Boston. Their goal is to create a network of congregations that are better equipped to respond to family violence.

- **Mental health providers:** Mental health providers include social workers, psychologists, psychiatrists, mental health counselors, psychiatric nurses, and marriage and family therapists. They help adults and children cope with the emotional experience of being exposed to violence.

- **Police:** The job of police is to keep people safe. Not only can they be helpful in relation to a crime but those departments with community policing programs are also very well informed about community resources. Some even have their own youth programs.

- **Domestic violence advocates:** Domestic violence advocates can be found in health centers and hospitals, mental health centers, courts, and battered women shelters. They are extremely knowledgeable about all aspects of domestic violence and can help navigate victims through many complex systems such as the courts. Many can assist victims of domestic violence help their children through direct service and referrals.

How to Support the Child

How to Support a Child Who Has Witnessed Violence

- **Healing begins with relationships:** The adult helping relationship is the most powerful tool we have to assist children in healing from traumatic events.

- **Help children know what to expect:** Provide a highly structured and predictable home and learning environment for children.

- **Let the child know that it is ok to talk about what has happened:** When children are ready, it helps to be able to talk about the violence in their lives with trusted adults.

- **Give parents support:** Help parents understand that young children think differently than adults and need careful explanations about scary events.

- **Foster children's self-esteem:** Children who live with violence need reminders that they are lovable, competent, and important.

- **Don't try it alone:** Identify and collaborate with other caregivers in the child's life.

- **Teach alternatives to violence:** Help children learn conflict resolution skills and about nonviolent ways of playing.

- **Model nurturing in your interactions with children:** Serve as role models for children in resolving issues in respectful and nonviolent ways.

Chapter 32

Interventions
and Help for Abusers

Chapter Contents

Section 32.1

What Abusers Can Do to Stop the Violence

If you're being abusive toward your partner, the first and hardest part of changing is admitting your behavior is wrong. It's very important to take responsibility for the problem and get help to end it. If you've already taken this step, you're on the right track.

What Do I Need to Know?

Changing abusive behavior is a long and hard process that you cannot do alone. Though you may not know it, you rely on your beliefs and attitudes to justify your abusive behavior. With help, you can change and learn how to treat your partner with true respect. It's extremely important that you get professional help through this process. Chat with a peer advocate to find services in your local area.

Remember that physical and sexual violence aren't the only types of abuse. You may be harming your partner in verbal or emotional ways, like through intimidation, threats, isolation, or other means of control. You should take steps to end *all* the types of abuse now. Addressing the roots of your behavior will take time, but if you want a healthy relationship, you need to make the commitment to change immediately.

What Can I Do?

- Remember, violence is always a choice. There are no excuses and no one else to blame for being abusive.

- Focus on how your abuse affects your partner, family, and children. Fully accept how seriously you have hurt the people you care about.

- Accept the consequences of your actions. Your partner has the right to get help from police or the courts. You may face legal consequences for being abusive, either with jail time or a restraining order.

- Remember you are not alone. Your friends and family can support you through the difficult process of changing.

- Get help from a program that focuses on abusive relationships. A good program will help you stop being abusive and create a better relationship for you and your partner.

- Respect your partner's right to be safe and healthy as you work toward change, even if it means you can't be together.

- Because change is hard, there may be times when you may justify your actions or feel like giving up. Remember your original commitment to change and you'll be more likely to succeed.

Section 32.2

History and Theories of Batterer Intervention Programs

"History and Theories of Batterers' Intervention Programs in the USA," updated October 2008. © The Advocates for Human Rights (www.stopvaw.org). All rights reserved. Reprinted with permission.

The first batterers' intervention programs (BIPs) in the United States were established thirty years ago in response to hotline calls from victims and offenders. As legal systems reformed to criminalize domestic violence and prosecution protocols were mandated, judges began to order offenders to attend BIPs. Early programs were often developed with substance abuse or mental health programs as guidance. But victim advocates soon raised serious concerns about program aspects which were counterproductive to victim safety and offender accountability. For example, confidentiality must not be extended to offenders during the process. If a batterer becomes angry and program moderators perceive a threat to the victim, they must be able to notify the victim of the potential danger.[1]

A BIP should be instituted only as a part of a coordinated and intensive response.[2]

Other aspects of a coordinated community response include victim services, civil court actions for orders for protection or child support, police and court enforcement of protective orders, and, possibly, psychological, drug, or alcohol treatment programs for the violent offenders.[3]

BIPs will be most effective if the programming reflects the root cause of domestic violence—a desire for power and control over one's female intimate partner. Effective batterer intervention programs work to alter men's beliefs and attitudes toward violence and personal responsibility.[4] Batterers will not change their behavior by participating in the group unless they are willing to change. Batterers must recognize and acknowledge their abusive behavior and fully understand the effect it has on their partners, their relationships, and themselves. Batterers must take responsibility for both the physical violence that they inflict on their partners as well as other forms of abuse such as sexual violence, psychological abuse, and economic coercion. Facilitators in BIPs often challenge men about their negative or sexist attitudes and beliefs, support for abusive behaviors, and denial of abuse. This kind of challenge helps men examine the origins of their beliefs and actions with the group and take responsibility for the abuse.

Batterer intervention programs should assist batterers in learning skills for nonviolence. Programs should teach offenders to monitor their actions and to understand the feelings they have when they become violent, such as anger, inadequacy, jealousy, or the need to control the situation. At the same time, however, programs should emphasize that while a batterer may feel angry or upset, he must still take personal responsibility for his actions. His use of violence or other forms of abuse is a personal choice.

In helping batterers to learn alternative behaviors, programs may have offenders draw the chain of events that lead to the abusive behaviors. In this way, programs help batterers to know when they are acting abusively and to recognize warning signs or cues that, for example, indicate that their anger is escalating and that they may become violent. If necessary, the batterers should temporarily withdraw from a situation of conflict. They should talk to someone who will support them in not using violence. When the batterer can react in a nonabusive manner, he should return to discuss the problem without using violence or other forms of abuse. As the intervention program continues, batterers should better understand their abusive behavior and develop alternative skills and methods of interacting with their partners that do not involve violence.

BIPs should not be designed as marriage or couples counseling. Batterers' intervention programs should focus on stopping the perpetrator's criminal conduct rather than keeping the couple together. Similarly, they are not substance abuse counseling. Treatment for alcohol and drug abuse should be addressed separately.

Notes

1. From: Adams, David, "Treatment Programs for Batterers," *Clinics in Family Practice,* Vol. 5 No. 1, March 2003. Program changes were made accordingly.

2. From: "Batterer Intervention Programs: Where Do We Go From Here?" by the U.S. Department of Justice Office of Justice Programs, U.S. Dept of Justice, June 2003.

3. From: Gondolf, Edward W., *Batterer Intervention Systems: Issues, Outcomes and Recommendations*, Thousand Oaks: Sage Publications, 2003.

4. From: Edelson, Jeffrey, and Tolman, Richard, *Intervention for Men Who Batter: An Ecological Approach* (1992).

Section 32.3

Types of Batterer Interventions

"Perpetrators of Violence/Batterers," reprinted with permission from the Global Virtual Knowledge Centre to End Violence Against Women and Girls, http://endvawnow.org. © 2012 UN Women (United Nations Entity for Gender Equality and the Empowerment of Women). All rights reserved.

What are the different types of perpetrator interventions and treatment approaches?

There is a commonly accepted belief that the most appropriate model for working with perpetrators is a broad cognitive-behavioral approach combined with gender analysis (Mullender and Burton 2000). Though this model is widespread in practice, there are other models that are widely implemented. In practice, however, many programs combine different approaches, thus the categories below are not necessarily mutually exclusive and can be considered in various combinations.

Cognitive-behavioral intervention: Cognitive-behavioral or psycho-educational approaches are the most prominent. These view violence as a learned behavior that can be unlearned (rather than as a consequence of individual pathology, stress, alcohol abuse, or a "dysfunctional" relationship). The approach aims to foster mutual respect and requires men to accept responsibility for their past actions and future choices. It requires regular group attendance and needs skilled group facilitators who can challenge denial and minimization and harness the dynamic of the group to do the same (Mullender and Burton 2000). This intervention has also been found to be the most appropriate for the majority of perpetrators (most perpetrators do not show evidence of psychological or personality disorders) and is less costly than others (Gondolf 2004).

Gender analysis: Gender analysis is thought to be an important element in the work with perpetrators of intimate partner violence. Gender analysis tackles the belief system that convinces male perpetrators that they have a right to control women in intimate relationships.

Failure to address this belief system means that men may simply switch from physical to emotional abuse, and women and children will continue to live in fear (Mullender and Burton 2000).

Duluth model: The Duluth model is a widely used approach that includes a component on working with perpetrators of violence. Though originally developed in Duluth, Minnesota (USA) it has been widely replicated. The Duluth model's underlying theory is that aggressors want to control their partners and that changing this dynamic is key to changing their behavior. Its curriculum uses a "power and control wheel" depicting tactics abusers use to control their partners. Themes counteracting these tactics are discussed in classes and group sessions that attempt to induce batterers to confront their attitudes and behavior (National Institute of Justice 2003).

Group practice: Another model, group practice, works from the premise that battering has multiple causes and is best addressed through a combined approach that includes an individual needs assessment. Proponents of these programs believe that a more long-term approach than the Duluth model is necessary (National Institute of Justice 2003).

Programs based on aggressors' typologies: Programs based on batterer typologies or profiles are gaining popularity. These interventions profile the batterer through a psychological assessment, and then classify him by level of risk, substance abuse, and other factors that may influence which intervention is most likely to work for him. Programs based on this approach are still relatively new and not fully evaluated (National Institute of Justice 2003).

Couples therapy: A controversial intervention is couples therapy, which views men and women as equally responsible for creating disturbances in the relationship. It is widely criticized for assigning the victim a share of the blame for the continuation of violence (National Institute of Justice 2003).

Section 32.4

Effectiveness of Batterer Intervention Programs

"Effectiveness of Batterers' Intervention Programs,"
updated October 2008. © The Advocates for Human Rights
(www.stopvaw.org). All rights reserved. Reprinted with permission.

In general, research has shown that batterers intervention programs (BIPs) are most effective when combined with a coordinated community response that includes accountability to judicial systems.[1]

Experts have conducted a variety of studies to determine the effectiveness of BIPs. Most agree that "effectiveness" means the cessation of abuse. This outcome has been measured in different ways, among them: no further complaints or arrests; the batterer's representations during treatment programs; the victim's reports to program officials. The studies concluded that BIPs have a "modest but positive" effect upon violence prevention. However, across all programs, men of color had a lower rate of program completion than white men, and thus experts agree that cultural competency is very important to program success.[2]

In a recent study, the Council of Europe agreed that "… the extent of behavioural change brought about by such programmes is modest. At best they control and reduce the danger of physical violence, but rarely eliminate the pattern of dominance behind it."[3]

A 2003 report by the World Health Organization, entitled *Intervening with Perpetrators of Intimate Partner Violence: A Global Perspective*, confirmed a moderate success rate, stating that reviews of BIPs in the United States and United Kingdom found that about two-thirds of people who complete BIPs remain nonviolent for up to three years. However, from 22 to 42 percent of abusers studied in the United States and in Canada failed to complete a program.

Other research indicates that BIPs have little effect on recidivism or attitudes of violent offenders. However, at least one study found that men who were required to attend longer programs had significantly fewer complaints lodged against them than those who completed an eight-week program.[4]

Additionally, shorter programs, with less time to change batterer attitude, may create more sophisticated batterers who learn to control their partner's behavior through methods of intimidation other than physical violence.

Notes

1. From: Adams, David, "Treatment Programs for Batterers," *Clinics in Family Practice*, Vol. 5 No. 1, March 2003.

2. From: Sullivan, Cris M., and Adams, Adrienne E., "A National Review of Outcomes and Indicators Used to Evaluate Domestic Violence Programs," prepared for United Way of Greater Milwaukee, February 2007.

3. From: Hagemann-White, Carol, and Bohn, Sabine, *Protecting Women against Violence: Analytical study on the effective implementation of Recommendation Rec (2002)5 on the protection of women against violence in Council of Europe member states*, Directorate General of Human Rights and Legal Affairs, Strasbourg, 2007.

4. From: National Institute of Justice, Special Report: Batterers Intervention Programs: Where Do We Go From Here? June 2003 at www.ojp.usdoj.gov/nij.

Chapter 33

Workplace Intervention

Chapter Contents

Section 33.1

Recognizing and Responding to Domestic Violence in the Workplace

"Desk Reference for Recognizing and Responding to Domestic Violence in the Workplace," reprinted with permission from the New York State Office for the Prevention of Domestic Violence (www.opdv.ny.gov), © 2012. The complete text of this document is available at http://www.opdv.ny.gov/professionals/workplace/deskref.html.

This section is designed to help you assess for domestic violence and provide appropriate assistance and referral for victims. Because the vast majority of victims of adult domestic violence are women who are abused by their male partners, this guide will refer to victims as female and abusers as male. The information, however, applies to all victims regardless of their gender or the gender of their partner, including gay, lesbian, and transgender victims and men who are abused by their female partners.

Possible Indicators

Victims of domestic violence may seek assistance for a wide variety of problems other than the violence itself. Possible indicators of domestic violence include:

- visible physical injuries, including bruises, lacerations, burns, human bite marks, and fractures (especially of the eyes, nose, teeth, and jaw); injuries during pregnancy, miscarriage, or premature births; injuries that are inconsistent with explanation; multiple injuries in different stages of healing; unexplained delay in seeking medical treatment for injuries;

- stress-related illnesses including headaches, backaches, chronic pain, gastrointestinal disorders, sleep disorders, eating disorders, fatigue, and anxiety-related conditions such as heart palpitations, hyperventilation, and panic attacks;

- marital or family problems;

- alcohol or other addictions;

- depression, suicidal thoughts or attempts;

- absenteeism, lateness, and leaving work early;

- changes in job performance such as difficulty concentrating, repeating errors, and slower work pace;

- unusual or excessive number of phone calls from family members, strong reactions to these calls; and

- disruptive personal visits to the workplace from employee's present or former partner or spouse.

Interviewing Guidelines

The best way to identify whether an employee is a victim of domestic violence is to *ask*. Recommended guidelines for assessing for domestic violence include:

- interview employee alone and in a private setting;

- inform employee of extent and limits of confidentiality;

- use direct observations in framing questions (e.g., "You seem very concerned that your husband will find out that you've been to see me. Are you afraid of your husband?");

- universalize (i.e., "Lots of women I see who miss a lot of work are having problems at home. Is someone or something at home making it difficult for you to come to work?");

- ask questions about all forms of coercive behavior, including physical, emotional, psychological, and economic abuse; and

- be direct, specific and concrete and avoid using jargon or labels. *Don't* ask, "Are you a battered woman?" or "Are you a victim of domestic violence?" *Do* ask, "Has your partner ever hit you or threatened to hit you?" or "Has your partner ever made threats or done other things that make you afraid?"

If an employee answers "Yes" to the assessment questions, the following steps are suggested:

- **Encourage her to talk about it:**
  - "Would you like to talk about what has happened to you?"
  - "How do you feel about it?"
  - "How can I help?"

- **Listen nonjudgmentally and actively:** If you actively listen, ask clarifying questions, and avoid making judgments and giving advice, you will most likely learn directly from her what it is she needs.

- Validate her experience: Victims of domestic violence are frequently not believed or not taken seriously, and the fear they report is minimized. You can express support through simple statements, as appropriate, such as:

  - "You are not alone. This happens to lots of women."

  - "You are not to blame. It's not your fault."

  - "You are not crazy. Your feelings are normal and reasonable for someone who's been through what you've been through."

  - "It sounds like you have good reason to be afraid."

  - "Help is available. I'd like to help if I can."

- **Explore options and make appropriate referrals:**

  - Elicit the options she has already identified.

  - Share information to expand her set of available options.

  - Understand her analysis of the risks attached to various options.

  - Offer new information and support.

  - Help with safety planning and problem solving.

- **Resources and options may include:**

  - Personal resources: Friends, family members, neighbors, and other social supports;

  - Workplace resources: Security, human resources, supervisor, and/or co-workers;

  - Domestic violence services: Emergency shelter, twenty-four-hour hotline, and full range of nonresidential services; and

  - Legal resources: Police, family court, and criminal court.

- **Resources should *not* include:**

  - Marriage counseling.

  - Couples or family counseling: Services that require victims to participate in joint sessions with their partners increase victim's risk of physical and emotional harm and are therefore not recommended for dealing with domestic violence.

- **Provide support for employee's decisions:** Don't judge the success of your intervention by the employee's action, and remember that there are risks attached to every decision a victim makes. Be patient and respectful of a victim's decisions, even if you don't agree with them.

If an Employee Answers "No" to the assessment questions, but there are clear indicators of domestic violence, you can:

- let her know that domestic violence happens to lots of people and that help is available if she ever needs it; and

- encourage her to take the local hotline number in case she or anyone she knows might need it.

Section 33.2

What to Do When a Colleague Discloses Abuse

"What to Do When a Colleague Discloses Abuse," reprinted with permission from the Colorado Bar Association Family Violence Program. © 2003 Colorado Bar Association. All rights reserved. For additional information, visit www.cobar.org. Information deemed accurate as of May 2012.

There is a wide range of responses that an employer or another employee can make when a fellow employee is in an abusive situation: some are general responses of support, others target specific actions (such as, safety planning).

Responses of Support and Concern

Support the person:

- Tell her/him that he/she is not alone and that he/she has your support.

- Express admiration for his/her courage in coming forth. Let her/him know that he/she is breaking down a wall of silence.

- Strongly communicate that you do not blame her/him for the abuse.

- Believe the person. Let him/her know you believe her/him and that domestic violence is illegal and unacceptable to you and to the company.

Listen in a nonjudgmental way:

- They are already being judged and criticized by their abuser.

- While we might have an opinion on how we would act or what we would say in a similar situation, we are not the person experiencing abuse and they are not us.

- Show respect for what she/he says even if you disagree.

- Express concern.

- "I am afraid/concerned for you."

- "You shouldn't have to be afraid."

- "It seems like your partner is controlling, overly jealous, etc."

- "You deserve to be treated well."

- Communicate that without intervention the abuse is not likely to stop but will probably get worse.

Assure the person of their rights:

- "It is not your fault. You do not deserve to be hit, put down, isolated, etc."

Ask questions:

- Ask about the abuse and encourage the person to discuss the abusive relationship in specific terms.

Listen and validate the person's experience and feelings:

- Encourage the person to express feelings about the abuse. That might include anger, shame, fear, guilt, confusion, and hopelessness.

- Acknowledge the validity of these complex feelings. Do not deny or minimize them.

Assure confidentiality:

- When a victim shares information about domestic violence with anyone, including an employer and co-workers, she/he assumes great risk. Assure her/him that what he/she says will remain confidential unless there is concern about welfare or safety of others, or unless it is legally required that the information be disclosed.

- Speak in settings that are comfortable, safe, and where the person can talk confidentially.

Assess needs:

- Ask the person how you can help. Does she/he need referrals for more information? A safe place to stay? Medical assistance? Help with children?

Take all necessary steps to protect employees:

- At the same time, don't coerce the victim to take actions she/he is not willing to take. She/he knows best how to judge the risks she/he faces and how the abuser may react. Remember, you are not available twenty-four hours a day to protect her/him.

Assess risk:

- Ask the person about the possibility of suicide or the risk of being killed by her/his partner.

- Ask the following:
  - "Are there weapons in the home?"
  - "Has the batterer made violent threats toward you or your children if you leave or say you are leaving?"
  - "How has the batterer reacted on any previous attempts to leave him/her?"
  - "Has the batterer been violent with anyone outside the home?"
  - "Have you ever gotten a protective or restraining order against the batterer?"

- If the person voices concerns that her/his partner may kill her/him, *believe her / him*. Abused people are the best judge of how dangerous their partners are.

- If you have not already done so, ask permission to contact a local family violence program and request their involvement.

- If there are direct threats made to hurt the employee at work, take immediate action to protect her/him and other employees.

- If there are no direct threats to hurt the employee at work, do not force the employee to participate in a workplace threat assessment process.

Act to empower the person:

- Successful intervention means helping the victim regain a sense of power and control over his/her own life.

- Avoid giving advice or making decisions for the person. You can make recommendations and assist in providing support, information, and referrals, but the person must make their own decisions. Avoid overwhelming the person with referrals and assignments.

- Ask questions instead of giving answers.

Avoid behaviors that are rescuing:

- Do not act skeptical or as if you do not believe the person.

- Do not tell her/him what she/he should do or make decisions for him/her.

- Do not make promises you cannot keep.

- Do not blame or criticize.

- Do not try to remake the person into who you think she/he should be or hurry the person's own decision-making process.

- Do not intervene beyond your own capabilities.

Avoid saying any of the following:

- "Things may get better over time."

- "This is really hard to believe."

- "He/she doesn't seem like that kind of person."

- "I can't believe you put up with this. Why don't you just leave?"

- "Why do you let her/him treat you like that?"

- "If you're still with him/her, it must not be that bad."

- "If you don't leave this person then you're going to be killed."

- "You can't stay in this situation."

- "You should just dump her/him."

- "Your partner doesn't love you or he/she wouldn't treat you like that."

- "You should . . ."

- "If I were you . . ."

Avoid asking any of the following:

- "Why do you stay with your partner?" The person's inability to leave is part of the crisis.

- "Are you a battered person?" No one likes to be labeled. To many women, especially, this is a shameful and self-blaming label. They are likely to deny or minimize the abuse they suffer and will not readily identify with this label.

- "What have you done to provoke the abuse?" "Why do you think your partner is abusing you?" Both of these questions imply that the person is to blame for the abuse she/he is suffering.

- "Why haven't you asked for help sooner?" This denies the fear, shame, and guilt that the person may be feeling.

Be there and be patient:

- Assure her/him that you are available when he/she wants to talk. Keep in touch, but move at the pace she/he sets.

- Coping with abuse takes time. She/he may not do what you expect her/him to do when you expect her/him to do it. If you think it is your responsibility to fix the problem, you may end up feeling frustrated. Instead, focus on building trust, and be patient.

- Each positive encounter you have with the person helps her/him to better take charge of his/her life, make informed decisions, and work toward positive change.

Action Responses

Suggest safety planning:

- Ask if the person would like help in creating a safety plan.

- If the person plans to continue living with the abusive partner, ask if she/he has thought about a safety plan to protect her/himself and children.

407

- If the person plans to leave the abusive partner, ask if he/she has thought about a safety plan to protect him/herself while at work. Violence often escalates when a victim leaves the abusive relationship or when the law enforcement become involved. Abused people are often at greatest risk when they leave or threaten to leave.

- Express concern for his/her safety if he/she stays in the abusive relationship, but do not criticize that decision. This is probably one of the most frustrating aspects of working with abused people, but it is crucial to successful intervention. They may believe they can still change the abusive partner or they worry that children will be hurt if they leave. Whether you agree with the person's decisions or not, talk to him/her in a supportive way. It is important to maintain a relationship with the person in order ultimately to provide help.

Offer referrals:

- Provide the person with as much information and as many referrals as you can without overwhelming her/him. Meet him/her "where she/he is" at the moment. Set up further meetings if necessary.

- Always ask the person if she/he would like the phone number of the local family violence program. That is a place where the person can get confidential counseling or the number for the National Domestic Violence Hotline which provides toll free, confidential information and referrals seven days a week, twenty-four hours a day (800-799-SAFE).

- Tell the person that services always are available, whether she/he leaves or stays with the abusive partner.

Section 33.3

What to Do When a Colleague Does Not Disclose Abuse but Abuse Is Suspected

"What to Do When a Colleague Does Not Disclose Abuse but Abuse Is Suspected," reprinted with permission from the Colorado Bar Association Family Violence Program. © 2003 Colorado Bar Association. All rights reserved. For additional information, visit www.cobar.org. Information deemed accurate as of May 2012.

It is likely that an abused colleague may not disclose the abuse directly. Here are suggestions that will assist you in confirming (or denying) whether the abuse you suspect is happening is actually happening and also assist you in supporting the suspected victim.

Ask direct questions in a nonjudgmental way:

- "I noticed that you have some bruises around your neck. How did this happen? Did someone do this to you?"

- "I am concerned for your safety. Do you have a safety plan?"

- "Is someone hurting you?"

- "You seem kind of uneasy around your partner, is everything okay?"

- "Is your partner hurting you?"

- "Are you ever afraid of your partner?"

- "Would it help to tell . . . ? To do . . . ?"

Ask direct questions when there is either evidence of abuse or a strong suspicion that the person is being abused. A private setting and appropriate circumstances are important:

- "Has your partner ever threatened to hurt you?"

- "Are you afraid of your partner when he/she gets mad?"

- "Does your partner try to control how you dress, who you see, or what you do?"

409

- "Has your partner ever threatened your children?"

- "Has your partner ever hit, pushed, shoved, punched, or kicked you?"

- "Has your partner ever hit, pushed, shoved, punched, or kicked your children?"

Ask indirect questions when there is no obvious evidence of abuse but when you suspect the person is a victim:

- "I talk to many people who have similar problems. Many of these people are being hurt by a loved one. Are you in this situation? Have you ever been in this situation?"

- "Many people I talk to are in relationships with someone who is hurting or controlling them. Are you in a relationship like this? Have you ever been in a relationship like this?"

Phrase questions in different ways to help the person recognize what is happening in their relationship:

- She/he might not equate what is happening to them with domestic violence.

Do not force people to disclose the abuse or require them to take particular steps to stop the abuse:

- Privacy rights need to be respected.

- A victim's silence may be due to cultural, racial, linguistic, or gender issues which make it difficult to talk about such personal experiences with co-workers from different backgrounds. Referrals can be made to agencies that are culturally appropriate.

If she/he denies any type of abuse in his/her relationship or says that everything is okay, accept what she/he is telling you:

- Keep the door of communication open by offering information if it is ever needed.

- Document your concerns.

Make every effort to include people trained in domestic violence intervention:

- Intervention by untrained staff can put a victim's life at risk or place co-workers in danger.

- It is often very difficult for a battered person to discuss the crisis. She/he may flatly deny the abuse or be afraid to provide information, fearing she/he will be fired, he/she will not be believed, or the abuser will retaliate with increased violence after learning that the victim disclosed the abuse.

Section 33.4

What to Do When a Colleague Is Abusive

"What to Do When a Colleague Is Abusive," reprinted with permission from the Colorado Bar Association Family Violence Program. © 2003 Colorado Bar Association. All rights reserved. For additional information, visit www .cobar.org. Information deemed accurate as of May 2012.

While reaching out to a suspected victim of domestic violence may be difficult, reaching out to a person suspected of being abusive is even harder. Calling someone on his or her abusive behaviors may be the hardest thing you ever have to do. It could also be the most compassionate. By addressing a friend, family member, or co-worker about abusive behaviors, you could save someone's life.

At work, a person who is abusive can:

- be invisible due to exemplary job performance;

- deny problems;

- blame others, especially the victim;

- gain sympathy by sharing convincing stories about his/her "difficult" partner, about how miserable he/she is and how hard it is for him/her;

- show defensive injuries (e.g., scratch marks, bite marks);

- seem reasonable;

- be knowledgeable about the system and use it to his/her advantage so it appears that he/she is the victim;

- be absent or late related to his/her actions toward the victim, or for court or jail time.

411

In speaking with a person who is abusive:

- Express empathy for difficulties he/she experienced/experiences.

- Do not blame the victim.

- Advise stopping the abuse (just as you would advise someone not to drive drunk).

- Do not ask how the victim provoked him.

- Do not encourage the person to find an attorney that will "fight this all the way";

- Maintain that there is no excuse for violence.

- Speak to the victim's reality as you know it, especially the extent of the victim's physical or emotional injuries.

- Do not presume that what the person tells you is the whole story. Seek outside sources, law enforcement reports, medical records, eyewitness reports, etc.

- Help the person understand that it is better to take responsibility for his/her actions and find help than obsess over the victim.

- Remind the person that only he/she controls his/her behavior. No one can make him/her be abusive or lose control.

- Provide the person with a list of certified treatment providers.

- Provide the individual with referral information to the employee assistance program if he/she is a co-worker.

- Make an effort to stay in touch with this person. The person who is abusive may be as isolated as the victim.

- Be persistent and realize you may have to take the initiative.

- Do not assume that the person understands the meaning of protective orders, no contact orders, restraining orders, child support orders, or other court orders.

- If the court has ruled on parenting privileges, remind the person that the purpose of parenting time is to maintain contact with the children, not the former partner.

- Explain that information will only be released on a need-to-know basis and as required by law.

- Help the person de-escalate by suggesting practical ways to comply with court orders.

- Do not be taken in by excuses.

- Do not assume the victim is safe if he/she says it won't happen again, even if the person who has been abusive is remorseful.

- Do not try to physically intervene. Rather, call the law enforcement.

- Do not feel guilty about calling the law enforcement. You might be saving someone's life.

If a colleague tells you that he/she has been violent at home, the following comments are helpful responses:

- "No matter how angry you are at your partner, there are ways to talk about that anger without being violent."

- "I know you believe she/he started it, but you chose to respond the way you did. No one can make you be violent or abusive."

- "It doesn't have to be this way. You can get help. You can learn to control the way you react. There are other people who have been where you are at and can help."

- "I'm concerned. It's clear that you feel a lot of anger and tension over this. What can we do to make sure nobody gets hurt?"

Don't condone the abuser's behavior or laugh with that person, if they try to make light of it.

When employers become aware that an employee has actually committed an act of domestic violence in the workplace, appropriate disciplinary action needs to be taken:

- Someone in authority can order an abuser to stay away from the workplace. Failure by the abuser to stay away can result in a charge of trespass.

- An abuser may commit other criminal violations on the premises of the workplace (e.g., stalking, assault, or carrying a concealed weapon). In these or similar situations, law enforcement should be called immediately.

- An employer can obtain a protective order against an abuser who stalks, threatens, or harasses the employees or customers of that business. With a protective order, law enforcement does not have to wait until some other crime (e.g., assault, harassment, or trespass) is committed before arresting. A disadvantage to protective orders is that they may only further infuriate the abuser and/or give the victim a false sense of security.

Section 33.5

What to Do When a Non-Employee Abuser Threatens the Employee in the Workplace

"What to Do When a Non-Employee Abuser Threatens the Victim in the Workplace," reprinted with permission from the Colorado Bar Association Family Violence Program. © 2003 Colorado Bar Association. All rights reserved. For additional information, visit www.cobar.org. Information deemed accurate as of May 2012.

If an employer becomes aware that an employee is being threatened or stalked and that the abuser intends to enter the workplace in order to harm the employee, the employer should take steps to guard the premises and protect employees from foreseeable violence.

If an employer believes an abuser's actions are disrupting or endangering the workplace, the abuser needs to be dealt with as would any other trespasser or harassing individual.

- Tell the abuser to leave the premises and make it clear that law enforcement has been called.

- Call law enforcement if danger appears imminent.

- Talk to the victimized employee. Find out what works best and discuss options, such as taking time off, going to a domestic violence program, filing criminal charges, changing location of work station, going to a friend or relative's house, seeing a lawyer about legal protection, or other strategy.

- If the victim has a protective order requiring the abuser to stay away from her/him or her/his workplace, keep a copy of the protective order in the office to show law enforcement when needed.

Someone in authority can order an abuser to stay away from the workplace. Failure by the abuser to stay away can result in a charge of trespass.

An abuser may commit other criminal violations on the premises of the workplace, e.g., stalking, assault, or carrying a concealed weapon. In these or similar situations, law enforcement should be called immediately.

An employer can obtain a protective order against an abuser who stalks, threatens, or harasses the employees or customers of that business. With a protective order, law enforcement does not have to wait until some other crime (e.g., assault, harassment, or trespass) is committed before arresting. A disadvantage to protective orders is that they may only further infuriate the abuser and/or give the victim a false sense of security.

Section 33.6

When the Abuser and Victim Are Both Employees

Excerpted from "Guidelines for Setting Up Security Measures to Stop Domestic Violence in the Workplace," © Centre for Research & Education on Violence against Women and Children, 2010. All rights reserved. Reprinted with permission. For additional information, visit www.makeitourbusiness.com

There are cases where both the victim and abuser work for you. If this happens, make sure that the abuser does not have access to the victim at work. This means keeping the victim's schedule, work hours, and location private. Do not schedule both employees to work at the same time. If possible, have them work at different sites. Limit their workplace access to scheduled work hours. You may also need to move the abuser (or victim if she desires) to another physical location.

Talk to the abuser's supervisor, the workplace coordinator, and Human Resources (union representative, work group, etc., as appropriate) about your safety plan. Let them know how they can help keep everyone safe.

Hold the abuser accountable for any unacceptable behavior in the workplace. Use disciplinary procedures to deal with abuse. If the abuser engages in violence or other criminal activity such as stalking or unauthorized electronic monitoring in the workplace, call the police.

Chapter 34

Preventing Workplace Violence

Chapter Contents

Section 34.1

When Does Domestic or Sexual Violence Become Workplace Violence?

Excerpted from "Workplace Violence: Issues in Response,"
Federal Bureau of Investigation, 2004. Reviewed by David A. Cooke,
M.D., FACP, July 2012.

Domestic violence is a pattern of behavior in which one intimate partner uses physical violence, coercion, threats, intimidation, isolation and emotional, sexual or economic abuse to control the other partner in a relationship.[1] Stalking or other harassing behavior is often an integral part of domestic violence.

According to one study, 5 percent of workplace homicides (that is, about one-third of homicides not associated with a robbery or other "stranger" crime) fall into this category.[2]

Homicides, of course, represent a tiny fraction of workplace incidents related to domestic violence. Far more frequent are cases of stalking, threats, and harassment. Often those acts are criminal offenses in their own right; however, even when harassment may not meet the legal standard for criminal penalties, it can be frightening and disruptive not just for the person who is the target, but for coworkers as well.

Frequently, employers are hesitant about involving themselves with an employee's personal relationships. Privacy is a legitimate concern, and finding the proper boundary between private and business affairs can be a difficult and sensitive matter. But domestic violence and stalking that come through the workplace door appropriately become the employer's concern too. Just as a business takes responsibility for protecting its workers from assaults or robberies by outsiders, it is also responsible for protecting them against stalking or other possible crimes by domestic partners. Studies have shown that the most common stalking situations that law enforcement has to deal with are those based upon some type of personal relationship, with women primarily being victimized by males as a result of this behavior. However, in a smaller percentage of cases, both men and women can be stalked and harassed by casual acquaintances or strangers.

The following observable behavior may suggest possible victimization:[3]

- Tardiness or unexplained absences
- Frequent—and often unplanned—use of leave time
- Anxiety
- Lack of concentration
- Change in job performance
- A tendency to remain isolated from coworkers or reluctance to participate in social events
- Discomfort when communicating with others
- Disruptive phone calls or e-mail
- Sudden or unexplained requests to be moved from public locations in the workplace, such as sales or reception areas
- Frequent financial problems indicating lack of access to money
- Unexplained bruises or injuries
- Noticeable change in use of makeup (to cover up injuries)
- Inappropriate clothes (e.g., sunglasses worn inside the building, turtleneck worn in the summer)
- Disruptive visits from current or former intimate partner
- Sudden changes of address or reluctance to divulge where she is staying
- Acting uncharacteristically moody, depressed, or distracted
- In the process of ending an intimate relationship; breakup seems to cause the employee undue anxiety
- Court appearances
- Being the victim of vandalism or threats

Domestic violence and workplace violence are also related in another way: the evolution of domestic violence during the last several decades as a specific legal, social, and law enforcement issue can provide a model for similarly identifying and developing responses to violence in the workplace.

A particular concern when domestic and workplace violence intersects is the possibility that the victim, not the offender, will end up being punished. All too frequently, when an employee is being stalked, harassed, or threatened at work, an employer will decide that the quickest and easiest solution is to kick the problem out the door and fire the employee, rather than look for ways to protect her and her co-workers. Though common, especially when low-status, low-paying jobs are involved, this practice raises obvious ethical questions—and possibly issues of legal liability as well.

As with any other threat, the first requirement for protecting employees from domestic violence and stalking at the workplace is finding out that the threat exists. This can be particularly difficult in domestic abuse cases, where abuse victims often remain silent out of shame, embarrassment, a sense of helplessness, and fear. Just as a supportive workplace climate makes employees feel safe in reporting other threats, an environment of trust and respect will make it easier for someone fearing domestic violence or stalking to tell an employer and seek assistance or protection.

Perhaps more than with any other risk, employees facing domestic threats may tend to confide most easily in co-workers, rather than supervisors, managers, or a company's security force. It is also co-workers who are most likely to sense that someone they work with may be at risk from an abusive relationship, even if the person doesn't say anything explicitly. Employers need to be careful about violating privacy or asking employees to break a co-worker's confidence, but it is entirely reasonable and justifiable to encourage disclosure when others in the workplace may also be in danger.

Beyond trying to create and maintain a generally supportive workplace atmosphere, employers can provide specific training to help the workforce to be more aware and sensitive to signs of possible domestic abuse. Training can also include teaching ways to persuade a reluctant co-worker to tell supervisors and accept help an employer may be able to offer. Although domestic violence and stalking are largely thought of as violence against women and thus as a "woman's problem," training and awareness programs should be directed at all employees, men and women alike.

For employees involved in security or who will take part in threat assessment and response, an employer can offer additional training focusing on how best to deal with domestic abuse victims. The same or similar training should be provided to anyone working with victims in a company's Employment Assistance Program. Both in training efforts and in providing help to at-risk workers, employers should draw on outside resources as well as their own: law enforcement, women's law and antiviolence advocacy groups, and social service agencies, for example.

When an employer becomes aware that an employee is being stalked, harassed, threatened, or abused and that the risk has or may come into the workplace, the threat should be subjected to the same evaluation procedure as any other violent threat, to assess the likelihood of violence and determine the best means of intervention. In almost all cases, employers should advise police of the circumstances, risk of violence, and possible criminal violations (of harassment or stalking laws, for instance) and involve law enforcement professionals in assessing and managing the threat. During and after the assessment, someone—from security, human resources, or a supervisor—should be responsible for keeping in close touch with the abuse victim, not only to help protect his or her safety and meet any needs that arise, but also to make sure of receiving any relevant information about the abuser (whom the victim, presumably, will know better than anyone else in her workplace).

Other steps include the following:

- Referring the employee for emotional, legal, or financial counseling, either through the company's own employee assistance structure or from outside practitioners (e.g., battered women's shelter or similar programs).

- Ascertaining if the employee has sought or obtained a protective "stay-away" court order against an abusive partner or other harasser.

- Adopting policies that will allow an abused worker time off for purposes such as going to court to seek a restraining order or appearing to testify at a criminal trial.

- Reviewing the employee's workspace and modifying it, if necessary, to make sure that a possible assailant cannot get there.

- Acting consistently with the employee's privacy rights and wishes and taking measures to inform other employees (security guards, secretaries, receptionists, and telephone operators, for instance) so they can block an abuser's calls or make sure he is kept out of the workplace.

Employers may consider other actions as well. One option would be to help an employee obtain a restraining order (or obtain one on its own to keep a harasser off company property). Another would be to extend protective measures away from the work site, looking at other places a worker may regularly go—such as a school or daycare facility where her children are enrolled, for example—and suggesting precautions that could be taken.

Notes

1. American Bar Association Commission on Domestic Violence, *A Guide for Employees: Domestic Violence in the Workplace* (Washington, D.C.: 1999), 11.

2. University of Iowa Injury Prevention Research Center, *Workplace Violence: A Report to the Nation* (Iowa City, Iowa: February 2001), 12.

3. American Bar Association Commission on Domestic Violence, *A Guide for Employees: Domestic Violence in the Workplace* (Washington, D.C.: 1999), 16.

Section 34.2

Stalking: Should Employers Be Concerned?

Stalking is a common problem. A National Violence Against Women Survey found that 8.1 percent of all women and 2.2 percent of all men surveyed were stalked at least once in their lifetime. This means that approximately one out of every twelve women and one out of every forty-five men in America has been stalked.

Since the workplace is the one venue where the stalker is sure of the victim's whereabouts, employers should be concerned about and aware of stalking as an issue.

What is stalking? Though most states define stalking as the willful, malicious, and repeated following and harassing of another person, some include such activities as lying in wait, surveillance, nonconsensual communication, telephone harassment, and vandalism. Most stalking laws require that the perpetrator make a credible threat of violence against the victim; others include threats against the victim's immediate family; and others require only that the course of conduct engaged in by the alleged stalker constitute an implied threat.

Who stalks whom? Female victims are significantly more likely than male victims to be stalked by spouses or ex-spouses. Male victims are significantly more likely to be stalked by acquaintances and strangers. The survey found that victims of stalking are primarily between the ages of eighteen to thirty-nine.

The link to domestic violence. The survey found strong evidence of a link between stalking and domestic violence. Eighty percent (80%) of women who were stalked by an intimate or former intimate partner reported being physically assaulted by that stalker. Survey results also indicate that in approximately 80 percent of the cases involving former intimate partners, the stalking either started or continued after the woman left the relationship.

Steps you can take to support employees in cases of domestic violence/stalking:

- Become familiar with stalking laws on a federal level, as well as the local and state laws in your area.

- Relocate the workstation of threatened employees.

- Alter employee work schedules.

- Provide photographs (or at a minimum, physical descriptions) of stalkers/perpetrators to receptionists and security personnel.

- Obtain a copy of the restraining order if one is issued

- Encourage law enforcement to enforce restraining orders.

- If needed, provide employees with leaves of absence.

- Limit information about employees that is disclosed by phone. Information that would help locate possible victims or which indicate what time he/she will return should not be provided. (You may want to consider this an appropriate policy to have in place at all times for all employees.)

- Provide the victim with the time off he/she may need to go to court, seek shelter, or connect with other resources.

- Above all, reassure employees that they can use company assistance and resources without their jobs being in jeopardy and that they can trust their employer.

Remember—when it comes to your workplace, you have a duty and a right to keep it safe and secure for all employees.

Section 34.3

Workplace Security and Safety Procedures

Excerpted and adapted from "Domestic Violence: A Workplace Issue," © 2011 State of Vermont Office of the Attorney General. All rights reserved. Reprinted with permission. To view the original version of this document, visit www.atg.state.vt.us.

Domestic Violence Doesn't Stay at Home When Victims Go to Work

Domestic violence occurs between people of all racial, economic, education and religious backgrounds; in heterosexual and same-sex relationships; while living together or separately, married or unmarried; and in short or long-term relationships:

- Nationally, one in five employed adults is the victim of domestic violence.

- One in four employees reports working with a co-worker who has been a victim of domestic violence.

- 74 percent of employed battered women say they are harassed by their partner at work.

- 94 percent of corporate security directors and 78 percent of human resource professionals consider domestic violence a critical workplace issue.

- Four out of five employees believe workplaces can make a difference by addressing domestic violence in the workplace.

- In a 2011 study, over 77 percent of Vermont offenders surveyed felt workplace policies addressing domestic abuse would be an effective deterrent to further violence.

Costs to Your Business

Loss of productivity or work time, absenteeism, employee turnover, and creating an actual or perceived unsafe or hostile work environment are common workplace impacts of domestic violence.

In a 2011 Vermont study of domestic violence offenders:

- 75 percent said they had a hard time concentrating at work because of their relationship issues.

- 80 percent felt their job performance was negatively affected.

- 55 percent used a cell phone to threaten, control, or abuse their partner during the workday.

- The 193 offenders surveyed reported a total of 52,731 days taken from work for domestic violence–related circumstances.

- Almost half of respondents reported that their partners took time off from work because of the domestic violence. Those partners lost an average of twenty workdays per person.

- 19 percent of respondents reported causing or almost causing an accident at work because they were distracted due to the domestic violence.

Nationally, domestic violence costs businesses nearly $6 billion in healthcare expenses and lost productivity every year.

Employers have been held liable for failing to adequately address domestic violence in the workplace. Recent jury awards to victims, co-workers, and their estates ranged from $25,000 to several million dollars.

A Safe and Secure Workplace

Security measures can play a critical role in protecting all employees at work. Consider these changes to your workplace:

- Provide front desk or security staff copies of court orders and abuser's identifying information, including photographs and description of car, if available.

- Relocate employee to safer workplace or workstation.

- Install buzzer system, panic button, or other security devices.

- Limit access to building and if feasible, use one entrance.

- Provide escorts to employee's parked car.

- Install lighting in parking lots, additional fencing, and cameras.

- Arrange priority parking spaces.

- Adopt phone security measures.

- Document harassing or abusive behavior.

- Assist in developing a safety plan course of action for employee. Call local domestic violence program for more information.

- Work with your staff and/or local law enforcement to develop a response plan.

Recommendations for All Employers

Employers can play an important role in providing clear guidelines and a supportive and productive workplace by implementing model practices and policies that respond to domestic violence:

- **Adopt:** Adopt a policy addressing domestic violence in the workplace. Implement leave, benefit, and referral initiatives.

- **Train:** Trainings for managers and supervisors raise awareness and sensitivity and make the workplace safer and more productive. In a 2011 study, 92 percent of Vermont domestic violence offenders surveyed said that a private discussion with a supervisor would be an effective deterrent.

- **Educate:** Educate staff through brown bag lunches, workshops, and newsletters. Post and distribute resource and referral information in areas of high visibility and on web pages. Seventy-two percent of offenders in a Vermont survey said that posters and brochures in the workplace would help prevent abuse from impacting the business.

- **Consider Security:** Review worksite security measures to protect all employees.

- **Connect:** Connect with local domestic violence service programs.

- **Support:** Perpetrators are solely responsible for domestic violence, but everyone can help support and protect survivors: join or donate to an organization working to prevent violence against women.

Section 34.4

Employer's Guide to Protection Orders

Your employee may, at some time, obtain a protection order to protect himself or herself from violence or one of your employees may be subject to a protection order for perpetrating violence. What does this mean to you as an employer?

What Is the Connection between Protection Orders and Your Workplace?

Workplace safety has been a concern for workers, the government, unions, law enforcement, and others for many decades. Workers should be able to earn a living free from hazards, threats, and other dangers arising from violent conduct. Beyond the traditional occupation-based threats to safety, employees experience very real threats to their safety from personal relationships or their status as victims of domestic violence, stalking, or sexual assault, including sexual harassment that occurs in the workplace. What can you do to assist those employees? What should you do?

It is absolutely within your best interest as an employer to promote a safe and secure workplace for employees. Safety and security at work encourages productive employees. And that is your concern:

- The Centers for Disease Control and Prevention estimates that the annual cost of lost productivity due to domestic violence equals $727.8 million, with more than 7.9 million paid workdays lost each year.[1]

- Women stalked by an intimate partner averaged the largest number of days lost from paid work (10.1).[2]

- Women raped lost an average 8.1 days from paid work.[3]

- Victims of intimate partner physical assault lost 7.2 days on average per victimization.[4]

Inevitably, an employee's concerns about personal violence or about violence and harassment may impact work productivity. But there are bigger concerns than the bottom line. There are a host of considerations that you as an employer have when it comes to one of your employees being victimized at home or at work, by an intimate partner, by an acquaintance, or by a stranger. The CDC report, Surveillance for Violent Deaths—National Violent Death Reporting System, 16 States (2007), found that 2.1 percent of domestic violence homicides take place at work in a commercial or retail setting. In the United States, it is estimated that ignoring problems of sexual harassment can cost the average company up to $6.7 million a year in low productivity, low morale, and employee turnover and absenteeism, not including litigation or other legal costs. Sexual violence in the workplace results in similar losses of productivity, absenteeism, and morale, in addition to higher healthcare costs for employers and employees alike.

In 2004, Shennel McKendall was murdered outside her workplace in Chapel Hill, North Carolina. Neither the campus police nor her workplace at the hospital knew of her troubles. She had not sought extra protection at work. She had a protection order, but no one at work knew about it.[5]

Definitions

Petitioner: A petitioner starts a civil or private (noncriminal) action by going to court and filing a request or petition. In this case, the petitioner is likely the victim of violence or stalking (but sometimes a perpetrator will initiate a petition and claim to be the victim). In some jurisdictions, such as in the State of California, the petitioner may also be the employer.

Respondent: A respondent "responds" to the petition, and in this case is the alleged perpetrator of violence or stalking. A respondent (called "defendant" in some jurisdictions, but that term is usually reserved for criminal actions) has a specific amount of time to answer the allegations of violence or stalking listed in the petition. The response can range from "I agree to stay away from this person" to "the violence never happened and I'm going to disagree with this petition and all allegations in it."

Injunction: An injunction is an order from a court directing one or more parties to refrain from committing certain acts, or directing them to do certain acts.

Protection order: A protection order is a form of injunction in which a civil or criminal court instructs a party to do or to stop doing something or else face civil or criminal penalties. In the present context, a victim of violence (known as the petitioner) requests that the court tell the alleged perpetrator (known as the respondent or defendant) to stop harassing, stalking, contacting, abusing, etc., the petitioner.

Ex parte: This means that only one party is present before the court. In seeking a protection order, initially only the petitioner is present, but the court may still order a temporary order, provided the respondent is given notice and the opportunity to appear in court and tell his or her side of the story.

Civil versus criminal proceeding: In a civil case, the petitioner generally determines whether the action will continue, and at any time can drop the action by filing a motion to withdraw. The state, tribe, or in some cases, the U.S. Attorney's Office, initiate criminal cases after someone has been arrested by the police and charged with a crime. The prosecutor determines whether or not to prosecute the defendant. Thus, in contrast to a civil action, the state, tribe, or the U.S. Attorney's Office are in charge of criminal cases, and victims of crimes are witnesses rather than parties to a case.

Contempt: A party or person before the court (e.g., as a witness) can be held in contempt for failure to follow the court's order or injunction. There are two kinds of contempt of court: civil and criminal. Civil contempt generally refers to a party's failure to perform an action that a court has ordered, such as pay child support, or to refrain from doing something the court has forbidden, like contacting another person. The damaged party (e.g., petitioner) can ask the court to punish the party who is causing the damage. For civil contempt, the court's goal is to make the petitioner whole, as if the harm had not been done. A contempt case ends when the offending party complies with the court's order.

Criminal contempt generally addresses actions or inactions in the court, such as a party's disruptive behavior or refusal to testify. But in some jurisdictions, the failure to comply with a protection order is criminal contempt and can result in a jail sentence. In criminal contempt, the court's motivation is to punish the offending party for his or her actions or inactions.

Protection Order Basics

How Much Time Away from Work Will My Employee Need to Get a Protection Order?

While the protection order process has been streamlined to make it as easy as possible for someone who has been victimized to get help from the court, the procedure is far from simple. In many cases, the petitioner will need several trips to the court over the course of several weeks or even months. To obtain and enforce an order, a petitioner must complete the following steps (depending on his or her specific circumstances and the laws in the jurisdiction where the person is requesting the order):

- Complete the forms, file the initial petition, and then wait to see a judge. This can take all day in some cases.

- Return to court for a hearing after a respondent has been given notice of the requested order.

- If a respondent cannot be reached with notice of the proceeding, the court might need to reschedule the hearing, sometimes more than once, requiring a petitioner's return to court.

- If a respondent violates an order, the petitioner may have to return to court to file a motion for contempt or testify in a criminal proceeding if the violation was a crime under the jurisdiction's law. A petitioner might need to return more than once to enforce other requirements of an order, such as payment of child support.

- If an order is about to expire, petitioner might need to ask for an extension of the protective provisions when the violence has not stopped or the petitioner still fears the respondent.

An employee will require time away from work for each trip to court to obtain or enforce a protection order. Courts are typically open only during normal business hours, and the amount of time away from work will depend on the facts of the particular case as well as the court's workload.

How May an Order of Protection Impact the Workplace?

This depends on the protection sought by the individual and the protections available under state, federal, local, and/or tribal law. A petition for a protection order generally includes a "stay-away" provision, prohibiting the respondent from coming within a certain number of feet of the victim. A civil protection order may also include a list of places where the respondent is prohibited from entering, under the logic that these are places where the petitioner frequents and the respondent does not have a necessity to visit. Examples include:

- the petitioner's home (if the respondent and the petitioner shared a home the order may require that the respondent vacate the home);

- petitioner's workplace;

- anywhere the petitioner might frequent on a regular basis.

In most jurisdictions, the petitioner may seek temporary custody of children, and if temporary custody is ordered, the order may also include stay-away provisions that apply to the children, including prohibiting the respondent from coming to the child's school or after school care program. In most jurisdictions, the courts will specify a certain distance the respondent must remain from the prohibited places, e.g., "respondent is prohibited from coming within five hundred feet of the petitioner's workplace located at 123 Main Street."

Additional relief provisions can also include:

- exclusive use of the parties' home (e.g., the offending party must leave the residence immediately; in some cases, law enforcement will evict the respondent);

- custody, visitation, possible safety provisions when parents exchange children at the beginning or end of visits, or independent supervision of a parent's visitation with children;

- child support;

- spousal maintenance (a.k.a. "alimony");

- bill payments (e.g., utilities);

- wage garnishment;

- rental or mortgage payments;

- forfeiture of guns or other weapons, etc.

My Employee Does Not Want to Seek a Protection Order. Should I Request One on His or Her Behalf?

This is a difficult question. Some jurisdictions permit an employer to petition for a general restraining order against a person, such as a disgruntled former employee or someone who causes disruptions or harasses employees at the workplace. However, some jurisdictions, including Arizona, Arkansas, and California[6], permit an employer to petition for a protection order on behalf of someone experiencing violence whether or not the employee requests an order.

While this tool might appear to enhance workplace safety under certain circumstances, it is vitally important to keep the victim/employee involved in all decisions regarding a protection order on his or her behalf. Moving ahead without regard to a victim's wishes in this context could pose a serious safety risk for him or her and potentially other employees. Before embarking on this legal option, it is strongly encouraged that you have a conversation with the victim, determine his or her wishes and concerns, consider safety risks and possible solutions in getting a protection order, and refer the victim to an expert to continue safety planning. No decision should ever be made to obtain a workplace order of protection without involving the victim. In North Carolina and Nevada, for example, the law requires an employer to notify or consult with the employee-victim prior to petitioning the court for a protection order on the employee's behalf.

Why Might It Be Dangerous for My Employee after He or She Receives a Protection Order, or If I Obtain One on His or Her Behalf?

A victim of domestic, sexual, or dating violence and stalking is always at risk. However, the victim's separation from an abuser (if the victim was in a relationship with the abuser) or a victim's initiative to hold a perpetrator accountable for the violence may greatly increase the risk of retaliation or additional violence against a victim. Consider:

- Over 70 percent of the women injured in domestic violence cases are injured after separation.[7]

- Estrangement, in addition to a past history of violence, is a leading predictor for lethality in intimate partner relationships.[8]

- A recent study found that the biggest risk factor for ongoing violence and protection order violations is the presence of stalking behaviors.[9] Stalkers often utilize the workplace to monitor and harass their victims.

My Employee Has Obtained a Protection Order. What Can I Do to Help? What Are My Responsibilities?

You have a vital role to play if an employee informs you that he or she has obtained a protection order due to domestic, sexual, dating violence, or stalking. If your employee chooses to share this information, your response and action are critical to enhancing your employee's safety and security:

- Listen
- Express concern
- Ask how you can help
- Discuss options that may assist the employee, such as time off or a reasonable accommodation in the workplace
- Respect your employee's personal choices

Do not penalize or judge a victim of domestic violence, dating violence, stalking, or sexual assault. Your support can substantially impact on your employee's life and work.

Every case is unique, and every employee faces different circumstances and needs. Remember to involve the victim/survivor in any decisions you make or actions you take on his or her behalf. Also, consider the following.

Job Duties

Talk with your employee and find out if the protection order terms and conditions affect his or her job duties in any way, or if the violence, stalking, or sexual assault necessitates a temporary or permanent revision of job duties. For example, if your place of employment is a public or retail establishment, and the employee is a greeter, receptionist, or someone who works on the floor of a retail establishment, consider a temporary reassignment of job duties to increase his or her safety. If the employee works at a desk, consider providing him or her with a new phone extension, or placing all calls into a voicemail system. Never give out an employee's home address, even to other colleagues.

Safety and Security

Protect your employee's privacy. Keep your employee's information confidential, unless the employee knowingly permits disclosure. Your employee may need accommodations to enhance his or her safety while at work. For example, you might arrange for an escort to walk your employee to the parking garage at night, if he or she feels at risk. Other options to consider with the employee include:

- Telecommuting

- Changes to direct deposits

- Schedule changes, such as fluctuating work hours

Information Collection/Documentation

With the input of the petitioner employee, you can assist in saving or archiving emails, voicemails, text messages, etc., that relate to contact by an alleged abuser. If a respondent violates a protection order on workplace property, you can help document the violation with the police or the courts. If you notice bruises or other forms of abuse, document them in a confidential manner and separate the information from the employee's employment file.

In New York State, Susan Still's employer dutifully jotted down on her calendar each indication of abuse she saw—bruises, calling in sick and showing up next with an injury, and harassing phone calls. That evidence helped convict Still's abuser and substantiated a thirty-six-year sentence, the longest sentence ever given for a crime of domestic violence in New York.

Safety Planning

Employers should encourage employees to speak with professionals who are trained in the dynamic process of safety planning. It is not expected that you as an employer can or should conduct safety planning; safety planning is an ongoing process, not a one-time event. The employee, in conjunction with an advocate or expert, should consider every aspect of his or her day to assess safety concerns. Through the safety-planning process, an employee may identify ways that the employer can help to make the employee's life safer, such as changes to schedule or other accommodations.

Many companies have restrictions on personal computer use; but it may be a safety risk for a victim of violence to use a personal computer to assist with safety planning. Abusers often download spyware without the victim's knowledge. Or, a victim of violence may not have the economic means to afford a computer. Consider permitting the victim to utilize company equipment, either during or off work time, to assist in safety planning.

434

Referral and Resources

Ensure that your human resources department, or the designated staff person identified in your Employer Policy on Domestic Violence, Sexual Violence, Dating Violence, and Stalking, maintains a list of local and national resources to assist victims.

My Employee Has Obtained a Protection Order against Another Employee. What Can I Do to Help? What Are My Responsibilities?[10]

This is a complex issue and it is important that your Employer Policy on Domestic Violence, Sexual Violence, Dating Violence, and Stalking include a provision on how to respond to perpetrators of violence in the workplace. Each situation will require an individualized response and you should consult with your attorney and consider:

- Is it feasible and safe to relocate the respondent to a new location that would not intersect with the victim?

- Is there information indicating that the respondent has used company time, materials, or resources to abuse, harass, or stalk the petitioner?

- Has the respondent, through his or her use of violence, violated any other company policy, such as a company sexual harassment policy?

- Is the respondent's work product suffering?

- How are the victim and other employees impacted by the respondent's presence in the workplace?

In 2001, the Massachusetts group Employers Against Domestic Violence found through a focus group of twenty-nine convicted batterers that time spent at work was consumed by monitoring their victims from afar, with several abusers making costly and dangerous mistakes on the job as a result.

One particularly difficult scenario arises if the respondent's work is stellar, and the petitioner's performance is suffering. In these circumstances, please consider:

- Economic abuse and employment sabotage are major forms of controlling behavior and tactics that abusers use.

- The victim may temporarily experience a range of post-trauma symptoms.

- Assisting the petitioner/employee to feel safe at work, through the measures suggested in this section, may improve the employee's performance.

- Consider the workplace culture you would like to create and sustain—one that is free of violence.

My Employee Has Had a Protection Order Issued against Him or Her. What Are My Responsibilities?

As an employer, it's unlikely you will know that an employee has a protection order against him or her unless the petitioner on the order informs you directly. If the petitioner does contact you, it may mean that a violation took place using company property or materials and the petitioner wants you to be aware of it. If that is the case, investigate the claims as you would any other claim of employee misconduct, follow your policies and procedures, and review the information in the preceding section, above.

Notes

1. U.S. Dept. of Health and Human Services, National Center for Injury Prevention and Control. March, 2003. Costs of Intimate Partner Violence Against Women in the United States. Atlanta, GA: Centers for Disease Control and Prevention.

2. Id.

3. Id.

4. Id.

5. Julia Lewis, "Estrange Couple Dead in Apparent Murder-Suicide on UNC Property," November 29, 2004. Available at www.wral.com/news/local/story/114166"Sexual Harassment in the Fortune 500", *Working Woman* (Dec. 19, 1988).

6. See State Law Guide: Workplace Restraining Orders at www.legalmomentum.org

7. Stark & Flitcraft (1988); Fox & Zawitz (1999); Statistics Canada (2001); Websdale (2003).

8. Campbell, J. C., et al. Risk Factors for Femicide in Abusive Relationships: Results from a Multi-site Case Control Study, *American Journal of Public Health*, 93, 1089–97.

9.   T K Logan, Ph.D., et al. The Kentucky Civil Protective Order Study: A Rural and Urban Multiple Perspective Study of Protective Order Violation Consequences, Responses, & Cost. National Institute of Justice (September 2009).

10.   If the employees are members of a union, the employer's options may be impacted, for example, if the respondent/member has seniority.

Section 34.5

The Facts on Workplace and Domestic Violence: Some Statistics

On average, four to five women a day are murdered by their husbands or boyfriends each day in the United States[1] and women experience two million injuries from intimate partner violence each year.[2] Domestic violence can follow victims to work, spilling over into the workplace when a victim is harassed, receives threatening phone calls, is absent because of injuries, or is less productive due to extreme stress. Domestic violence is a serious, recognizable, and preventable problem, similar to other workplace health and safety issues that affect businesses and their bottom lines.

Prevalence

- Women are much more likely than men to be victims of on-the-job intimate partner homicide. Spouses, boyfriends/girlfriends and ex-boyfriends/ex-girlfriends were responsible for the on-the-job deaths of 321 women and 38 men from 1997 to 2009, according to the U.S. Department of Labor, Bureau of Labor Statistics.[3]

- In 2008, relatives and other personal acquaintances committed 28 percent of all workplace homicides in which women were victims, and just 4 percent of all workplace homicides in which men were victims.[4]

- According to a 2006 study from the U.S. Bureau of Labor Statistics, nearly one in four large private industry establishments (with more than one thousand employees) reported at least one incidence of domestic violence, including threats and assaults, in the past year.[5]

- A 2005 phone survey of 1,200 full-time American employees found that 44 percent of full-time employed adults personally experienced domestic violence's effect in their workplaces, and 21 percent identified themselves as victims of intimate partner violence.[6]

Toll on Productivity

- A 2005 study using data from a national telephone survey of eight thousand women about their experiences with violence found that women experiencing physical intimate partner violence victimization reported an average of 7.2 days of work-related lost productivity and 33.9 days in productivity losses associated with other activities.[7]

- About 130,000 victims of stalking in a twelve-month period from 2005 to 2006 reported that they were fired or asked to leave their job because of the stalking. About one in eight employed stalking victims lost time from work because of fear for their safety or because they needed to get a restraining order or testify in court. More than half these victims lost five days or more from work.[8]

- A 2005 study of female employees in Maine who experienced domestic violence found that: 98 percent had difficulty concentrating on work tasks; 96 percent reported that domestic abuse affected their ability to perform their job duties; 87 percent received harassing phone calls at work; 78 percent reported being late to work because of abuse; and 60 percent lost their jobs due to domestic abuse.[9]

- In a 2005 telephone survey from the Corporate Alliance to End Partner Violence, 64 percent of the respondents who identified themselves as victims of domestic violence indicated that their ability to work was affected by the violence. More than half of domestic violence victims (57 percent) said they were distracted, almost half (45 percent) feared getting discovered, and two in five were afraid of their intimate partner's unexpected visit (either by phone or in person).[10]

Costs

- The Centers for Disease Control and Prevention estimates that the cost of intimate partner rape, physical assault, and stalking totaled $5.8 billion each year for direct medical and mental healthcare services and lost productivity from paid work and household chores. Of this, total productivity losses account for nearly $1.8 billion in the United States in 1995.[11] When updated to 2003 dollars, the cost of intimate partner rape, physical assault, and stalking is more than $8.3 billion.[12] And in 2010 dollars, it would be considerably more. Much of these costs are paid for by the employer.

- The Centers for Disease Control and Prevention estimates the annual cost of lost productivity due to domestic violence is $727.8 million (in 1995 dollars), with more than 7.9 million paid workdays—the equivalent of more than thirty-two thousand full-time jobs—lost each year.[13]

- The Tennessee Economic Council on Women estimates that domestic violence costs Tennessee approximately $174 million per year. This 2006 report considers costs in lost wages, productivity, sick leave, absenteeism and costs to the medical, legal, and social services systems.[14]

Employer's Perspectives

- Nearly two in three corporate executives (63 percent) say that domestic violence is a major problem in our society and more than half (55 percent) cite its harmful impact on productivity in their companies, but only 13 percent of corporate executives think their companies should address domestic violence.[15]

- Nine in ten employees (91 percent) say that domestic violence has a negative impact on their company's bottom line. Just 43 percent of corporate executives agree. Seven in ten corporate executives (71 percent) do not perceive domestic violence as a major issue at their company.[16]

- More than 70 percent of United States workplaces do not have a formal program or policy that addresses workplace violence. Programs or policies related to workplace violence are more prevalent among larger private establishments or governments.[17]

Notes

1. Catalano, S., Smith, E., Snyder, H., Rand, M. 2009. Female Victims of Violence. U.S. Department of Justice, Bureau of Justice Statistics. Available at: http://bjs.ojp.usdoj.gov/content/pub/pdf/fvv.pdf.

2. U.S. Centers for Disease Control and Prevention. 2008. Adverse Health Conditions and Health Risk Behaviors Associated with Intimate Partner Violence. *Morbidity and Mortality Weekly Report*, 57(05);113–17. Available at: http://www.cdc.gov/mmwr/preview/mmwrhtml/mm5705a1.htm.

3. U.S. Department of Labor, Bureau of Labor Statistics. 2010. Occupational Homicides by Selected Characteristics, 1997–2009. Available at: http://www.bls.gov/iif/oshwc/cfoi/work_hom.pdf.

4. U.S. Department of Labor, Bureau of Labor Statistics. 2010. Workplace Shootings Fact Sheet. Available at: http://www.bls.gov/iif/oshwc/cfoi/osar0014.htm#1.

5. U.S. Department of Labor, Bureau of Labor Statistics. 2006. Survey of Workplace Violence Prevention, 2005. Washington, DC. Available at: http://www.bls.gov/iif/oshwc/osnr0026.pdf.

6. CAEPV National Benchmark Telephone Survey. 2005. Bloomington, IL: Corporate Alliance to End Partner Violence. Available at: http://www.caepv.org/getinfo/facts_stats.php?factsec=3.

7. Arias I, Corso P. 2005. Average Cost Per Person Victimized by an Intimate Partner of the Opposite Gender: a Comparison of Men and Women. *Violence and Victims*, 20(4):379–91.

8. Baum, Katrina, Catalano, Shannan, Rand, Michael and Rose, Kristina. 2009. Stalking Victimization in the United States. U.S. Department of Justice Bureau of Justice Statistics. Available at: http://www.ovw.usdoj.gov/docs/stalking-victimization.pdf.

9. Ridley, E, Rioux, J, Lim, KC, Mason, D, Houghton, KF, Luppi, F, Melody, T. 2005. Domestic Violence Survivors at Work: How Perpetrators Impact Employment. Maine Department of Labor and Family Crisis Services. Available at: http://mainegov-images .informe.org/labor/labor_stats/publications/dvreports/survivor study.pdf.

10. CAEPV National Benchmark Telephone Survey. 2005. Bloom-ington, IL: Corporate Alliance to End Partner Violence. Avail-able at: http://www.caepv.org/getinfo/facts_stats.php?factsec=3.

11. Costs of Intimate Partner Violence Against Women in the United States. Centers for Disease Control and Prevention, National Center for Injury Prevention and Control. 2003. Available at: http://www.cdc.gov/violenceprevention/pdf/ IPVBook-a.pdf.

12. Max, W, Rice, DP, Finkelstein, E, Bardwell, R, Leadbetter, S. 2004. The Economic Toll of Intimate Partner Violence Against Women in the United States. *Violence and Victims*, 19(3) 259–72.

13 Costs of Intimate Partner Violence Against Women in the United States. Centers for Disease Control and Prevention, National Center for Injury Prevention and Control. 2003. Available at: http://www.cdc.gov/ncipc/pub-res/ipv_cost/ IPVBook-Final-Feb18.pdf.

14. Tennessee Economic Council on Women, The Impact of Domes-tic Violence on the Tennessee Economy: A Report to the Ten-nessee General Assembly, January, 2006.

15. Corporate Leaders and America's Workforce on Domestic Violence Survey. 2007. Safe Horizon, the Corporate Alliance to End Partner Violence and Liz Claiborne Inc. Available at: http://www.caepv.org/about/program_detail.php?refID=34.

16. Ibid.

17. U.S. Department of Labor, Bureau of Labor Statistics. 2006. Survey of Workplace Violence Prevention, 2005. Washington, DC. Available at: http://www.bls.gov/iif/oshwc/osnr0026.pdf.

Chapter 35

Intervention by Faith Communities

Chapter Contents

Section 35.1

Responding to Domestic Violence: Guidelines for Religious Leaders

"Suggestions for Clergy and Faith Community Leaders and Members Responding to Victims and Survivors of Intimate Partner Abuse," © 2012 Safe Havens Interfaith Partnership Against Domestic Violence (www.interfaith partners.org). All rights reserved. Reprinted with permission.

Safety Is the First Priority—Support the Victim's Right to Safety

- Intimate partner abuse can be dangerous and even deadly. Maintain confidentiality. Do not disclose information to anyone without the survivor's permission. Never reveal a victim's location.

- Refer the survivor to appropriate medical services. Offer to go with her or him.

- Refer the survivor to services in your community, including shelters, domestic violence service providers, police, legal advocacy, hotlines, and support groups.

- Respond to faith questions about divorce, forgiveness, suffering, etc. with faith-based resources that condemn violence and oppression and affirm God's vision of safety and peace for all.

- Remind the victim that abusers do not end the violence on their own. Without professional intervention, the abuse will escalate over time.

- Do not use couples' counseling if you know or suspect that abuse is present.

- Discuss the impact of the abuse on the children. Children usually see and know more than their parents think. Living in a violent household is a form of abuse with severe effects on children.

Be Victim Centered

- Take the survivor's story seriously. Allow the victim time to tell the story in his or her own words.

- Bear witness to the abuse and its consequences. Acknowledge that what happened is abusive.

- Stay focused on the survivor. Let him or her set the agenda. Practice active and empathetic listening. Celebrate every small step toward safety and wholeness.

Do Not Blame the Victim

- *No one deserves to be abused.* Victims often feel that they have failed as spouse or partner, or that their behavior provokes the abuse. Emphasize that the abuse is the fault of the abuser, not the victim. Conflict is normal; abuse is not.

- Abusers often undermine the victim's self-esteem. Victims may not believe that they can care for their children, that they are worthy of a better life. Help victims identify their skills and strengths. Celebrate the courage that it took to ask for help. Lift the burden of shame and guilt from the victim.

- Do not use stress, unemployment, alcoholism, a difficult child-hood, or anything else as excuses for the abuser's behavior. There is no excuse for abuse. Affirm that the person who abuses breaks the covenant of marriage, not the person who reaches out for help.

- Recognize that the stigma of domestic abuse falls on the victim, not the abuser.

Do Not Tell the Victim What to Do

- Respect every decision victims and survivors make, and do not make decisions for them. Let them know that your support is available no matter how they decide to handle the situation. It is normal for them to feel confused and to change their minds. Continue to provide support.

- Recognize that victims may feel ambivalent about the abuser. Victims often still love their abusers, who can be good parents and providers. Never speak negatively or angrily about the abuser.

Section 35.2

What the Religious Community Can Do in Response to Domestic Violence

Religious communities provide a safe haven for women and families in need. In addition, they exhort society to share compassion and comfort with those afflicted by the tragedy of domestic violence. Leaders of the religious community have identified actions to create a unified response to violence against women.

Become a safe place: Make your church, temple, mosque, or synagogue a safe place where victims of domestic violence can come for help. Display brochures and posters which include the telephone number of the domestic violence and sexual assault programs in your area. Publicize the National Domestic Violence Hotline: 800-799-SAFE (7233), 800-787-3224 (TDD).

Educate the congregation: Provide ways for members of the congregation to learn as much as they can about domestic and sexual violence. Routinely include information in monthly newsletters, on bulletin boards, and in marriage preparation classes. Sponsor educational seminars on violence against women in your congregation.

Speak out: Speak out about domestic violence and sexual assault from the pulpit. As a faith leader, you can have a powerful impact on people's attitudes and beliefs.

Lead by example: Volunteer to serve on the board of directors at the local domestic violence/sexual assault program or attend a training to become a crisis volunteer.

Offer space: Offer meeting space for educational seminars or weekly support groups or serve as a supervised visitation site when parents need to safely visit their children.

Partner with existing resources: Include your local domestic violence or sexual assault program in donations and community service projects. Adopt a shelter for which your church, temple, mosque or synagogue provides material support, or provide similar support to families as they rebuild their lives following a shelter stay.

Prepare to be a resource: Do the theological and scriptural homework necessary to better understand and respond to family violence and receive training from professionals in the fields of sexual and domestic violence.

Intervene: If you suspect violence is occurring in a relationship, speak to each member of the couple separately. Help the victim plan for safety. Let both individuals know of the community resources available to assist them. Do not attempt couples counseling.

Support professional training: Encourage and support training and education for clergy and lay leaders, hospital chaplains, and seminary students to increase awareness about sexual and domestic violence.

Address internal issues: Encourage continued efforts by religious institutions to address allegations of abuse by religious leaders to insure that religious leaders are a safe resource for victims and their children.

Chapter 36

Intervention by Healthcare Providers

Chapter Contents

Section 36.1

Documenting Domestic Violence: How Healthcare Providers Can Help Victims

Excerpted from "Documenting Domestic Violence: How Health Care Providers Can Help Victims," U.S. Department of Justice, September 2001. Reviewed by David A. Cooke, M.D., FACP, May 2012.

Physicians and other healthcare providers know that often the first thing victims of domestic violence need is medical attention. They also know they may have a legal obligation to inform the police when they suspect the patient they are treating has been abused. What they may not know is that they can help the patient win her case in court against the abuser by carefully documenting her injuries.[1]

In the past decade, a great deal has been done to improve the way the healthcare community responds to domestic violence. One way that effort has paid off is in medical documentation of abuse. Many healthcare protocols and training programs now note the importance of such documentation. But only if medical documentation is accurate and comprehensive can it serve as objective, third-party evidence useful in legal proceedings.

For a number of reasons, documentation is not as strong as it could be in providing evidence, so medical records are not used in legal proceedings to the extent they could be. In addition to being difficult to obtain, the records are often incomplete or inaccurate and the handwriting may be illegible. These flaws can make medical records more harmful than helpful.

Healthcare providers have received little information about how medical records can help domestic violence victims take legal action against their abusers. They often are not aware that admissibility is affected by subtle differences in the way they record the injuries. By making some fairly simple changes in documentation, physicians and other healthcare professionals can dramatically increase the usefulness of the information they record and thereby help their patients obtain the legal remedies they seek.

Why Thorough Documentation Is Essential

The victim's attorney, or the victim acting on her own behalf as a pro se litigant, can submit medical documentation as evidence for obtaining a range of protective relief (such as a restraining order). Victims can also use medical documentation in less formal legal contexts to support their assertions of abuse. Persuasive, factual information may qualify them for special status or exemptions in obtaining public housing, welfare, health and life insurance, victim compensation, and immigration relief related to domestic violence and in resolving landlord-tenant disputes.

For formal legal proceedings, the documentation needs to be strong enough to be admissible in a court of law.[2] Typically, the only third-party evidence available to victims of domestic violence is police reports, but these can vary in quality and completeness. Medical documentation can corroborate police data. It constitutes unbiased, factual information recorded shortly after the abuse occurs, when recall is easier.

Medical records can contain a variety of information useful in legal proceedings. Photographs taken in the course of the examination record images of injuries that might fade by the time legal proceedings begin, and they capture the moment in a way that no verbal description can convey. Body maps[3] can document the extent and location of injuries. The records may also hold information about the emotional impact of the abuse. However, the way the information is recorded can affect its admissibility. For instance, a statement about the injury in which the patient is clearly identified as the source of information is more likely to be accepted as evidence in legal proceedings. Even poor handwriting on written records can affect their admissibility.

Overcoming Barriers to Good Documentation

There are several reasons medical record keeping is not generally adequate. Healthcare providers are concerned about confidentiality and liability. They are concerned about recording information that might inadvertently harm the victim. Many are confused about whether, how, and why to record information about domestic violence, so in an effort to be "neutral," some use language that may subvert the patient's legal case and even support the abuser's case.

Some healthcare providers are afraid to testify in court. They may see the risks to the patient and themselves as possibly outweighing the benefits of documenting abuse. Even healthcare providers who are reluctant to testify can still submit medical evidence. Although the hearsay rule prohibits out-of-court statements, an exception permits testimony about diagnosis and treatment. In addition, some states also allow the diagnosis and treatment elements of a certified medical record to be entered into the evidentiary record without the testimony of a healthcare provider. Thus, in some instances, physicians and other healthcare providers can be spared the burden of appearing in court.

The patient's "excited utterances" or "spontaneous exclamations" about the incident are another exception to the prohibition of hearsay. These are statements made by someone during or soon after an event, while in an agitated state of mind. They have exceptional credibility because of their proximity in time to the event and because they are not likely to be premeditated.

Excited utterances are valuable because they allow the prosecution to proceed even if the victim is unwilling to testify. These statements need to be carefully documented. A patient's report may be admissible if the record demonstrates that the patient made the statement while responding to the event stimulating the utterance (the act or acts of abuse). Noting the time between the event and the time the statements were made or describing the patient's demeanor as she made the statement can help show she was responding to the stimulating event. Such a showing is necessary to establish that a statement is an excited utterance or spontaneous exclamation, and thus an exception to the hearsay rule.[4]

What the Records Lack

It appears that at present, many medical records are not sufficiently well documented to provide adequate legal evidence of domestic violence. A study of 184 visits for medical care in which an injury or other evidence of abuse was noted revealed major shortcomings in the records:

- For the ninety-three instances of an injury, the records contained only one photograph. There was no mention in any records of photographs filed elsewhere (for example, with the police).

- A body map documenting the injury was included in only three of the ninety-three instances. Drawings of the injuries appeared in eight of the ninety-three instances.

- Doctors' and nurses' handwriting was illegible in key portions of the records in one-third of the patients' visits in which abuse or injury was noted.

- All three criteria for considering a patient's words an excited utterance were met in only twenty-eight of the more than eight hundred statements evaluated (3.4 percent). Most frequently missing was a description of the patient's demeanor, and often the patient was not clearly identified as the source of the information.

On the plus side, although photographs and body maps documenting injuries were rare, injuries were otherwise described in detail. And in fewer than 1 percent of the visits were negative comments made about the patient's appearance, manner, or motive for stating that abuse had occurred.

What Healthcare Providers Can Do

Medical records could be much more useful to domestic violence victims in legal proceedings if some minor changes were made in documentation. Clinicians can do the following:

- Take photographs of injuries known or suspected to have resulted from domestic violence.

- Write legibly. Computers can also help overcome the common problem of illegible handwriting.

- Set off the patient's own words in quotation marks or use such phrases as "patient states" or "patient reports" to indicate that the information recorded reflects the patient's words. To write "patient was kicked in abdomen" obscures the identity of the speaker.

- Avoid such phrases as "patient claims" or "patient alleges," which imply doubt about the patient's reliability. If the clinician's observations conflict with the patient's statements, the clinician should record the reason for the difference.

- Use medical terms and avoid legal terms such as "alleged perpetrator," "assailant," and "assault."

- Describe the person who hurt the patient by using quotation marks to set off the statement. The clinician would write, for example: "The patient stated, 'My boyfriend kicked and punched me.'"

- Avoid summarizing a patient's report of abuse in conclusive terms. If such language as "patient is a battered woman," "assault and battery," or "rape" lacks sufficient accompanying factual information, it is inadmissible.

- Do not place the term "domestic violence" or abbreviations such as "DV" in the diagnosis section of the medical record. Such terms do not convey factual information and are not medical terminology. Whether domestic violence has occurred is determined by the court.

- Describe the patient's demeanor, indicating, for example, whether she is crying or shaking or seems angry, agitated, upset, calm, or happy. Even if the patient's demeanor belies the evidence of abuse, the clinician's observations of that demeanor should be recorded.

- Record the time of day the patient is examined and, if possible, indicate how much time has elapsed since the abuse occurred. For example, the clinician might write, "Patient states that early this morning his boyfriend hit him."

Notes

1. Although men as well as women are victims of domestic violence, terms referencing women are most often used in this report because women are more frequently injured, in heterosexual relationships.

2. The evidentiary laws of each state define the scope and degree of use of medical records in legal proceedings.

3. A "body map" is a drawing of the human figure used by physicians. In domestic violence protocols, body maps are used to mark the locations, size, and age of injuries observed during a medical examination.

4. The rules of evidence adopted in most states include this exception to the general rule that statements made outside the courtroom are inadmissible. The exception is premised on the notion that if a speaker makes a statement while responding to an exciting or emotionally charged experience, that substantially reduces the likelihood that the speaker had time to fabricate the statement. This makes the statement more reliable.

Section 36.2

Screening for Abuse in Pregnant Women

Healthcare professionals providing prenatal and perinatal care for
pregnant women can and should screen routinely for the possibility
for abuse—ongoing woman abuse, past woman abuse sexual violence,
or a history of childhood sexual abuse. The information and resources
in this section will help explain why and how to screen for abuse, as
well as how to respond to disclosures of abuse that women may make
in response to the screening process.

Routine Screening

Many health professionals are reluctant to routinely, universally
screen for abuse in pregnancy even though there is widespread recognition that abuse has devastating physical and emotional effects on
the lives of women and their children. Professionals commonly cite the
following reasons for not screening:

- Inadequate resources
- Lack of training
- "Not my scope of practice"
- No time, large patient/client load
- Lack of knowledge about how to respond to disclosures of abuse
- Fear of making patients/clients uncomfortable
- Fear of retaliation from abuser

However, women repeatedly shared with us that if only someone had
asked them in a caring and supportive manner, they may have found their
voice to share what was happening to them. Specifically, women have
shared their perspective that, during their pregnancies, caregivers had a

responsibility to their unborn baby to look for signs of abuse, explain in a nonthreatening way the impact of abuse on their health, and be knowledgeable about services that could offer support or counseling.

Please note that current research is underway looking at the impacts of Universal Screening practices on women and whether or not it is successful in reducing violence against women or if it could cause more harm.[1] However, universal screening remains in the clinical guidelines for the American Medical Association, Society of Obstetricians and Gynaecologists of Canada, the American College of Obstetricians and Gynecologists, and the American Academy of Pediatrics.

We recognize the importance of evidence-based practice and eagerly await the outcomes of this research to help guide us in our practice of screening and responding to women who are experiencing abuse.

Asking Women about Abuse

Routine Universal Screening involves taking the time to create an atmosphere of trust. Women require privacy from their partners and family members in order to safely disclose abuse. It is dangerous and insensitive to make any assumption about who in your practice may have experienced abuse and who has not. Once privacy is assured, you must provide adequate time to screen for abuse and respond in a way that is supportive and knowledgeable about issues related to abuse. Make eye contact and demonstrate your willingness to listen through your body language.

What Questions Should I Ask?

You may ask questions about her understanding of abuse:

- "Some people think that in order to be considered abused, a person has to have been physically or sexually hurt. Are you aware of the other ways in which women can be abused?"

- "In your past and/or present relationship(s), were there times when you wondered whether or not your partner was being abusive?"

You might ask questions about how she and her partner work through disagreements:

- "Could you tell me how you feel after you and your partner argue?"

- "When you and your partner argue, do you feel listened to or silenced?"

456

- "Have you ever felt afraid during an argument?"

You might want to include questions about childhood sexual abuse and link it with present concerns related to abuse and pregnancy:

- "Many women that I work with have experienced abuse in their lives. Some women experienced sexual abuse in their childhood or in their teenage years. Other women have been hurt or abused in an adult relationship. In pregnancy, there can be reminders about past abuse that can show up and have a negative impact. If you have experienced an event in your life that you are worried may resurface in pregnancy, labor and birth, or postpartum, please know that I am a safe person for you to talk to and I am aware of other community resources that may be useful for you should you wish to connect with them."

However you choose to ask a woman about her past, please remember that the most important thing you may be doing is helping her to break the silence. By choosing to tell you about her experiences, she may learn that there is help available and that she is not alone.

Written Questionnaire or Face-to-Face Screening?

While results of a recent study indicate that women who were being abused preferred written questionnaires over face-to-face screening (*JAMA*, 2006), we have found a high degree of disclosures of past abuse in face-to face screening. However, this could be attributed to the fact that a relationship of trust has been established over time with our clients, all persons asking have been trained specifically to screen and respond to disclosures of abuse, our clients tend to be seeking out services that offer them greater control (midwives, doulas), and survivors may, for this reason, be overrepresented in the client population of midwifery and doula practices.

We have also heard feedback from survivors of abuse that one of the main problems with written disclosure was that they were not often followed up with support or referrals by a caregiver. Therefore, it is important that, regardless of the method used, disclosures be honored with the suggestions provided.

Why Ask Specifically about a History of Abuse?

Universal screening for abuse should not be about reading off a checklist of abusive behaviors or including just one question lumped in with other clinical questions. Women have repeatedly stated that having an abuse question grouped with questions about weight gain, diabetes, etc., is insulting and minimizes the significance of abuse in relation to their physical, emotional, and spiritual well-being.

Women have shared with us that it was important that caregivers asked specifically about abuse issues. They felt that by using the language of abuse (and not dancing around it) caregivers demonstrated an understanding about abuse issues and therefore were better prepared to hear their disclosures. This didn't necessarily mean that they told the person asking the questions, but they knew that the person at least cared on some level about abuse and its impacts.

Some women will not identify with being in an abusive relationship if they are not made aware of the many forms abuse can take. It can be a powerful education tool to display power and control wheels (charts) in a visible place and/or show them to her with an explanation of what is represented.

For many women it may not be enough to just ask, "Is there anything about your past that you wish to share with me?" This is often too broad and vague to capture that you are inquiring about abuse. They may not feel that this is what you are asking (the question could mean the death of a loved one), and therefore wouldn't want to catch you off guard. Other women felt like abuse was the "elephant in the room." They felt that there were so many obvious signs (bruises, aggressive partner, missing multiple appointments, etc.) that they resented that their doctor/midwife either didn't notice or didn't "care to ask."

What Is the Connection between Childhood Sexual Abuse and Abuse Later in Life?

Children who were abused may have a difficult time as adults setting and sticking to boundaries that keep them safe. Children learn about boundaries as they grow up and are able to say "no," asserting their own needs in ways that are developmentally appropriate, and having that "no" respected by those in caregiving roles. They communicate to the adults around them their wants and/or needs for physical space and hopefully this is respected and nourished. However, adults who sexually abuse children send different messages, such as: It doesn't matter what you want, your body belongs to me for my amusement, I/we own you, you are to blame. To cope with severe abuse, children learn to detach (also called dissociate), and this skill that assisted them to survive childhood abuse transfers into adulthood. Routinely detaching can make it challenging for women to get to know themselves, *their wants, their needs*. Even when the adult survivor is clearly being abused, he or she may have a very difficult time speaking out. Often the low self-worth, self-blame, and shame that results from earlier abuse sets adult survivors up for further revictimization. It is therefore imperative that people understand the link between earlier experiences of abuse and the likelihood that childhood sexual abuse survivors may have ongoing abuse issues in their current relationships. Just as important is recognizing that a woman who is in a current abusive relationship may also have a history of childhood abuse. Understanding this link may assist you in offering more appropriate referrals so that she can examine how the messages she learned early in her life are impacting her as an adult.

However, much more research is needed to look at the ramifications of women disclosing abuse, such as the involvement of child protection or reprisal abuse for a woman who leaves and then returns to an abusive partner. Due to the dynamics of abuse, particularly when children are involved, it often takes many attempts for a woman to leave an abusive relationship. You need to consider how the information could be used against her in court in such matters as child custody. It is advisable that you seek training or information on documentation related to the abuse of women and what your professional standards require.

Before you ask, please be sure to inform her:

- that you are about to ask her some questions that you ask *all* your clients;

- that the reason you ask is because you care about your clients and would have information and supports available to her should she need them;

- that you ask because you know that many women live with abuse and are afraid to tell;

- that her information will be kept confidential except in certain circumstances;

- what those circumstances are, such as duty-to-report obligations of your provincial or state child protection agencies or if you were subpoenaed to court;

- that she has the right not to answer at the present time but you would be available at a future time should she wish to speak with you.

Your Own Safety

Be aware of the potential risks to your own safety when working with women who are being abused. Adopt personal work habits that optimize your safety and lobby your workplace to implement security measures and protocols accordingly.

If you are in private practice or work unpredictable hours (doula, midwife), think about meeting in a place other than a client's home for the first visit, let someone know where you are going and when you are expecting to return, carry a cell phone, ask hospital security to escort you to your car at night, and at all times be aware of your surroundings (nearest exit, phone, etc.).

Who should screen for abuse?

"Should I be the one to ask about her past?"
Ask yourself:

- Do I have professional guidelines to follow?

- Do I have the skills and resources to respond to a disclosure?

- Do I have the time to provide support?

- Could the answer help me to provide her with better support or services?

- What obstacles prevent me from asking/responding?

- Are there any foreseeable negative consequences for my client/ patient for which I do not feel I could provide assistance (in the form of safety planning, referrals)?

If you answered "No" to some of these questions, it could mean you need more supervision, training, or information on how to best meet the needs of women in your care who may be experiencing abuse. Speak with a colleague, supervisor, or community organization for local training opportunities.

If You Are a Care Provider Who Has Experienced Abuse

How you bring awareness about the impacts of abuse to your patients/ clients may be shaped by your own abuse history. If you have experienced abuse we strongly recommend counseling before you start screening women so that you are not inadvertently transferring your own survivor issues onto the women you are working with. Recognize that your ability to empathize with women who have been abused can be very powerful but also self-destructive if you do not receive proper support, supervision, and collaboration.

Reference

1. Harriet L. MacMillan and C. Nadine Wathen, "Violence against women: integrating the evidence into clinical practice, Commentary, *Canadian Medical Association Journal*, www.cmaj.ca/cgi/content/full/169/6/570.

Further Suggested Reading

Felitti, V., Anda, R., Nordenberg, D., Williamson, D., Spitz, A., Edwards, V., Koss, M., Marks, J. (1998) Relationship of childhood abuse and household dysfunction to many of the leading causes of death in adults. The Adverse Childhood Experiences (ACE) Study, *American Journal of Preventive Medicine, 14,* 245–58

Hobbins, D. (2005). Survivors of childhood sexual abuse: Implications for perinatal nursing care. *JOGNN, 33,* 485–97.

Lavell-Harvard, D. M., & Corbiere Lavell, J. (Eds.). (2006). *Until our hearts are on the ground: Aboriginal mothering, oppression, resistance, and rebirth.* Toronto, Canada: Demeter Press.

Leeners, B., Richter-Appelt, H., Imthurn, B., & Rath, W. (2006). Influence of childhood sexual abuse on pregnancy, delivery, and the early postpartum period in adult women. *Journal of Psychosomatic Research, 61,* 139–51

Kendall-Tackett, K. (1998). Literature review: breastfeeding and the sexual abuse survivor. *Journal of Human Lactation, 14,* 125–33.

Seng, J. S. (2002). A conceptual framework for research on lifetime violence, posttraumatic stress, and childbearing. *Journal of Midwifery & Women's Health, 47*(5), 337–46.

Simkin, P. (1994). Effect of childhood sexual trauma on the childbearing woman: Memories that really matter. *Childbirth Instructor Magazine,* 20–23.

Part Five

Emergency Management, Moving Out, and Moving On

Chapter 37

Why Do Victims Stay with Their Abusers?

Chapter Contents

Section 37.1

Barriers to Leaving

The most common question asked about domestic violence victims is "Why does she stay?"

The question shows the misunderstanding of the dynamics of domestic violence. It also reveals a tendency to blame the victim. A more appropriate question would be:

"Why does he abuse her?" or "Why can't he be stopped from hurting his family?"

The question—"Why does she stay?"—puts the responsibility back on the victim, and is often followed with the statement, "She must like it."

Women stay in abusive relationships for many reasons. They do not stay because they "want to be abused."

A battered woman may believe:

- his violence is temporary;

- with loyalty and love, she can make him change;

- his promises that it will "never happen again";

- it's her responsibility to keep the family together;

- there will be more good times.

She may tell herself:

- He's had a hard life.

- He needs me.

- All men are violent; it is to be expected.

She may deny or minimize the violence. She may believe her abuser when he tells her that his abuse is "her fault."

Many women do not want the relationship to end; they want the violence to end.

Fear is a major factor.

Many women believe their abusers' threats. She believes he will kill her if she leaves him.

She may fear:

- more severe abuse;

- retaliation if he finds her;

- destruction of her belongings or home;

- harm to her job or reputation;

- stalking;

- charging her with a crime;

- harming children, pets, family, or friends;

- his committing suicide;

- court or police involvement.

At times, women may leave the relationship. She may return when he begs her to come back, or when she cannot find the resources to live on her own. She may return because she loves him.

The average battered woman leaves seven to eight times before permanently leaving a relationship.

There are many other reasons women stay in relationships. Some include:

- Economics:
  - Few job skills.
  - Limited education or work experience.
  - Limited cash.
  - No access to bank account.
  - Fear of poverty.

- Pressure from community of faith/family:
  - Family expectation to stay in marriage "at any cost."
  - Family denial of the violence.
  - Family blame her for the violence.
  - Religion may disapprove of divorce.
  - Religious leader may tell her to "stay and pray."

- Guilt/self-doubt:
  - Guilt about failure of the relationship.
  - Guilt about choosing an abuser.
  - Feelings of personal incompetence.
  - Concern about independence.
  - Loneliness.
- Concern for children:
  - Abuser may charge her with "kidnapping" or sue for custody.
  - Abuser may abduct or abuse the children.
  - Questions whether she can care for and support children on her own.
  - Fears losing custody of her children.
  - Believes children need a father.
- Lack of community support:
  - Unaware of services available to battered women.
  - Lack of adequate child care.
  - Few jobs.
  - Negative experiences with service providers.
  - Lack of affordable housing.
  - Isolated from community services.
  - No support from family and friends.

Many women in abusive relationships ask these questions:

- **Will it get better?** Studies show that over time, without intervention, abuse in the home gets more frequent and more violent.
- **Is it my fault?** No. Abuse is always wrong. In fact, abuse in the home is a crime. The victim is never to blame. There is no excuse for domestic violence.
- **Can I fix it?** No. Only the abuser can stop his violent behavior. Qualified batterer intervention programs may provide knowledge and skills to stop his violent behavior, but only the abuser can decide whether he will use them or not.

- **Will Alcoholics Anonymous or Narcotics Anonymous keep him from hitting me?** No. While your partner may need treatment for alcohol or drug abuse, the abusive behavior can continue even if he becomes sober or stops abusing drugs. It is recommended that an abuser get treated for his violence in a specialized intervention program, as well as for drug and alcohol abuse through substance abuse programs.

- **What can I do?** Take care of yourself by asking for help. Remember: No one deserves to be abused.

Section 37.2

Stages of Leaving

Reprinted with permission from Mecklenburg County Community Support Services Women's Commission, © 2012. For additional information, visit http://CSS.CharMeck.org and click on Women's Commission.

Denial

The abused:

- does not admit there is a problem;
- will excuse the abuser's violent behavior;
- believes that each incident is the last.

Guilt

The abused:

- begins to know that there is a problem but believes it is her fault;
- believes she deserves to be beaten;
- thinks if she had done this or that, he wouldn't have had to hit her;
- believes something is wrong with herself, not the abuser or relationship.

Enlightenment

The abused:

• no longer assumes responsibility for the violence;

• realizes no one deserves to be beat;

• is still committed to the relationship;

• believes if she stays, they can work things out.

Responsibility

The abused:

• accepts that the abuser will not change;

• accepts that the violence will not stop;

• decides not to "put up" with the abuse;

• leaves the relationship to start a new life.

Some victims may go back and forth between stages. A victim cannot be pushed from one stage to the next. She will, through her own experience, move on to each stage when she can.

Chapter 38

Staying Safe with an Abuser

No one deserves to be abused. Our hope is that if you are being abused, you will be able to find a way to safely get out of the abusive relationship. However, the reality is that for many different reasons, some victims are not able to leave an abusive relationship once the abuse begins. If you're in a physically abusive relationship, please consider the following tips to help try to keep you and your children safe until the time comes when you are able to leave.

Following these suggestions (often known as a safety plan) can't guarantee your safety, but it could help make you safer. However, it is important that you create a safety plan that it right for you. Not all of these suggestions will work for everyone, and some could even place you in greater danger. You have to do what you think is best to keep yourself and your children safe.

During the Violence

- The abuser may have patterns to his/her abuse. Try to be aware of any signs that show s/he's about to become violent so that you can assess how dangerous the situation may be for you and your children.

- If it looks like violence may happen, try to remove yourself and your children from the situation before the violence begins if you can.

- Be aware of anything the abuser can use as a weapon. If you can, try and keep any sharp or heavy objects that s/he may use to hurt you, like a hammer or an ice pick, out of the way.

- Know where guns, knives, and other weapons are. If you can, lock them up or make them as hard to get to as you can.

- Figure out where the "safe places" are in your home—the places where there aren't weapons. If it looks like the abuser is about to hurt you, try to get to a safe place. Stay out of the kitchen, garage, or workshop. Try to avoid rooms with tile or hardwood floors.

- If the abuser does start to harm you, don't run to where the children are; the abuser may hurt them too.

- If there's no way to escape the violence at that moment, make yourself a small target. Dive into a corner and curl up into a ball. Protect your face and put your arms around each side of your head, wrapping your fingers together.

- Try not to wear scarves or long jewelry. The abuser could use these things to strangle you.

What to Tell Your Children

- Create a plan with your children for when violence happens. Tell them not to get involved if the abuser is hurting you, since that may get them hurt. Decide on a code word to let them know that they should leave the house and get help. If the abuser won't let them leave the house safely, figure out with them where would be a safe place for them to go within the house where they can call for help (such as a room with a lock and a phone). Make sure they know that their first priority is to stay safe, not to physically protect you.

- Practice different ways to get out of your house safely. Practice with your children as well.

- Plan for what you will do if your children tell your partner about your plan or if your partner finds out about your plan some other way.

- Tell your children that violence is never right, even when someone they love is being violent. Tell them that the violence isn't their fault or your fault. Tell them that when anyone is being violent, it is important to keep safe.

Ways to Get Help

- If you need help in a public place, yell *"Fire!"* People respond more quickly to someone yelling "fire" than to any other cry for help.

- If you can, always have a phone where you know you can get to it. Know the numbers to call for help such as 911 or the National Domestic Violence Hotline at 800-799-SAFE (7233). Know where the nearest pay phone is in case you have to run out of the home without your cell phone. Know your local battered women's shelter number.

- Let friends and neighbors who you trust know what is going on in your home. Make a plan with them so that they know when you need help and so they know what to do (such as calling the police or banging on your door). Make up a signal with your neighbors, like flashing the lights on and off or hanging something out the window, which will alert them that you need help.

- Make a habit of backing the car into the driveway (so you can quickly pull out) and having a full tank of gas. Keep your car keys in the same place so you can easily grab them. If you would be leaving by yourself (if you don't have children), you might want to even keep the driver's door unlocked (and the other car doors locked) so that you are prepared to make a quick escape if you have to.

- Keep a copy of important papers with you or in your car, such as your and your children's birth certificates, passports, immigration papers, and Social Security cards, in case you have to leave in a hurry.

- If you can, call a domestic violence hotline from time to time to discuss your options and to talk to someone who understands you, even if you feel that you are not ready to leave. One number you can call is the National Domestic Violence Hotline at 800-799-SAFE.

- Think of several reasons for leaving the house at different times of the day or night that the abuser will believe, in case you feel that the violence is about to erupt and you need an excuse to get out.

Chapter 39

Managing a Domestic Violence Emergency

Chapter Contents

Section 39.1

Calling the Police

Sometimes the best way to keep yourself safe is to call the police—especially if you feel like you're in immediate danger, your restraining order has been violated, or you've been injured by your partner. If you have any doubt about safety, you can call the police—even if you haven't been physically hurt or touched in any way.

What can the police do?

While you may be hesitant or afraid to call the police, they may be able to help and protect you when you need it the most. Police may:

- stop the abuse long enough for you to escape to a safe place;

- give you a temporary restraining order, or if not, refer you to the right court agency where you can ask for one, depending on your state;

- arrest your abusive partner for hurting you or violating your restraining order;

- help you document the abuse, including taking pictures of your injuries and interviewing witnesses;

- help you find further assistance in your community by connecting you to a local domestic violence shelter or agency.

What can I do?

If the police are contacted, remember these important tips:

- When you call 911 or your local police department, tell them you're in danger and need help immediately. If the police don't come soon, call again and tell them that it's your second call.

- If you have a restraining or protective order, tell them about it when you call.

- Once the police arrive, show them the protective order.

- Get the officers' *names* and *badge numbers*.

- Ask the police to take pictures of your injuries and interview any witnesses.

- Show the police any threatening text messages or emails from your abusive partner.

- Allow the police to listen to any harassing voicemails left on your phone.

- Insist they file a report and get its number. If they refuse to take a report, go to your local police department and file one yourself that day or the next business day.

- If you believe you'll be unsafe once the police leave, get information from them about local agencies you can go to for help. You can also ask about getting an emergency restraining order that can help protect you immediately.

- On the next business day, call the police department to get the name and phone number of the detective or investigator assigned to your case. Call them to get more information.

Section 39.2

Preserving and Collecting Forensic Evidence after a Sexual Assault

In the immediate aftermath of a sexual assault, the most important thing is for the victim to get to a safe place. Whether it be the victim's home, a friend's home, or with a family member, immediate safety is what matters most. When a feeling of safety has been achieved, it is vital for the victim to receive medical attention, and strongly recommended for the victim to receive a forensic examination.

Preserving deoxyribonucleic acid (DNA) evidence can be key to identifying the perpetrator in a sexual assault case, especially those in which the offender is a stranger. DNA evidence is an integral part of a law enforcement investigation that can build a strong case to show that a sexual assault occurred and to show that the defendant is the source of biological material left on the victim's body.[1]

Victims should make every effort to save anything that might contain the perpetrator's DNA, therefore a victim should not:[1]

- bathe or shower;
- use the restroom;
- change clothes;
- comb hair;
- clean up the crime scene;
- move anything the offender may have touched.

Even if the victim has not yet decided to report the crime, receiving a forensic medical exam and keeping the evidence safe from damage will improve the chances that the police can access and test the stored evidence at a later date.

What does a forensic medical exam entail?

A forensic medical exam may be performed at a hospital or other healthcare facility, by a sexual assault nurse examiner (SANE), sexual assault forensic examiner (SAFE) or another medical professional. This exam is complex and on average, takes three to four hours. While this may seem lengthy, medical and forensic exams are comprehensive because the victim deserves and needs special attention to ensure that they are medically safe and protected. In addition, it is important to collect evidence so that if the victim chooses to report the crime to the police, they can access the stored evidence.[1]

1. To start, the medical professional will write down the victim's detailed history. This sets a clear picture of existing health status, including medications being taken and preexisting conditions unrelated to the assault.

2. Next there is a head-to-toe, detailed examination and assessment of the entire body (including an internal examination). This may include collection of blood, urine, hair, and other body secretion samples, photo documentation of injuries (such as bruises, cuts, and scraped skin), and collection of clothing (especially undergarments).

3. Finally, the medical professional will speak about treatment for sexually transmitted infections (STIs) that may have been exposed during the assault. Depending on the hospital and state, the victim may receive prophylaxis as well as referrals for follow-up counseling, community resources, and medical care.

Note: The victim has the right to accept or decline any or all parts of the exam. However, it is important to remember that critical evidence may be missed if not collected or analyzed.

After the forensic medical exam is performed and the evidence is collected and stored in the kit, the victim will be able to take a shower, brush their teeth, etc.—all while knowing that the evidence has been preserved to aid in a criminal prosecution if so desired.

What is a "rape kit"?

The sexual assault forensic exam kit (commonly referred to as a "rape kit") is the collection of DNA and other forensic evidence, which is then kept by the SANE or medical provider until picked up by law enforcement or the crime lab. It is then stored until the victim determines whether or not to pursue a case. The kit itself is generally a large envelope or cardboard box, which can safely store evidence collected from your body or clothing. While the contents of a sexual assault forensic exam may vary by state and jurisdiction, it may include items, such as:

- instructions;
- bags and sheets for evidence collection;
- swabs;
- comb;
- envelopes for hair and fibers;
- blood collection devices;
- documentation forms.

Under the Violence Against Women and Department of Justice Reauthorization Act of 2005, states may not:

> require a victim of sexual assault to participate in the criminal
> justice system or cooperate with law enforcement in order to
> be provided with a forensic medical exam, reimbursement for
> charges incurred on account of such an exam, or both.

Under this law, a state must ensure that victims have access to an exam free of charge or with a full reimbursement, even if the victim decides not to cooperate with law enforcement investigators. (Previously, states were required to ensure access to exams free of charge, but could put conditions on the exam, such as cooperating with law enforcement officials.)[2]

Essentially, this law allows victims time to decide whether to pursue their case. A sexual assault is a traumatic event and some victims are unable to decide in the immediate aftermath. Because forensic evidence can be lost as time progresses, A "Jane Doe Rape Kit" enables a victim to have forensic evidence collected without revealing identifying information. For instance, in some states, victims are given a code number they can use to identify themselves if they choose to report the crime at a later date.[1]

Each state has determined different time frames for the storage of a kit. The victim should be informed at the time of the exam as to the length of time the kit will be retained, as well as the disposition of the kit. A local crisis center can help explain all of the options moving forward.

Processing the evidence collected may take only a few weeks, but many areas of the country have significant backlogs. So the wait to have your evidence tested could range from a few weeks to a few months, or even longer.

Note: To find a local hospital or healthcare facility that is equipped to collect forensic evidence, contact the National Sexual Assault Hotline (800-656-HOPE). The hotline will connect callers to their local crisis center, which can provide information on the nearest medical facility, and in some instances, send an advocate to accompany victims through the evidence collection process.

Endnotes

1. DNA & Crime Victims: What Victims Need to Know. The National Center for Victims of Crime. 2008. http://www.ncvc.org/ncvc/main.aspx?dbID=DB_DNAResourceCenter240

2. Anonymous Reporting and Forensic Examinations. Department of Justice: Office on Violence Against Women. 2008. http://www.ovw.usdoj.gov

Section 39.3

Documenting Abuse

The warning signs of dating violence aren't always dramatic, but if you keep track of incidents of abuse, you can better identify red flags, take steps to prevent future abuse, and be prepared if you ever do decide to seek legal remedies. Detailed documentation is important, especially if the incident took place in a private setting or was repeated in a distinct pattern.

Ways to Document Abuse

- Keep a journal about what you're going through. Include:
  - Any incidents of abuse.
  - Statements you, your partner, or any witnesses made about what happened.
  - The date and time of each incident.
  - A description of any injuries, no matter how small. Take pictures if you can store them safely.
  - A description of the scene. For example, is the furniture overturned? Are any items thrown around? Again, take pictures if you can.
  - How the incident made you feel.
- Seek medical care, even if there are no visible injuries. Just because you don't have any cuts or bruises doesn't mean you weren't physically harmed.
- File a report with the police.

Digital Abuse Counts Too

In abusive relationships, threats and controlling behavior often occur by phone or over the internet. On occasion, your partner will even admit to the abuse or an element of it in a message or online post. You may be hesitant to report this type of unwanted contact or even recognize it as abuse, but it counts in a court of law.

Digital evidence is often fleeting and can be deleted, accidentally or intentionally, very easily. For this reason, it's important to secure evidence quickly:

- Print out all emails that contain any evidence or information about the incident. Make sure the printout includes the sender, recipient, date, and time.

- If possible, print out text messages. If not, take a picture of the cell phone displaying the message, contact information, date, and time.

- If possible, print out your call log. If not, take a picture of the cell phone displaying the contact information, date, and time.

- Print screen shots of social networking sites that contain evidence, such as admissions of abuse, threats of violence, or pictures that you didn't consent to. Remember to check both your and your partner's site.

- Record voicemails onto a digital recorder and include the time and date of the message.

Try to save all future abusive electronic communications using these same methods.

Chapter 40

Getting Help in
the Aftermath of Abuse

Chapter Contents

Section 40.1

Sources of Help for Victims of Domestic Violence

Excerpted from "The Greatest Escape: Special for Victims of Domestic Violence," © 2010 Marie De Santis, Women's Justice Center, www.justicewomen.com. Reprinted with permission.

The following is a description of some of the professionals and officials whose job it is to help you get safely free of domestic violence, to help you get justice, and to help you put together a new life. As you make your way out of domestic violence, you're going to be dealing with one professional after another. Many will be very helpful, but along the way you're bound to run into one or two who may treat you with disregard. When you come across a professional or official who is not treating your situation seriously, don't give up. And don't accept mistreatment. Get help from others, so they can work with you to get the situation corrected. You have a constitutional right to equal protection of the laws.

Victim Advocates

The victim advocate's job is to help victims like you by being supportive, by answering your questions, by helping you find counseling, explaining to you how the system works, helping you get restraining orders, accompanying you to official interviews and to the court, fighting for your rights, listening to your problems, informing you of your options, and giving you advice. In other words, the victim advocate should be like a trained best friend, someone who is knowledgeable and on your side.

The law in most states (including in California) says that victim advocates must keep everything you say completely confidential. Advocates cannot talk about your case with anyone unless you give permission. In fact, victim advocates should not take any action on your case until you give them permission to act. (The one exception to this rule is that victim advocates who specialize in domestic violence are usually mandated to report suspected child abuse.)

486

Calling and connecting with a victim advocate is a good place to start getting out of domestic violence because you can discuss all your doubts, fears, and questions with the advocate and be completely assured that the advocate will keep your conversations confidential. You can find victim advocates by calling your local woman's shelter, your local rape crisis center, local victim assistance centers, or by calling the police or the office of the district attorney. Most victim's centers have advocates available to talk with you twenty-four hours a day. Also most victim centers (at least in California) have advocates who speak the most common languages in your area in addition to English.

There are a couple other things you should know about victim advocates. Advocates have no official powers. They can't take any official action on your case such as filing charges against the perpetrator or making an arrest or approving a restraining order. However, because of their knowledge of the system some victim advocates are very effective at pressuring the system to get you the justice and protection you deserve. Some are not. As with all other persons you go to for help, if you're not getting what you need from your victim advocate, you should seek another who will help you.

The 911 Operator

The 911 operator is much more than a telephone operator. 911 operators are trained to handle your emergency domestic violence call. They are trained to help you stay calm. They are trained to ask you the critical questions, to give you emergency advice, to quickly access important documents in your case, such as restraining orders. And they are trained to get you the help you need as soon as possible. 911 operators also have immediate access to professional interpreters in close to one hundred different languages.

So when you call 911, stay on the line with the 911 operator as long as you safely can. Try to stay on the line until the police arrive at your door. Listen carefully to her or his voice. Answer all the operator's questions completely. Tell the operator as much as you can about the abuser's violence and threats. Tell the operator about any weapons available to the perpetrator. Tell the operator if the abuser has been violent in the past. Tell the operator your fears. Keep talking! And if you have to run or leave the phone for your safety, don't hang up!

Here is some other important information you should have about your 911 call:

- All 911 calls are tape-recorded and saved as evidence. The tape recording of your 911 call is frequently a key piece of evidence in your case. So keep talking! Don't hang up! Talking and staying on the line is especially important if you don't speak English. Remember that if you don't speak English a professional interpreter will quickly come on the 911 call with you and with the operator. Tell as much of your story as you can to the 911 operator and interpreter, because the officer who arrives on the scene may not speak your language. And though the police should also get you a professional interpreter, some do not. So your 911 call may be the best opportunity you'll have to get across an accurate account of your story. Also remember, the information you give the interpreter will be passed on to the officer who's coming to your call.

- At the same time that the 911 operator is asking you questions, she or he is also summarizing your call to the officer en route to the scene.

- If you dial 911 but for some reason you can't speak, or if you have to stop speaking, don't hang up! Just by having dialed 911, the 911 system automatically finds your address. In addition, by leaving the phone open even if you have to run, the 911 operator can gain critical information about what's going on just by listening to the sounds in the background of the call.

Police

Over the last ten years police have been given extensive new powers to help and protect domestic violence victims. New laws encourage police to make arrests in domestic violence cases. In most states police can also write you an emergency protective order on the spot. Using these emergency orders, police can kick the abuser out of the home, give you temporary legal custody of children, and order the abuser to stay away from you and your children. In addition, most all police have been given specialized training in the dynamics and investigation of domestic violence. Detailed police department policies generally mandate that police carry out thorough and clearly defined investigations on all domestic violence calls, mandate that police provide you with extensive follow-up information, and mandate that police offer you a range of services for your safety.

Here are some other things you should know in order for you to get the best help possible from police.

Police can only use their powers when they suspect a crime has occurred or is about to occur. So when you deal with the police it's very important to focus on telling the police about the abuser's

488

criminal behavior towards you. In domestic violence, examples of criminal acts are physical violence, sexual violence, threats of violence, vandalism, kidnapping, holding you against your will, and violation of restraining orders.

Your experience of domestic violence probably includes much more than these criminal acts, such as the abuser's insults, his lying, his foul language in front of the children, emotional betrayals, and more. But these things are not criminal. It's very hard for most domestic violence victims to separate it all out, since all of it, the criminal and the noncriminal acts, are damaging and painful to you. But when you are talking with police, try to stay focused on the abuser's criminal acts, and to give the officer as much evidence of those acts as you can.

As a victim of domestic violence, you can report to police at any time. Though it's always better to call police right away after an attack because evidence is fresh, you can go to police the next day, the next week, or the next month. You can dial 911 if you have an emergency, or you can walk into the police station and request an officer at any time.

Don't hold back! Tell the officer everything! The domestic violence crime report that police write following your call is usually the single most powerful document you will have in determining your future safety, your access to justice, your access to victim assistance, and more. The domestic violence crime report written by police can also be the most significant document in a contested restraining order hearing, contested child custody, and in any other legal problem you may have with the abuser. The police report can also be extremely helpful to you in any related problems you may have with your landlord, your job, your family, with immigration, and more.

So don't hold back. Tell the officer everything. Tell the officer the details of the most recent incident. Tell the officer about any evidence or witnesses you can think of. Tell the officer the specific threats the abuser has made to you. Tell the officer if you are afraid for your or your children's life or safety, and tell the officer why you are afraid. Show the officer all your injuries. Tell the officer about any weapons the abuser has used or has access to. Tell the officer what you know about the abuser's criminal history.

And more, tell the officer the history of the abuse. Tell the officer about the worst incident that has occurred. Tell the officer if the abuser has ever forced you to have sex. Tell the officer if the abuser has ever hurt the children. Encourage your children to tell the police what they know too.

If after the officer has left, you remember important information that should be in the officer's report, take out a piece of paper and write out the information. Take your written statement to the police station as soon as possible and ask the front desk person to please have the statement added to the report on your case.

If you get a police officer who responds badly to your case or an officer who doesn't do a complete job, do not give up! Unfortunately, despite the training and new laws, there are still too many officers who don't take domestic violence seriously. The bad attitudes and behavior of these officers are extremely dangerous to women. If this is the kind of officer who responds to your call, it is not your fault, it is the officer's fault, and you deserve much better.

Here are some things you can do:

- Take a few pieces of paper and write out your story yourself as best you can. Take it to the police station and ask the person at the front desk to add this statement to your police report.

- Or you can call the 911 operator and tell him or her that you still need help, or that important information was left out of your case.

- Or you can call the police station and ask to speak to the sergeant on duty, and tell the sergeant that important information was left out of your case.

Domestic Violence Shelters and Programs

If you fear for your life and feel that the protection of police and courts is not sufficient to protect you, you should call the domestic violence shelter in your area and ask for shelter. If the shelter is full, most shelters will refer you, and help you get to a shelter in a neighboring county.

In addition to providing safe housing, domestic violence shelters generally also have victim advocates, counselors, support groups, children's programs, and other programs available to help you. You can use these professionals and their programs whether or not you are staying at the shelter.

Domestic violence shelters also have twenty-four-hour crisis lines where you can call and talk with a domestic violence counselor day or night. The counselors on these crisis lines will be sympathetic and supportive. They are good listeners, and can inform you about the services available to you.

Don't be afraid to call domestic violence crisis lines any time of day or night. All your communication with the crisis line counselor will be completely confidential. And if you're still worried about the privacy of your story, use a false name when you make the call. The phone number for the crisis line in your area is probably in the front of your phonebook, or can be obtained by calling the telephone operator.

Rape Crisis Centers

Sexual abuse and rape are a very common part of domestic violence. Many women find it very difficult to talk about this aspect of domestic violence. And though domestic violence advocates may have some training in sexual violence, you may feel more comfortable talking about these things to an advocate who deals specifically with sexual assault.

Like domestic violence centers, rape crisis centers have confidential twenty-four-hour crisis lines, support groups, advocates, and other services to help you.

Victim Assistance Centers

Most states have established state monetary funds to help crime victims by paying for your counseling needs, medical expenses, emergency needs related to the crime, and by making up for wages you may have lost as a result of the crime. These state agencies usually have local offices. Ask your police department or domestic violence crisis line counselor for the location of the victim assistance office nearest you.

To be eligible for the victim assistance funds you need to have made a crime report to police. Then you need to fill out the necessary forms at your victim assistance center.

The County Jail

Though it may seem strange to think of your county jail as a source of help, once your partner is arrested, the jail is one of the first places you'll probably want to call. The jail can give you critical information about your partner's status, and, if you request it, the jail can notify you if they are about to release your partner. Most jails can be called twenty-four hours a day.

So if your partner has been arrested, call the jail and give them the full name of the person arrested and their date of birth if you have it. The jail can then tell you (in fact, they are obligated to tell you) if that person is currently in the jail. They can tell you the amount of bail, the booking charges, and the person's next court date, time, and courtroom. This information can be invaluable for many reasons. If you suddenly wake up in the middle of the night afraid and wondering if your partner has gotten out of jail, a call to the jail can reassure you and make it possible for you to go back to sleep.

Knowing the amount of your partner's bail can help you evaluate whether or not he's likely to get out. And if you feel the bail amount is too low, you can call the prosecutor (the district attorney) on your case, or write a note to the judge, and ask that the bail be raised.

When someone is "booked" into jail, the jail records the crimes the police suspect he has committed. These are called the "booking charges." These booking charges are not necessarily the charges the district attorney will file against your partner, but these booking charges do give you a general idea of what the final charges may be. In regard to your partner's next court date and time, this is information you can usually obtain from a number of sources. But very often the fastest way to get the information is by making a call to the jail. Remember, the jail won't have any of this information if your partner never went to jail or if he has bailed.

There is one other very important thing the jail can do for you if you request it. If you are a victim of domestic violence or sexual assault, the jail can notify you if your abuser is about to be released. You should keep in mind, however, that if the jail attempts to get ahold of you because they are about to release your abuser, and they can't find you, the jail will probably release the abuser anyway.

District Attorney's Office

When the police finish writing the report on your domestic violence case, they send the crime report to district attorney's office. After reading the report, the district attorney's office decides whether or not to file formal charges against your partner, and they decide what those charges will be.

If the district attorney decides not to file charges, that will be the end of the criminal case against the abuser, unless you object, and usually you'll have to object strongly.

If the district attorney does file charges, you'll want to know what those charges are, who the district attorney is who is assigned to the case, and when and if you'll need to testify. Usually you can get the answers to these questions by simply asking the district attorney office receptionist who answers your phone call.

As the case progresses, you'll likely have many more questions for which you should definitely get answers. Your first stop in getting these answers is to again call the district attorney's office. Or ask a victim advocate or smart friend to make the call for you.

Remember: The thoughts and sources of help we've laid out here are just to get you started on your struggle to be free of domestic violence. As you set out on your own unique path, you're going to have many more questions and needs along the way. Ask questions. Ask for help. Don't give up if someone gets in your way. You deserve peace, happiness, freedom, and justice, and all the help that's needed to get you there.

Section 40.2

Shelters and Safehouses

Excerpted from "Shelters and Safehouses," updated February 2006, © The Advocates for Human Rights (www.stopvaw.org). All rights reserved. Reprinted with permission. Although there may have been more recent studies on certain aspects of domestic violence since these pages were originally published, the Advocates for Human Rights has expressed confidence that the principles and concepts remain accurate as of 2012.

The Shelter and Safehouse Movements

The shelter and safehouse movement in the United States began in the early 1970s. Two of the earliest shelters were Women's Advocates in Minnesota and Transition House in Boston. Women who were concerned about domestic violence or were themselves victims of domestic violence came together and decided that one of the most critical issues facing victims was the absence of alternative housing. Many of these early groups began by housing women in advocates' own homes for one or two days. Safehouse networks continue to this day, and are a viable alternative to temporary housing when establishing a shelter is not feasible.

Shelters in the United States and in Great Britain have historically operated under one or more founding philosophies: philanthropic, bureaucratic, therapeutic, and activist. Shelters having a philanthropic approach often grew out of movements to address poverty

493

and homelessness and are focused on providing individuals with the basic necessities of food, shelter, and clothing. Shelters with a more bureaucratic approach mirror civil service organizations and are focused on coordinating the various agencies that deliver services to battered women. Shelters with a therapeutic approach are more closely tied to a mental health model and focus on providing battered women with therapy and counseling. Shelters with an activist approach take a broader view of the problem of domestic violence and are concerned not only with the physical and emotional needs of individual battered women but also with the societal structures that allow the continuation of wife abuse.[1]

Shelters in the United States have taken different approaches to solve some of the challenges they face in their day-to-day operations.

Funding

Locating funding for a shelter is a priority at the shelter's founding and throughout its life. Women's Advocates, for example, began fundraising in 1973 with a letter campaign; the women in the group mailed letters to friends and acquaintances, outlining the plans for the shelter and asking for donations or monthly pledges. The response to this mailing of approximately four hundred letters generated almost $700 a month. Women's Advocates then began to submit funding proposals and grant applications to local and state governments and private foundations; the shelter received a grant the following year for staff salaries and grants from foundations in subsequent years.

Women's Advocates also asks residents for small contributions to their room and board. Because even a few dollars a day can present a real hardship to some women, the shelter also makes it clear that women will not be turned away if they cannot pay. In general, the shelter has found that women do what they can to meet the cost of staying at the shelter. Women's Advocates also sought contributions from local welfare agencies, but negotiated with the local government to ensure that women were not later penalized for these payments from the government to the shelter.

Length of Stay

Some shelters have limits on how long a woman can stay, some do not. The longer a woman is allowed to stay, the more time she has to gather the resources that she will need to protect herself. At the same time, however, the longer the women stay, the fewer women who can be housed in times of crisis.

Shelters that do not limit the length of a stay note that most women will return home or find alternate accommodation when the crisis has passed. Other shelters limit the length of a resident's stay, or reach individual length-of-stay agreements with residents based on the resident's needs and how quickly she anticipates being able to find other housing.

Some shelters are able to combine temporary shelter with transitional housing options; women stay in the temporary shelter at first, but move, after a time, to longer-term transitional housing where they may stay for a year or two until they find permanent alternate housing.

Finally, a shortage of housing may simply make it too difficult to provide temporary shelter to women in crisis. Many advocacy groups operate crisis centers and hotlines as alternative ways to provide assistance to women in crisis.

Shelter Policies

Developing policies that both ensure the residents' autonomy and also foster order within the shelter can be difficult. Where necessary for the shelter's existence and residents' well-being and safety, rules are entirely appropriate.

At the same time, however, rules should not be so restrictive as to endanger women or undermine their ability to protect themselves. The residents have likely just left relationships in which they did not have control or autonomy; it is critical that the shelter does not replicate that dynamic by trying to control all aspects of the residents' conduct or denying them the ability to make choices about their lives. Rules that severely restrict resident autonomy do not empower women to evaluate their options and make the decisions they need to make about their lives.

Residents of a shelter often contribute to the shelter's maintenance. Some shelters develop rules that require certain levels of participation while others seek women's participation on their own terms. Women's Advocates addresses resident participation by developing a task list and then asking each woman to choose a task that she prefers to do; she is not assigned a responsibility by someone else.

Linda A. Osmundson, executive director of Florida's Center Against Spouse Abuse, provides a thoughtful discussion of these issues in her article, "Shelter Rules: Who Needs Them?" Based on her experience in running a shelter, she cautions against overly stringent rules. She maintains that before instituting new rules, shelter staff should ask: "Is this rule respectful?" and "Does this rule increase safety?" The rule should be instituted only if the answer to both questions is "yes."

Address Policies

Some shelters work to ensure resident security by keeping the shelter's location a secret; residents and staff are instructed not to reveal the address of the shelter. Many women are stalked and killed by their former partners after they leave. Being able to keep their location a secret not only protects women from these batterers but can also enhance their feeling of being safe.

Efforts to maintain an unknown address can be difficult, however, and are often frustrated by outside parties. Some government agencies where women go to seek financial or other assistance may not keep the address a secret. Some schools, after receiving the address where the woman and her children are staying, have policies of calling the woman's husband to inform him of his wife and children's location. Attempting to keep the shelter location a secret can also be difficult for children, who may not understand why they cannot say where they are living. The logistics of a secret address are also difficult for the residents; they may have to walk a number of blocks before they may call a cab or access public transportation in order to avoid revealing the location of the shelter.

Other shelters have adopted an open address strategy. Women's Advocates, for example, switched from a secret to an open address. They believed that maintaining an unknown address increased residents' feelings of insecurity and powerlessness. Another shelter in Minnesota adopted an open address policy because they had found that keeping the location a secret reinforced residents' feelings of shame and humiliation in connection with the violence. The positive relationship Women's Advocates has developed with its neighbors also helps to further resident safety; the shelter's neighbors are aware of the residents' security concerns and often inform the shelter if they notice suspicious activity.

In open address shelters, while residents do not generally reveal their location to their husbands, the shelter's address is listed in the local phone directory and on shelter brochures. Some shelters that have the advantage of being a part of a network of shelters can move a resident from one shelter to another if her batterer discovers her location. In these networks, while the locations of the individual shelters are known, the locations of the victims are not. Other shelters that do not have the advantage of working in a network will move a woman to safe locations (i.e., safehouses), such as an advocate's apartment, if she is located by her abuser.

The actual location of the shelter, however, is critical. A location near public transportation lines allows women to visit the necessary agencies or law enforcement offices. Not all shelters should be located in large cities; rural women often suffer from severe isolation, may not be aware of the existence of shelters in the city, or may not be able to reach them.

Security and Confidentiality

Shelter security is a vital issue for the residents; women may be in serious danger of being found and harmed by their partners. Security concerns can be addressed in a number of ways. First, shelters should take precautions to protect residents' safety and confidentiality, such as not disclosing information about residents to anyone and restricting access to resident files. (Residents should be able to access their own files, however.)

Where funding is available, shelters have installed electronic security systems. Women's Advocates, for example, has a security system that can be activated from any floor of the house. Yet security systems are only as useful as the police that respond to alarms, and like domestic violence victims, shelters may not receive adequate protection from police. Women's Advocates, for example, found that the police arrived thirty to forty minutes after they were called because their calls were classified as "domestic disturbances." The women met repeatedly with the local police department in order to obtain a more immediate response to its calls for assistance. Although these meetings were unsuccessful, the shelter eventually obtained better responses from the police department by lobbying the mayor's office.

Finally, to increase resident safety, Women's Advocates also worked with a city attorney to create an agreement between the city and the shelter that stated that the shelter had the right to deny fathers access to the property even though their children were staying at the shelter.

Children

Shelters in the United States focused on supporting and assisting battered women and did not initially pay much attention to the needs of the children who arrived with these women. Gradually, however, they learned more about the effects of domestic violence on children, and began developing special advocacy and support programs designed for children.

Internal Structure

Different shelters organize themselves in different ways; the organization of a shelter should be driven by the shelter's specific needs.

For example, Women's Advocates operates as a collective; there is no hierarchical division of labor, and all staff members participate in decisions equally. In its first few years of operation, all staff participated in all tasks equally; now, the shelter's work is organized by task forces for business and administration, children's programs, and women's programs. Women's Advocates notes that while the task force structure has increased internal efficiency, it has reduced the flow of information within the organization. In addition, the new structure does not allow (or require!) staff to develop new skills as readily as was possible when all staff participated in all tasks.

Other shelters have a board of directors that makes the long-term, directional decisions for the shelter, while day-to-day decisions are made by staff (either in a collective or hierarchical structure). Often, this board is structured to reflect the ethnic composition of the community served by the shelter, to ensure that decisions are attentive to the needs of the clients. Other shelters have combined a board composed of residents and staff that makes long-term decisions with another board that provides guidance but has no decision-making authority.

Staffing

Some shelters require staff to have professional training, some do not. Most, however, provide on-the-job training for both staff and volunteers. Staff and volunteers generally receive training when they start working at the shelter; most shelters also provide "in-service" training at monthly, quarterly, or bi-yearly intervals. Shelters also provide staff and volunteers with opportunities to exchange information and experiences; these opportunities should happen more often than training, and can, for example, be part of a weekly or bi-weekly staff meeting. Training is also vital in ensuring continuity of information; while this may not be as crucial if there is low turnover, such efforts are absolutely necessary when new staff is beginning to make sure institutional knowledge is not lost. Ensuring that staff have opportunities to exchange experiences with one another also helps to guard against staff burnout.

Record Keeping

Adequate record keeping can serve a number of functions for shelters and safehouses (as well as for hotlines). First, an initial description of a new resident's situation can be made available to staff members, so that staff members who may not have been present when the woman arrived do not need to ask the resident again about her situation. Second, this information helps advocates remain up-to-date on the needs of battered women in the community. Third, these records can be an important advocacy tool. Documenting the number of women who use the service, for example, can help establish a need for the service that can be used in funding applications. Statistics can also be useful in conducting community education efforts; they can help to further the public's awareness of the prevalence and seriousness of the problem.

Additional Services

Different shelters offer different services; some offer solely temporary housing, while others also provide healthcare services, legal advice, job training, and counseling. Most offer women assistance in obtaining social and medical services.

Adapted from Women's Advocates, The Story of a Shelter (1980); National Coalition Against Domestic Violence, *Guidelines for Starting a Shelter.*

Notes

1. From R. Emerson Dobash & Russel P. Dobash, *Women, Violence and Social Change* 76–77 (1992).

Section 40.3

What to Expect If You Contact a Program, Shelter, or Advocate

Excerpted from "Get Help Now," © 2012 Washington State
Coalition Against Domestic Violence (www.wscadv.org). All rights
reserved. Reprinted with permission.

What to Expect If You Call a Program

- **A caring listening ear:** All programs have people who can listen and help you sort out options.

- **Advocacy services:** Most programs have specially trained advocates who can help with welfare, child protective services (CPS), disability services, immigration, housing, employment protections, and more.

- **Emergency shelter:** Many programs offer shelter or safe homes.

- **Transitional housing:** Some programs have longer-term housing for survivors.

- **Support groups:** Some programs run groups for children, youth, and adults.

- **Legal advocacy:** Most programs offer information about protection orders and other civil matters. Most do not provide legal counsel, but can refer you to free or low-cost attorneys.

- **Crisis services:** Many programs offer twenty-four-hour crisis services.

What to Expect If You Go to a Shelter

Every shelter is different, but usually you can expect that:

- Shelters are free — no fees are charged to stay.

- Most shelters have shared kitchens, common areas, and bathrooms.

500

- If you have children, you will probably all share one bedroom.

- If you are alone, you may have to share a room.

- You are responsible for taking care of your own children.

- All shelters must welcome service animals.

- However, most shelters cannot accommodate pets. They will work with you to make arrangements to have your pets cared for elsewhere.

- Shelters have laundry facilities and supply linens (sheets, towels, and blankets).

- They usually have emergency food, clothing, and toiletries available for the first few days of a stay.

- Shelters can be stressful—this is group living with others who are experiencing tough times.

- You will be asked to honor the privacy of other residents by not discussing their names or situations with anyone else.

- Shelters are concerned about everybody's safety, so you may be asked to keep the location a secret.

- Visitors are generally not allowed.

Some shelters:

- allow you to bring your pets;

- have computers you can use to check your email and access online resources;

- offer free cell phones for 911 calls only.

Before you call a shelter, think about the things that are of biggest concern to you. Ask for all the details you need so you'll feel as comfortable as possible making your important decisions.

What to Expect If You Call a Legal Advocate

When you talk to a legal advocate, you can expect that:

- services are offered free of charge:

- legal advocates are not attorneys and will be unable to give legal advice;

- advocates can offer a range of services that might include:
  - accompanying you to court;
  - helping you fill out paperwork;
  - helping you understand the civil or criminal process;
  - outlining or prioritizing the legal options that are available;
  - informing you about what actually goes on in court;
  - preparing you for a hearing or trial, and giving support before, during, and after;
  - referring you to low or no-cost lawyers.

Chapter 41

Safety Planning for Victims of Domestic Violence

Chapter Contents

Section 41.1

Personal Safety Planning

The following strategies can be used to prepare for the possibility of further violence. Although you do not have control over your partner's violence, you do have a choice about how to respond and how to get yourself and your children/pets to safety. Remember, leaving an abusive relationship is the most dangerous time for a survivor. Take all threats of harm seriously and follow precautions if and when you are leaving or ending the relationship.

Safety Strategies When Living in a Violent Atmosphere

Try some or all of these safety strategies to leave safely or get help quickly:

- Place your purse, wallet, and keys in a safe and accessible place to leave quickly.

- As difficult as it may seem, inform family, friends, and neighbors about the violence and request that they call the police if they hear or see suspicious behaviors.

- Teach your children how to contact the police and the fire department. Be careful about placing responsibility on the children.

- Choose a code word for friends and children to communicate to them you need help.

- When you sense you are in danger, *get out*! You can go back later if you wish. You have the right to change your mind.

Safety When Preparing to Leave

When you decide to leave, it must be done with a careful plan in order to increase your personal safety. Abusers often become violent when they believe their partner is leaving the relationship. Try some or all of these strategies to get out safely and quickly:

- Store copies of important documents (medical records, birth certificates, social security cards, bank statements, etc) in a safe place.

- Make copies of vehicle and house keys.

- Open an individual savings account for financial independence and establishing credit.

- Keep your vehicle's fuel tank full.

- Pack a bag of belongings and store it in a safe location.

- Keep important phone numbers and addresses with you at all times.

- Pay attention to the abusive person's behavior during violent episodes to determine the best place to store your items in order to make a quick exit.

- Get involved with a domestic violence program in your community for support and counseling.

- Encourage the abusive person to consider counseling at a certified Batterer's Intervention and Prevention Program (BIPP) or similar program. Caution: Couples' counseling is *not* appropriate for violent couples. This can be dangerous for the nonabusive partner. Anger management classes alone will not end the abuse.

- Build a strong support system. Educate yourself about resources in the community and become educated on finances.

- Let family and friends know what is happening. Learn to feel good about yourself and your ability to handle this difficult situation.

- Treat yourself kindly. Be positive about yourself.

- Define and develop a healthy relationship to practice on yourself and your children.

- Remember you are never to blame for the abuse and violence in the relationship.

- Teach children nonviolent problem solving.

- Be honest with your children. Let them know that what is happening is wrong. Tell them they are not responsible for the abusive behavior. Let them know that staying does not condone the violence.

- Accept the abuse as real and dangerous. Minimizing it may cost you your life.

- Use these ideas to develop an action plan with goals, strategies, and time frames for achieving each goal. Write your plan down and be specific and realistic.

Safety When Establishing a New Residence

Try some or all of these strategies when establishing your own residence. When renting, speak with the landlord to see if he or she will install some or all of the security options. While not all strategies may be financially realistic for you, try to adopt similar precautionary measures when possible:

- Make sure the area around your home is well lit at night. If not, install outside motion detector lighting that turns on when a person approaches.

- Make sure the front of your residence is visible during the daytime.

- Install additional security systems, including deadbolt locks, poles to wedge against doors, and/or an electronic monitoring system.

- Purchase fire ladders if you live on or have a second floor. Fire ladders are available at hardware and discount stores.

- Vary your route to and from work, shop at different stores, and alter your daily routines to reduce your chances of being stalked.

- Purchase an answering machine, caller ID, or voicemail to screen calls. Block unidentified numbers and your abuser's telephone number.

- Keep a phone log. If the abuser calls you, save the messages left by him or her.

- Tell your children's caretakers who has permission to pick them up and that your partner is not permitted to do so.

- Ask the police department to perform a home safety check for recommendations.

Safety Planning for Your Pets

Pets can be used as leverage by the abusive person to keep you from leaving; plan for your pet's safety:

- Take the dog for a daily walk, if possible, to learn the layout of the neighborhood.

- Collect these items and store in a safe place for quick access when you leave: proof of legal ownership of the animal, a leash and/or carrier container, animal's medications, a favorite blanket and toy, and an information sheet with important facts about the animal and its needs.

- Tell anyone sheltering your animals to keep their location secret.

- Feminists for Animal Rights Companion Animal Rescue Effort (C.A.R.E.) operates a nationwide free foster home program.

Section 41.2

Safety Packing List

Excerpted from "Safety Planning for Abusive Situations," U.S. Department of Health and Human Services Office on Women's Health, May 18, 2011.

If you are leaving an abusive situation, take your children and, if possible, your pets. Put together the items listed below. Hide them someplace where you can get them quickly, or leave them with a friend. If you are in immediate danger, though, leave without these items.

Safety Packing List

- Identification for yourself and your children

- Birth certificates

- Social Security cards (or numbers written on paper if you can't find the cards)

- Driver's license

- Photo identification or passports
- Welfare benefits card
- Green card

Important Papers

- Marriage certificate
- Divorce papers
- Custody orders
- Legal protection or restraining orders
- Health insurance papers and medical cards
- Medical records for all family members
- Children's school records
- Investment papers/records and account numbers
- Work permits
- Immigration papers
- Rental agreement/lease or house deed
- Car title, registration, and insurance information
- Records of police reports you have filed or other evidence of abuse

Money and Other Ways to Get By

- Cash
- Credit cards
- Automated teller machine (ATM) card
- Checkbook and bankbook (with deposit slips)
- Jewelry or small objects you can sell

Keys

- House
- Car
- Safety deposit box or post office box

Ways to Communicate

- Phone calling card
- Cell phone
- Address book

Note: Don't share a calling card or cell phone plan with an abuser, because they can be used to find you. And if you already have a shared card or phone plan, try not to use them after you've left.

Medications

- At least one month's supply for all medicines you and your children are taking
- A copy of any prescriptions

Things to Help You Cope

- Pictures
- Keepsakes
- Children's small toys or books

Section 41.3

Child Safety Planning

When you're a parent in an unhealthy or abusive relationship, it makes a difficult situation even harder. Not only do you have to worry about your safety, but you also have to consider your child's well-being.

Witnessing domestic and dating violence can have a huge impact on children, both physically and psychologically. They may grow up believing that domestic violence is normal and mimic the behaviors they witnessed in their parents' relationship. If you're involved in an unhealthy or abusive relationship, it's important to get help.

What Can I Do?

Making the decision to leave is very hard, especially if you have a child with your abusive partner. Whether or not you are ready or able to leave, you can take steps to help keep you and your child safe. If you stay:

- Prepare a safety plan with your child and try to follow it whenever possible. Arrange a safe place for your children to go and plan a code word to let them know when they should leave and where to get help. It's also important to tell them that their job is to stay safe, not protect you.

- Make sure your child knows the abuse isn't their fault and violence is never ok, even when someone they love is being abusive.

- Pack a bag you can take with you in an emergency—be sure to include important documentation for you and your children and anything your kids may need (formula, medicine, diapers, birth certificates, immigration papers). Keep the bag hidden in a safe place or leave it with someone you trust.

- Memorize all important numbers in case you have to leave without your phone.

If You Leave

- Talk to an attorney about your state's custody laws. Consider getting a protection order. It may award you temporary custody of your children and help with your longer-term plans.

- Call the police if you and your children need immediate protection. Be sure to get a police report to use as evidence in your custody case.

You know what is best for your child. If you can't leave your partner because you fear for your or your child's safety, you should contact a resource in your community to discuss your options right away.

Section 41.4

Safety in Court

"Safety in Court," reprinted with permission from www.WomensLaw.org. © 2012 National Network to End Domestic Violence. All rights reserved. Citations in the original WomensLaw.org content were omitted for this reprinting. For additional information and resources, visit http://www.womens law.org or http://nnedv.org.

After you have left an abusive relationship, there may be many occasions where you will have to see the abuser in court to deal with a protection order, custody, child support, divorce, or criminal proceedings. Since you are in a courthouse surrounded by people and even court officers, you may feel like it is okay to let your guard down. However, please remember that any time you come into contact with the abuser, you have to take steps to protect yourself. Here are some tips to help keep you as safe as possible.

Following these suggestions (often known as a safety plan) can't guarantee your safety, but it could help make you safer. However, it is important that you create a safety plan that is right for you. Not all of these suggestions will work for everyone, and some could even place you in greater danger. You have to do what you think is best to keep yourself and your children safe.

Getting to the Courthouse

- Try to get to court at a different time than you think the abuser will arrive to avoid seeing him/her on the street or in line to enter the court. If the abuser is always late, try arriving early. If the abuser always arrives early, try arriving closer to your hearing time or come with a friend. Remember: make sure to leave plenty of time to get through the lines, metal detectors, etc., so that you get to the hearing on time. If you are late, the case may be called without you and dismissed. Finding a domestic violence advocate to go with you can really help with safety. Call the National Domestic Violence Hotline (800-799-SAFE) to find help near you.

- See if your police department or sheriff's department will take you to the courthouse. Meet them somewhere other than the courthouse and then ask the officer to walk you inside. Have the officer wait with you until you find the bailiff or courthouse security and let them know your situation. Try to sit near the court officers or security guards if you can.

- Bring a friend or family member with you so you won't have to be alone at all during the day.

- If your friend or family member cannot spend the day in court with you, ask that person to drive you to court. It's best to get someone whose car the abuser doesn't know. Ask him/her to drop you off at the courthouse entrance so you don't have to walk alone through the parking lot.

- If you have to drive yourself, try to make your car unrecognizable. If you can, borrow or rent a car that the abuser doesn't know. If you drive your own car, you might want to consider covering it with a protective car-cover, if this is a popular thing to do in your neighborhood. (However, if your car is the only one covered, it may actually draw the abuser's attention to it, which is the opposite of what you want.)

Once You're Inside the Courthouse

- Stay together with whoever came with you while inside the courthouse. Ask your friend/family member person to keep an eye on the surroundings and pay attention to safety considerations. If you need to use the bathroom and it has a lot of stalls, ask your friend/ family member to come into the bathroom with you. If your friend/ family member is the opposite sex than you, ask him/her to wait outside the bathroom for you.

- Find someone who knows the courthouse well, like a domestic violence worker or someone who works at the courthouse. Ask them about safe places you can sit where you will be close to courthouse security but where you will still hear your name called when they call your case. Ask them where all the exits are, in case you have to leave in a hurry. Besides the main exit, there may be exits through the courtrooms, side exits, or fire exits that you could use in an emergency.

- Ask the bailiff or courthouse security to keep the abuser away from you. Let the bailiff or courthouse security know if the abuser sits near you or tries to harass you. If you have a restraining order, remember that the order is still in effect while you are in the courthouse. If the abuser violates the order while in the waiting room or in line to the courthouse, you can report it to a court officer or call the police.

Leaving the Courthouse

- At the end of your hearing, ask the judge or the court officer/ bailiff to "detain" the abuser. In other words, to hold him/her until you can leave.

- If the judge doesn't detain the abuser, think about letting the abuser leave the courthouse first, then wait a long time before leaving and try to leave out of a different exit than the main exit. However, even if you wait a long time, be aware that the abuser could still be out there waiting for you, so be observant.

- Have a police officer or sheriff walk out of the courthouse with you and walk you to your car.

- Have a friend pick you up at the exit or if you had a friend/family member come with you, make sure that s/he walks to your car with you.

513

Chapter 42

Protecting Your Pet

Chapter Contents

Section 42.1

Understanding the Link between Domestic Violence and Animal Abuse

Excerpted from "Understanding the Link Between Animal Abuse and Family Violence," © 2012 American Humane Association (www.american humane.org). All rights reserved. Reprinted with permission.

What Is the Link?

A correlation between animal abuse, family violence, and other forms of community violence has been established. Child and animal protection professionals have recognized this link, noting that abuse of both children and animals is connected in a self-perpetuating cycle of violence. When animals in a home are abused or neglected, it is a warning sign that others in the household may not be safe. In addition, children who witness animal abuse are at a greater risk of becoming abusers themselves.

How Serious Is It?

A survey of pet-owning families with substantiated child abuse and neglect found that animals were abused in 88 percent of homes where child physical abuse was present (DeViney, Dickert, & Lockwood, 1983). A study of women seeking shelter at a safe house showed that 71 percent of those having pets affirmed that their partner had threatened, hurt, or killed their companion animals, and 32 percent of mothers reported that their children had hurt or killed their pets (Ascione, 1998). Still another study showed that violent offenders incarcerated in a maximum-security prison were significantly more likely than nonviolent offenders to have committed childhood acts of cruelty toward pets (Merz-Perez, Heide, & Silverman, 2001).

What's Being Done?

In many communities, human services, animal services, and law enforcement agencies are sharing resources and expertise to address violence. Professionals are beginning to engage in cross-training and cross-reporting through inter-agency partnerships. Humane societies are also teaming with domestic violence shelters to provide emergency shelter for pets of domestic violence victims. In addition, some states have strengthened their animal-cruelty legislation and taken other measures to address the link. These state-level actions permit earlier intervention and send a clear message that all forms of violence are taken seriously. For example:

- There are now felony-level penalties for animal cruelty in nearly all states.

- Several states require veterinarians to report suspected animal abuse and offer veterinarians who report cruelty immunity from civil and criminal liability.

- Some states require animal control officers to report suspected child abuse or neglect and receive training in recognizing and reporting child abuse and neglect.

- A few states permit child and adult protection workers to report suspected animal abuse or receive training on identifying and reporting animal cruelty, abuse, and neglect.

- Nearly half the states call for psychological counseling for individuals convicted of animal cruelty.

References

Ascione, F. R. (1998). Battered women's reports of their partners' and their children's cruelty to animals. *Journal of Emotional Abuse*, 1(1), 119–33.

DeViney, E., Dickert, J., & Lockwood, R. (1998). The care of pets within child abusing families. In R. Lockwood & F. R. Ascione, (Eds.), *Cruelty to animals and interpersonal violence*. West Lafayette, IN: Purdue University Press. (Reprinted from *International Journal for the Study of Animal Problems*, 4, (1983) 321–29.)

Merz-Perez, L., Heide, K. M., & Silverman, I. J. (2001). Childhood cruelty to animals and subsequent violence against humans. *International Journal of Offender Therapy and Comparative Criminology*, 45(5), 556–73.

Resources

American Humane's National Resource Center on the Link. www.americanhumane.org/link or 800-227-4645.

Ascione, F. R. (2001). Animal abuse and youth violence. *OJJDP Juvenile Justice Bulletin.*

Ascione, F. R., & Arkow, P. (Eds.). (1999). *Child abuse, domestic violence, and animal abuse: Linking the circles of compassion for prevention and intervention.* West Lafayette, IN: Purdue University Press.

Barnard, S. (1999). Taking animal abuse seriously: A human services perspective. In F. R. Ascione & P. Arkow (Eds.), *Child abuse, domestic violence, and animal abuse: Linking the circles of compassion for prevention and intervention* (pp. 101–8). West Lafayette, IN: Purdue University Press.

Boat, B. W. (1999). Abuse of children and abuse of animals: Using the links to inform child assessment and protection. In F. R. Ascione & P. Arkow (Eds.), *Child abuse, domestic violence, and animal abuse: Linking the circles of compassion for prevention and intervention* (pp. 83–100). West Lafayette, IN: Purdue University Press.

Lockwood, R., & Ascione, F. R. (Eds.). (1998). *Cruelty to animals and interpersonal violence: Readings in research and application.* West Lafayette, IN: Purdue University Press.

PSYETA AniCare and AniCare Child models of treatment of animal abuse. http://www.psyeta.org/

Section 42.2

Facts about Animal Abuse and Domestic Violence: Some Statistics

Why it Matters

- Seventy-one percent of pet-owning women entering women's shelters reported that their batterer had injured, maimed, killed, or threatened family pets for revenge or to psychologically control victims; 32 percent reported their children had hurt or killed animals.

- Sixty-eight percent of battered women reported violence towards their animals. Eighty-seven percent of these incidents occurred in the presence of the women, and 75 percent in the presence of the children, to psychologically control and coerce them.

- Thirteen percent of intentional animal abuse cases involve domestic violence.

- Between 25 percent and 40 percent of battered women are unable to escape abusive situations because they worry about what will happen to their pets or livestock, should they leave.

- Pets may suffer unexplained injuries, health problems, or permanent disabilities at the hands of abusers, or disappear from home.

- Abusers kill, harm, or threaten children's pets to coerce them into sexual abuse or to force them to remain silent about abuse. Disturbed children kill or harm animals to emulate their parents' conduct, to prevent the abuser from killing the pet, or to take out their aggressions on another victim.

- In one study, 70 percent of animal abusers also had records for other crimes. Domestic violence victims whose animals were abused saw the animal cruelty as one more violent episode

519

in a long history of indiscriminate violence aimed at them and their vulnerability.

- Investigation of animal abuse is often the first point of social services intervention for a family in trouble.

- For many battered women, pets are sources of comfort, providing strong emotional support: 98 percent of Americans consider pets to be companions or members of the family.

- Animal cruelty problems are people problems. When animals are abused, people are at risk.

Did You Know?

- More American households have pets than have children. We spend more money on pet food than on baby food. There are more dogs in the United States than people in most countries in Europe—and more cats than dogs.

- A child growing up in the United States is more likely to have a pet than a live-at-home father.

- Pets live most frequently in homes with children: 64.1 percent of homes with children under age six, and 74.8 percent of homes with children over age six, have pets. The woman is the primary caregiver in 72.8 percent of pet-owning households.

- Battered women have been known to live in their cars with their pets for as long as four months until an opening was available at a pet-friendly safe house.

State Animal Cruelty Laws

Anti-cruelty laws exist in all U.S. states and territories to prohibit unnecessary killing, mutilating, torturing, beating, neglecting, and abandoning of animals, or depriving them of proper food, water, or shelter. Animal cruelty cases may be investigated by a local humane society, Society for the Prevention of Cruelty to Animals (SPCA), or animal control agency or, in areas where these organizations are not present, by police or sheriff's departments. When an investigation un-covers enough evidence to warrant prosecution, charges may be filed by the local district or state's attorney. Often, only the most serious cases generate sufficient sympathy and evidence to warrant prosecu-tion, and gaining convictions may be very difficult.

If You Need Help

Contact your local humane society, SPCA, animal control agency, or veterinarian to see if they have temporary foster care facilities for pets belonging to battered women.

What You Can Do

- Have your pets vaccinated against rabies, and license your pets with your town or county; make sure these registrations are in your name to help prove your ownership.

- Consider and plan for the safety and welfare of your animals. Do not leave pets with your abuser. Be prepared to take your pets with you: many women's shelters have established "safe haven" foster care programs for the animal victims of domestic violence.

- Alternatively, arrange temporary shelter for your pets with a veterinarian, family member, trusted friend, or local animal shelter.

What Advocates Can Do for Battered Women with Pets

- Add questions about the presence of pets and their welfare to shelter intake questionnaires and risk assessments.

- Work with animal shelters, veterinarians, and rescue groups to establish "safe haven" foster care programs for the animal victims of domestic violence; some women's shelters have building kennels at their facilities.

- Include provisions for pets in safety planning strategies.

- Help your clients to prove ownership of their animals.

- Help victims to retrieve animals left behind.

- Include animals in abuse prevention orders.

- Help victims find pet-friendly transitional and permanent housing.

- When victims can no longer care for their pets, make referrals to animal adoption agencies.

- Establish community coalitions against family violence that include humane societies, SPCAs, animal control agencies, and veterinarians. Invite representatives from these agencies to train your staff on how animal abuse cases are investigated and prosecuted: offer to train their staffs and volunteers about domestic violence issues.

Resources

Arkow, P. (2003). *Breaking the Cycles of Violence: A Guide to Multidisciplinary Interventions. A Handbook for Child Protection, Domestic Violence and Animal Protection Agencies*. Alameda, CA: Latham Foundation.

Ascione, F.R. (2000). *Safe Havens for Pets: Guidelines for Programs Sheltering Pets for Women Who Are Battered*. Logan, UT: Utah State University. FrankA@coe.usu.edu

Ascione, F. R., & Arkow, P. (eds.) (1999). *Child Abuse, Domestic Violence and Animal Abuse: Linking the Circles of Compassion for Prevention and Intervention*. West Lafayette, IN: Purdue University Press, 1999.

Duel, Debra (2004). *Violence Prevention & Intervention: A Directory of Animal-Related Programs*. Washington, DC: Humane Society of the U.S.

Maxwell, M. S. & O'Rourke, K. (2000). *Domestic Violence: A Competency-Based Training Manual for Florida's Animal Abuse Investigators*. Tallahassee: Florida State University Institute for Family Violence Studies.

National Crime Prevention Council (2003). *50 Strategies to Prevent Violent Domestic Crimes: Screening Animal Cruelty Cases for Domestic Violence*. Washington, DC.

Sources

1. Ascione, F.R., Weber, C. V. & Wood, D. S. (1997). The abuse of animals and domestic violence: A national survey of shelters for women who are battered. *Society & Animals* 5(3), 205–18.

2. Quinlisk, J.A. (1999). Animal Abuse and Family Violence. In, Ascione, F. R. & Arkow, P., eds.: *Child Abuse, Domestic Violence, and Animal Abuse: Linking the Circles of Compassion for Prevention and Intervention*. West Lafayette, IN: Purdue University Press, pp. 168–75.

3. Humane Society of the U.S. (2001). 2000 Report of Animal Cruelty Cases. Washington, DC.

4. Arkow, P. (2003). *Breaking the cycles of violence: A guide to multi-disciplinary interventions. A handbook for child protection, domestic violence and animal protection agencies.* Alameda, CA: Latham Foundation.

5. McIntosh, S. (2001). Calgary research results: Exploring the links between animal abuse and domestic violence. *Latham Letter* 22(4), 14–16.

6. Arkow, P. (1994). Animal abuse and domestic violence: Intake statistics tell a sad story. *Latham Letter* 15(2), 17.

7. Jorgensen, S. & Maloney, L. (1999). Animal abuse and the victims of domestic violence. In, F. R. Ascione & P. Arkow, eds.: *Child Abuse, Domestic Violence, and Animal Abuse: Linking the Circles of Compassion for Prevention and Intervention.* West Lafayette, IN: Purdue University Press, pp. 143–58.

8. Loar, L. (1999). "I'll only help you if you have two legs," or, Why human services professionals should pay attention to cases involving cruelty to animals. In, Ascione, F. R. & Arkow, P., eds.: *Child Abuse, Domestic Violence, and Animal Abuse: Linking the Circles of Compassion for Prevention and Intervention.* West Lafayette, IN: Purdue University Press, 1999, pp. 120–36.

9. Ascione, F. R. (2005). *Children and Animals: Exploring the Roots of Kindness and Cruelty.* West Lafayette, IN: Purdue University Press, 2005.

10. Luke, C., Arluke, A., & Levin, J. (1998). *Cruelty to Animals and Other Crimes: A Study by the MSPCA and Northeastern University.* Boston: MSPCA.

11. American Veterinary Medical Association (2003): *U.S. Pet Ownership & Demographics Sourcebook.* Schaumburg, IL: AVMA.

12. Arkow, P. (1996). The relationships between animal abuse and other forms of family violence. *Family Violence & Sexual Assault Bulletin* 12(1–2), 29–34.

13. American Pet Products Manufacturers Association: Industry Statistics & Trends (http://www.appma.org/); Baby Food & Drink US (http://www.marketresearch.com/); Annie E. Casey Foundation/Kids Count Census Data Online (http://www.aecf.org/)

14. Melson, G.F. (2001). *Why the Wild Things Are: Animals in the Lives of Children.* Cambridge: Harvard University Press.

15. Kogan, L.R., McConnell, S., Schoenfeld-Tacher, R., & Jansen-Lock, P. (2004). Crosstrails: A unique foster program to provide safety for pets of women in safehouses. *Violence Against Women* 10, 418–34.

16. Lacroix, C. A. (1999). Another weapon for combating family violence: Prevention of animal abuse. In, F. R. Ascione & P. Arkow, eds.: *Child Abuse, Domestic Violence, and Animal Abuse: Linking the Circles of Compassion for Prevention and Intervention.* West Lafayette, IN: Purdue University Press, pp. 62–80.

17. Frasch, P. D., Otto, S. K., Olsen, K. M., & Ernest, P. A. (1999). State animal anti-cruelty statutes: An overview. *Animal Law* 5, 69–80.

Section 42.3

Frequently Asked Questions about Animal Abuse and Domestic Violence

Excerpted from "The Connection between Domestic Violence and Animal Cruelty," copyright 2012 The American Society for the Prevention of Cruelty to Animals (ASPCA). All rights reserved.

Why Do Abusers Batter Animals?

- To demonstrate power and control over the family
- To isolate the victim and children
- To enforce submission
- To perpetuate an environment of fear
- To prevent the victim from leaving or coerce her to return
- To punish for leaving or showing independence

What Can Law Enforcement Do?

It is imperative that first responders understand the connection between animal abuse and family violence. When responding to domestic calls it is imperative to be alert for signs that children and/or pets might be victimized. Children may be more willing to discuss what has happened to a pet than their own victimization.

Victims and their children should be asked:

- Do you have any pets?

- Has the batterer or anyone else threatened to harm your pet?

- Will you need assistance in finding a safe place for the pet if you leave?

Be sure to document any signs of animal abuse and report it to the appropriate agency empowered to investigate animal cruelty. Many victims will not go forward with the prosecution of their abuser. However, prosecution on animal cruelty charges can result in incarceration or treatment equivalent to what might result from a domestic violence prosecution.

What Can Victim Advocates and Domestic Violence Shelters Do?

- Work with victims to be sure they include pets in their safety planning.

- Include questions about any threats or injuries to pets on your intake questionnaires.

- Work with legislators to insure that pets can be included in orders of protection and educate judges about the necessity to do so.

- Work with your local humane organizations or animal control to establish programs for the emergency housing of pets coming from homes experiencing violence.

What Can Animal Shelters and Humane Organizations Do?

- Reach out to local domestic violence shelters and establish programs for emergency housing of pets from homes with domestic violence.

- If no space is available, work with animal foster care agencies to establish a network of homes that might provide emergency care for these pets.

- Incorporate information on these connections in school programs, particularly those that might reach children at risk of family violence.

Legal Protections for Animal Victims of Domestic Violence

Sadly, victims of domestic violence often remain in dangerous or dysfunctional relationships to protect their pets. A study of women seeking temporary "safe haven" shelter showed that 71 percent of those having companion animals reported that their partners had threatened, hurt, or killed their animals. It is likewise well documented that many more abuse victims never even go to a shelter because they fear for the safety of the pets they must leave behind.

In recognition of this phenomenon, several states have passed laws that (1) empower judges to include pets in court-issued orders of protection; and/or (2) include the harm or threat of harm to animals in the state's legal definition of "domestic violence."

Conclusion

Animal cruelty is increasingly viewed as a serious issue by professionals in law enforcement and mental health—as well as by the general public. The effective prosecution of animal abuse has many benefits. It can provide an early and timely response to those who are, or who are risk of becoming, a threat to the safety of others. It can provide an added tool for the protection of those who are victims of family violence. Finally, it can bring personal satisfaction in developing new skills and new understanding, and helping build a truly compassionate society.

Section 42.4

How to Report Animal Cruelty

Find out who is responsible for investigating and enforcing the anti-cruelty codes in your town, county, and/or state. These people typically work for your local humane organization, animal control agency, taxpayer-funded animal shelter, or police precinct.

If you run into trouble finding the correct agency to contact, you should call or visit your local police department and ask for their help in enforcing the law. If your local police department is unable to assist, ask your local shelter or animal control agency for advice. To find contact information for your local shelter, visit the ASPCA's searchable database of nearly five thousand organizations at http://www.aspca .org/adoption/shelters.

Section 42.5

Protection for Pets in Domestic Violence Protection Orders

"Domestic Violence and Pets: List of States that Include Pets in Protection Orders," © 2012 Reprinted with permission from Michigan State University College of Law, Animal Legal and Historical website, www.animallaw.info, researched by Rebecca Wisch.

Note that twenty-two states (as well as D.C. and Puerto Rico) to date (2012) have enacted legislation that includes provisions for pets in DV protection orders.

Arizona

AZ ST § 13-3602; A. R. S. § 13-3602
This Arizona law provides that, if a court issues an order of protection, the court may grant the petitioner the exclusive care, custody, or control of any animal that is owned, possessed, leased, kept, or held by the petitioner, the respondent, or a minor child residing in the residence or household of the petitioner or the respondent, and order the respondent to stay away from the animal and forbid the respondent from taking, transferring, encumbering, concealing, committing an act of cruelty or neglect in violation of section 13- 2910, or otherwise disposing of the animal.

Arkansas

AR ST § 9-15-205; A.C.A. § 9-15-205
Upon a finding of domestic abuse, a court may "[d]irect the care, custody, or control of any pet owned, possessed, leased, kept, or held by either party residing in the household" in an order for protection filed by a petitioner.

California

CA FAM § 6320–6327; West's Ann. Cal. Fam. Code § 6320–6327

528

On a showing of good cause, the court may include in a protective order a grant to the petitioner of the exclusive care, possession, or control of any animal owned, possessed, leased, kept, or held by either the petitioner or the respondent or a minor child residing in the residence or household of either the petitioner or the respondent.

Colorado

CO ST § 18-6-800.3; C. R. S. A. § 18-6-800.3

"Domestic violence" also includes any other crime against a person, or against property, including an animal, or any municipal ordinance violation against a person, or against property, including an animal.

District of Columbia (D.C.)

DC ST § 16-1005; DC CODE § 16-1005

This D.C. law provides that if, after a hearing, the judicial officer finds that there is good cause to believe the respondent has committed or threatened to commit a criminal offense against the petitioner or against petitioner's animal or an animal in petitioner's household, the judicial officer may issue a protection order that directs the care, custody, or control of a domestic animal that belongs to petitioner or respondent or lives in his or her household.

Connecticut

CT ST § 46b-15; C. G. S. A. § 46b-15

Under this Connecticut law, any family or household member who has been subjected to a continuous threat of present physical pain or physical injury by another family or household member or person in, or has recently been in, a dating relationship who has been subjected to a continuous threat of present physical pain or physical injury by the other person in such relationship may apply to the Superior Court for an order of protection. The court may also make orders for the protection of any animal owned or kept by the applicant including, but not limited to, an order enjoining the respondent from injuring or threatening to injure such animal.

Hawaii

HI ST § 586-4; H R S § 586-4

In Hawaii, the ex parte temporary restraining order may also enjoin or restrain both of the parties from taking, concealing, removing, threatening, physically abusing, or otherwise disposing of any animal identified to the court as belonging to a household, until further order of the court.

Illinois

IL ST CH 725 § 5/112A-14; 725 I.L.C.S. 5/112A-14

This Illinois law allows a court to issue an order of protection if the court finds that petitioner has been abused by a family or household member. It also allows for the protection of animals in domestic violence situations. The court can "[g]rant the petitioner the exclusive care, custody, or control of any animal owned, possessed, leased, kept, or held by either the petitioner or the respondent or a minor child residing in the residence or household of either the petitioner or the respondent and order the respondent to stay away from the animal and forbid the respondent from taking, transferring, encumbering, concealing, harming, or otherwise disposing of the animal."

Louisiana

LA R.S. 46:2135; LSA-R.S. 46:2135

This Louisiana law allows a court to enter a temporary restraining order, without bond, as it deems necessary to protect from abuse the petitioner. Among the provisions is one that allows the court to grant ". . . to the petitioner the exclusive care, possession, or control of any pets belonging to or under the care of the petitioner or minor children residing in the residence or household of either party, and directing the defendant to refrain from harassing, interfering with, abusing or injuring any pet, without legal justification, known to be owned, possessed, leased, kept, or held by either party or a minor child residing in the residence or household of either party."

Maine

ME ST T. 19-A § 4007; 19-A M. R. S. A. § 4007

This Maine law concerning personal protection orders in cases of abuse was amended in March of 2006 to include companion animals in protection orders. The new language specifies that a court may enter an order directing the care, custody, or control of any animal owned, possessed, leased, kept or held by either party or a minor child residing in the household.

Maryland

MD FAMILY § 4-501, 504.1; MD Code, Family Law, § 4-501, 504.1

This Maryland law amended in 2011 allows an interim protective order to award temporary possession of any pet (defined in § 4-501 as a domesticated animal except livestock) to the person eligible for relief or the respondent).

Minnesota

MN ST § 518B.01; M.S.A. § 518B.01

This law reflects Minnesota's provision for restraining orders in cases of domestic abuse. An amendment in 2010 concerns the care and keeping of a companion animal owned by either petitioner or respondent, and has a provision to allow the court to prevent harm to such animal. As stated in the law, "The order may direct the care, possession, or control of a pet or companion animal owned, possessed, or kept by the petitioner or respondent or a child of the petitioner or respondent. It may also direct the respondent to refrain from physically abusing or injuring any pet or companion animal, without legal justification, known to be owned, possessed, kept, or held by either party or a minor child residing in the residence or household of either party as an indirect means of intentionally threatening the safety of such person."

Nevada

NEV. REV. STAT. §33.018; NV ST §33.018

In Nevada, a knowing, purposeful or reckless course of conduct intended to harass the other, such as injuring or killing an animal, is included in their definition of domestic violence. A victim can then get a protection order and enjoin the adverse party from physically injuring, threatening to injure, or taking possession of any animal that is owned or kept by the applicant or minor child, either directly or through an agent.

New Jersey

On January 17, 2012, Governor Christie signed the Domestic Violence Pet Protection Law. The law authorizes courts to include pets in domestic violence restraining orders. The court is allowed to enter an order "prohibiting the defendant from having any contact with any animal owned, possessed, leased, kept or held by either party or a minor child residing in the household."

New York

NY FAM CT § 842; McKinney's Family Court Act § 842

This New York law pertains to the issuance of protection orders. In July of 2006, the amendment that allows companion animals owned by the petitioner of the order or a minor child residing in the household to be included in the order was signed into law. The law specifically allows a court to order the respondent to refrain from intentionally injuring or killing, without justification, any companion animal the respondent knows to be owned, possessed, leased, kept, or held by the petitioner or a minor child residing in the household.

North Carolina

NC ST § 50B-3; N.C.G.S.A. § 50B-3

This North Carolina law reflects the state's provision for protective orders in cases of domestic abuse. A protective order may provide for possession of personal property of the parties, including the care, custody, and control of any animal owned, possessed, kept, or held as a pet by either party or minor child residing in the household. The court may also order a party to refrain from cruelly treating or abusing an animal owned, possessed, kept, or held as a pet by either party or minor child residing in the household.

Oklahoma

OK ST T. 22 § 60.2; 22 Okl. St. Ann. § 60.2

This Oklahoma law reflects the state's provision for protective orders in cases of domestic abuse. The person seeking a protective order may further request the exclusive care, possession, or control of any animal owned, possessed, leased, kept, or held by either the petitioner, defendant, or minor child residing in the residence of the petitioner or defendant. The court may order the defendant to make no contact with the animal and forbid the defendant from taking, transferring, encumbering, concealing, molesting, attacking, striking, threatening, harming, or otherwise disposing of the animal.

Puerto Rico

PR ST T. 5 § 1678; 5 L.P.R.A. § 1678

This Puerto Rico law provides that, in all cases in which a person is accused of domestic violence or child abuse, the court shall, by petition of party, issue a protection order for the petitioner so that he/she be the sole custodian of the animal. The court shall order the accused to keep far away from the animal and prohibit contact of any kind. Violation is a fourth-degree felony.

Tennessee

TN ST §36-3-601; T. C. A. § 36-3-601
Tennessee's domestic abuse definition includes inflicting, or attempting to inflict, physical injury on any animal owned, possessed, leased, kept, or held by an adult or minor.

Vermont

VT ST T. 15 § 1103; 15 V.S.A. § 1103
Vermont law was amended to allow a court to include an order relating to the possession, care, and control of any animal owned, possessed, leased, kept, or held as a pet by either party or a minor child residing in the household in a domestic violence situation.

Washington

WA ST 26.50.060; West's RCWA 26.50.060
This Washington law reflects the state's provision for protective orders in cases of domestic abuse. In addition to other forms of relief, a court may also order possession and use of essential personal effects. Personal effects may include pets. The court may order that a petitioner be granted the exclusive custody or control of any pet owned, possessed, leased, kept, or held by the petitioner, respondent, or minor child residing with either the petitioner or respondent and may prohibit the respondent from interfering with the petitioner's efforts to remove the pet. The court may also prohibit the respondent from knowingly coming within, or knowingly remaining within, a specified distance of specified locations where the pet is regularly found.

West Virginia

WV ST § 48-27-503; W. Va. Code, § 48-27-503
In West Virginia, the terms of a protective order may include awarding the petitioner the exclusive care, possession, or control of any animal owned, possessed, leased, kept, or held by either the petitioner or the respondent or a minor child residing in the residence or household of either the petitioner or the respondent and prohibiting the

respondent from taking, concealing, molesting, physically injuring, killing, or otherwise disposing of the animal and limiting or precluding contact by the respondent with the animal.

Chapter 43

Issues in Internet Safety

Chapter Contents

Section 43.1

Cyberstalking

"Cyberstalking is threatening behavior or unwanted advances directed at another using the internet and other forms of online and computer communications."

Brief Overview

The internet is another form of communication vulnerable to abuse by stalkers. Cyberstalking can take forms such as:

- threatening/obscene emails;
- live chat harassment or flaming (online verbal abuse);
- harassment through texting;
- hacking and/or monitoring a victim's computer and internet activity;
- forming a website in honor of a victim;
- can include offline stalking/harassments such as following a victim or actual physical contact between a stalker and his/her victim.

While cyberstalking is a specific kind of stalking, the possible severity of its emotional and physical threat is similar to the fear caused by offline stalking, with the same potential consequences. As a result of their victimization, many victims have physical and emotional reactions such as:

- changes in sleeping and/or eating patterns;
- experiencing nightmares;

- feeling anxious or helpless;
- fearing for one's safety.

The use of technology to stalk is increasing due to the rapid development of technology in today's world. Like offline stalking, cyberstalking is a form of personal terrorism. Similarly, cyberstalking may precede offline stalking, sexual assault, physical violence, or even murder.

Cyberstalking Laws

Forty-six states have laws that explicitly include electronic forms of communication within stalking or harassment laws. New Jersey, New Mexico, Nebraska, Kentucky, and the District of Columbia do not have cyberstalking laws.

Prevention Tips

- Do not share personal information in public spaces anywhere online.
- Do not use your real name or nickname as your screen name or user ID. Pick a name that is gender- and age-neutral.
- Do not post personal information as part of any user profiles (i.e. Facebook, Myspace, Twitter).
- Use a "nonsense" password that has no relation to you as a person; use a combination of numbers, symbols, and letters and make sure it is at least six characters long. Also, try to change your password frequently and avoid using the same password for multiple accounts.
- Be *very* cautious about meeting online acquaintances in person. If you choose to meet, do so in a public place and take along a friend.
- Make sure that your internet service provider (ISP) and internet relay chat (IRC) network have an acceptable user policy that prohibits cyberstalking.
- If a situation online becomes hostile you should log off or surf elsewhere.
- Do not share passwords to email or social networking sites with friends or acquaintances.
- Activate password protection on cell phones.
- If a situation places you in fear, contact a local law enforcement agency.

What to Do If You Are Being Cyberstalked

- If you are receiving unwanted contact, make clear to that person that you would like him or her not to contact you again.

- Save all communications for evidence. Do not edit or alter them in any way. Also, keep a record of your contacts with internet system administrators or law enforcement officials.

- You may want to consider blocking or filtering messages from the harasser. Although formats differ, a common chat room command to block someone would be to type: /ignore (without the brackets). However, in some circumstances (such as threats of violence), it may be more appropriate to save the information and contact law enforcement authorities.

- If harassment continues after you have asked the person to stop, contact the harasser's internet service provider (ISP). Often, an ISP can try to stop the conduct by direct contact with the stalker or by closing their account. If you receive abusive e-mails, identify the domain (after the "@" sign) and contact that ISP. Most ISP's have an e-mail address such as abuse@ or postmaster@ that can be used for complaints. If the ISP has a website, visit the site for information on how to file a complaint.

- Contact your local police department and inform them of the situation in as much detail as possible.

- To obtain more information on how to report an internet crime such as stalking, harassment, or exploitation, visit the U.S. Department of Justice website Computer Crime and Intellectual Property Section.

Section 43.2

Internet Safety Tips

Browsing the web safely and privately is concern for many people. A good general rule is that nothing online is private. Another general rule is that you can't be completely anonymous online. However, you can take steps to prevent sensitive and personal information from making its rounds on the web.

E-mail

- Have more than one e-mail account and use them for different purposes.

- Create e-mail addresses that don't contain your full name since that can be identifying.

Passwords

- Safest passwords contain letters, numbers, and symbols. Avoid words that are in a dictionary and any important dates.

- Try not to have the same password for every account. Come up with a system that's easy to remember but will enable you to have a different password for each account.

Social Networks

- Check out the privacy settings and make sure it's set to the level of privacy you want. Keep in mind that even if you set your social network page to private, it doesn't guarantee that your information is completely private.

- Don't forget that your friends' friends may be able to see your posts and pages even though you are not friends with them.

- Be thoughtful about who's on your friend list when you post or link to certain things.

- Read the social network's privacy policy and find out who else has access to your information, such as advertisers, third parties, apps, and games developers, etc.

Online Accounts

- Read the privacy policy. When you create an online account, whether it's to buy things, to join a group, or open an account, you should know what that site does with the information you share.

- Pay attention when creating an account. Oftentimes, this is when you can opt out of sharing personal information beyond what's necessary to create an account.

- Click "no" when it offers to check your e-mail address book to find your "friends." Some illegitimate sites have used this option by sending spam and viruses to everyone in your address book.

- Try not to use your name or a combination of your name as your username.

- When filling out account profiles, for increased privacy give no or very minimal information and opt out of joining the site's directory.

- For more privacy, try not to use too many applications with one account username/password. If someone guesses your username or password, they'll have access to all your applications.

- Log off when you're not using an account and do not choose to have the computer remember your passwords.

Friends and Family

- Talk to your friends and family about what they can post online about you.

- Don't forget that employers, churches, sport teams, groups, and volunteer organizations that you are a part of may share your personal information online.

Safe Web Browsing

- Make sure you are running anti-virus and anti-spyware software and make sure that definitions are updated.

- Periodically run scans on your computer, separate from your regular antivirus/antispyware.

- Periodically delete history, cookies, temporary internet files, and saved forms and passwords from your web browser.

- For added privacy, use anonymizers when you browse the web.

- Most search engines keep records of search terms, so when using search engines, avoid searching your full legal name with information you don't want linked together, such as your social security number or driver's license number.

Section 43.3

Social Networking Safety

Excerpted from "Staying Safe on Social Network Sites," United States Computer Emergency Readiness Team, 2011.

What Are Social Networking Sites?

Although the features of social networking sites differ, they all allow you to provide information about yourself and offer some type of communication mechanism (forums, chat rooms, e-mail, instant messenger) that enables you to connect with other users. On some sites, you can browse for people based on certain criteria, while other sites require that you be "introduced" to new people through a connection you share. Many of the sites have communities or subgroups that may be based on a particular interest.

How Can You Protect Yourself?

Limit the amount of personal information you post: Do not post information that would make you vulnerable, such as your address or information about your schedule or routine. If your connections post information about you, make sure the combined information is not more than you would be comfortable with strangers knowing. Also be considerate when posting information, including photos, about your connections.

Remember that the internet is a public resource: Only post information you are comfortable with anyone seeing. This includes information and photos in your profile and in blogs and other forums. Also, once you post information online, you can't retract it. Even if you remove the information from a site, saved or cached versions may still exist on other people's machines.

Be wary of strangers: The internet makes it easy for people to misrepresent their identities and motives. Consider limiting the people who are allowed to contact you on these sites. If you interact with people you do not know, be cautious about the amount of information you reveal or agreeing to meet them in person.

Be skeptical: Don't believe everything you read online. People may post false or misleading information about various topics, including their own identities. This is not necessarily done with malicious intent; it could be unintentional, an exaggeration, or a joke. Take appropriate precautions, though, and try to verify the authenticity of any information before taking any action.

Evaluate your settings: Take advantage of a site's privacy settings. The default settings for some sites may allow anyone to see your profile, but you can customize your settings to restrict access to only certain people. There is still a risk that private information could be exposed despite these restrictions, so don't post anything that you wouldn't want the public to see. Sites may change their options periodically, so review your security and privacy settings regularly to make sure that your choices are still appropriate.

Be wary of third-party applications: Third-party applications may provide entertainment or functionality, but use caution when deciding which applications to enable. Avoid applications that seem suspicious, and modify your settings to limit the amount of information the applications can access.

Use strong passwords: Protect your account with passwords that cannot easily be guessed. If your password is compromised, someone else may be able to access your account and pretend to be you.

Check privacy policies: Some sites may share information such as e-mail addresses or user preferences with other companies. This may lead to an increase in spam. Also, try to locate the policy for handling referrals to make sure that you do not unintentionally sign your friends up for spam.

Keep software, particularly your web browser, up to date: Install software updates so that attackers cannot take advantage of known

542

problems or vulnerabilities. Many operating systems offer automatic updates. If this option is available, you should enable it.

Use and maintain anti-virus software: Anti-virus software helps protect your computer against known viruses, so you may be able to detect and remove the virus before it can do any damage. Because attackers are continually writing new viruses, it is important to keep your definitions up to date.

Section 43.4

Check-Ins Safety Tips

"Check-Ins," © 2012 LoveisRespect.org. All rights reserved. Reprinted with permission. Additional information and resources are available at www.loveisrespect.org.

There are many situations where it's not only fun but practical to check-in with Gowalla, foursquare, Facebook, etc. As useful as this technology is, did you ever stop to wonder, is it safe?

For someone in or getting out of an abusive relationship, the answer is often no. It can be dangerous if your abusive partner only has to log in to foursquare or Facebook to see where you are, what you're doing, and who you're with.

So try to be mindful of how to use check-ins—whether you're in a healthy relationship or not. If you or a friend are in an unhealthy relationship, consider the following before checking in.

Always Ask

Always ask everyone if it's alright to check them in, even if you are sure it was ok a week ago. If anyone in your group says no, consider playing it safe and not checking in at all. You don't want an abusive partner figuring out who else is there based on the group you posted.

Update Your Privacy Settings

Facebook, foursquare, and Gowalla all let you control who sees your check-ins, but they default to making your account public. Consider adjusting your settings so only your friends, not the general public, can see your check-ins. Remember, though, that abusive partners may find a way around your settings.

Know Your Networks

Just because you're not friends with the abusive person doesn't mean you're not friends with their friends. If you think sensitive information could be accessed by your contacts a few friends away, just side with caution and don't post.

Pay Attention to Statuses and Tweets Too

Be aware that tagging someone in a status or tweet could create problems for them too, especially if you give away their location.

Wait Until After the Event

If you're posting about a one-time event that you really want to celebrate online, give it a day or two until you mention it. That way, the abusive person is less likely to use the information against you and your friends.

Chapter 44

Navigating the Legal System

Chapter Contents

Section 44.1

Questions to Ask Before You Hire an Attorney

General Questions about Divorce or Custody Cases

- Have you or any members of your firm ever represented my partner or anyone associated with my partner?

- Do you handle divorce or custody cases?

- How many of these cases have you handled?

- How many of them were contested?

- How many of them went to trial?

- Did any of the cases involve expert witnesses?

- How many were before the judge(s) who will hear my case?

- What kind of decisions does this judge usually make?

- Have you ever appealed a case, and if so, what were the issue(s) appealed? How many of these appealed cases did you win? (Remember that even excellent attorneys lose cases.)

Questions about Attorney Fees and Costs

- What are your fees? What work do these fees cover? Is this an hourly fee or a flat fee for the entire case?

- Is there an additional charge for appearing in court?

- Do you ever charge less for people who do not have much money?

- Do you charge a retainer? How much?

- What does it cover? Do you refund all or part of the retainer if my case ends up being dropped or not taking much time? (Attorneys should be willing to refund any part of the retainer not spent.)

- Are there other expenses which I may have to pay? What are they and how much are they likely to be?

- Will you be the only person working on my case? What will other people do? How will I be charged for their work? Will I be charged for speaking to your secretary? Your receptionist?

- Are there ways that I can assist you so as to keep down my costs?

- Will you send me a copy of letters, documents, and court papers that you file or receive regarding my case?

- Do you charge extra if the case gets more complicated or we have to go back to court?

- Will you require that I have paid everything that I owe you before you will go to court with me or finish my case? (Many attorneys do this. They may also refuse to return your original papers or copies of your file, and in some states this may be legal. Therefore you should insist on getting a copy of any paper filed with the court or given or received from another party or otherwise relevant to your case. Be sure to keep all of them in a safe place, in case you ever need them.)

- Are you willing to work out a payment plan with me?

- Will you put our agreement about fees and what work you will perform in writing?

Section 44.2

Restraining Orders

Restraining order or protective order laws are state laws and each state has a different law (also called a statute).

A restraining order or protective order is a legal order issued by a state court which requires one person to stop harming another person. It is also sometimes called a protection order, an injunction, an order of protection, or some other similar name.

Below is general information explaining what restraining orders are and how they can help you.

In general, domestic violence restraining order laws establish who can file for an order, what protection or relief a person can get from such an order, and how the order will be enforced. While there are differences from state to state, all protective order statutes permit the court to order the abuser to stop hurting or threatening you ("cease abuse" provisions). The majority of states' orders can also instruct the abuser to stay away from you, your home, your workplace, or your school ("stay away" provisions). You generally also can ask the court to order that all contact, whether by telephone, notes, mail, fax, e-mail, or delivery of flowers or gifts, is prohibited ("no contact" provisions).

Some statutes also allow the court to order the abuser to pay you temporary child support or continue to make mortgage payments on a home owned by both of you ("support" provisions), to award you sole use of a home or car owned by both of you ("exclusive use" provisions), or to pay you for medical costs or property damage caused by the abuser ("restitution" provisions).

Some courts might also be able to order the abuser to turn over any guns, rifles, and ammunition s/he has ("relinquish firearms" provisions), attend a batterers' treatment program, appear for regular drug tests, or start alcohol or drug abuse counseling.

Many jurisdictions also allow the court to make decisions about the care and safety of your children. Courts can order the abuser to stay away from and have no contact with your children's doctors, daycare, school, or after-school job. Most courts can make temporary custody decisions, although many courts are very reluctant to do so. Some can issue visitation or child support orders. You can also ask the court to order supervised visitation, or to specify a safe arrangement for transferring the children back and forth between you and the abuser ("custody, visitation and child support" provisions).

When the abuser does something that the court has ordered him/her not to do, or fails to do something the court has ordered him/her to do, s/he may have violated the order. The victim can ask the police or the court, or both, depending on the violation, to enforce the order. The police can generally enforce the stay away, no contact, cease abuse, exclusive use, and possibly custody provisions—those that need immediate response. If you are unable to call them when the violation occurs, they should take a report if you call them soon afterwards. These types of violations can also later be addressed by the court, and it is often a good idea to bring them to the court's attention.

Other violations are not easily enforced by the police, such as failure to pay support or attend treatment programs—those are better enforced by the court. If you file a "motion for contempt" explaining how the abuser violated the order, the court will hold a hearing to determine if the facts prove that the abuser violated the order. If the court finds a violation did occur, the judge will determine a penalty. Depending upon the laws of your jurisdiction and the nature of the violation, the penalty might be a finding of civil or criminal contempt, which could result in a fine, jail time, or both. The violation might also be a reason for the order to be extended or modified in some way. In some cases, it might result in a misdemeanor or felony criminal conviction and punishment.

Section 44.3

Protective Orders for Minors

"Legal Information on Teen Dating Violence," reprinted with permission from www.WomensLaw.org, © 2012 National Network to End Domestic Violence. All rights reserved. Citations in the original WomensLaw.org content were omitted for this reprinting. For additional information and resources, visit http://www.womenslaw.org or http://nnedv.org.

What is a restraining order and what does it do?

A restraining order (also known as a protective order, order of protection, or many other names) is a court order requiring that your boyfriend or girlfriend, past or present, stop "abusing" you. The order may also state that your boyfriend or girlfriend cannot contact you, has to stay away from you, and may include many other protections. The requirements for getting a restraining order, exactly what protections you can get from a restraining order, and how "abuse" is defined differ in each state. In addition, not all states allow people under age eighteen permission to get a restraining order on their own without an adult's help.

Am I eligible for a restraining order even though I am under eighteen?

In many states, you can apply for a restraining order even if you are under eighteen, but you may need an adult (usually a parent or legal guardian) to file the order on your behalf. Other states allow minors to file on their own without involving your parent or another adult. Most states that allow minors to apply for restraining orders on their own require that you are at least sixteen years old. A few, however, let minors of any age, or sometimes minors twelve or older, go to court without an adult.

Even if your state requires an adult to assist you in applying for an order, but you don't want to get your parent/guardian involved or she or he will not help you file for the order, you may still have some other options. In some states, the law allows what is referred to as a "next friend" to apply for you, which could be a trusted adult other than a parent/guardian. In other states, a judge may appoint what is called a "guardian ad litem," which is someone to represent your interests during the litigation (court proceeding). It could be a lawyer or a non-lawyer. In some states a judge must approve of the adult who you choose to go to court with you instead of your parents (called a guardian ad litem).

For help, you may want to contact a domestic violence organization or a lawyer. There are free legal services available through different organizations, and many states have specific organizations that represent only teens. Another idea is that you may want to call the clerk of the court in your county and ask what the procedure is for a minor filing an order and if she or he can file alone.

Section 44.4

Suing Your Abuser

"Suing Your Abuser," reprinted with permission from www.WomensLaw .org. Copyright 2012 National Network to End Domestic Violence. All rights reserved. Citations in the original WomensLaw.org content were omitted for this reprinting. For additional information and resources, visit http://www.womenslaw.org or http://nnedv.org.

You may have a right to seek justice from an abuser through the court system where you live.

When people are injured by others, they are permitted to seek what the law refers to as "damages," in the form of money, for such things as medical bills, lost wages or employment, physical and emotional pain and suffering, and, in some cases, to punish the abuser. Each state has its own laws on these subjects, but, for the most part, they are very similar when it comes to injuries from abuse.

Small Claims Court

If your damages are below a certain amount, you may be able to file on your own in small claims court. Small claims court is a less formal type of court, and many people are able to go to small claims court without the help of an attorney. Ask the clerk of court for more information on small claims court in your area. However, it may be important to talk to an attorney to find out what the statute of limitations are for the type of case that you are bringing. Basically, the statute of limitations set a time frame for how long after an incident or crime a person can be sued. Once the statute of limitations runs out, you can no longer sue the abuser.

Finding a Lawyer

To sue someone for damages (not in small claims court), you will most likely need the help of a lawyer. Some lawyers will take a case like this for a "contingent fee." That means the lawyer doesn't get paid for his or her time and labor unless you win in court, and then she or he takes some percentage, usually a third, of whatever damages the judge orders. (However, you may still have to pay court costs and other costs such as fees for mailing, copying, etc.) Sometimes the judge will order the defendant to pay for your attorney's fees if you win the case at trial.

Chapter 45

Identity Protection for Abuse Victims

Chapter Contents

Section 45.1

Tips for Protecting Your Identity

Identity theft is rampant in the United States. Survivors of domestic violence must take extra precautions to protect themselves from abusers who use identity as a means of power and control. Abusers may use survivors' credit cards without their permission, open fraudulent new credit cards in survivors' names (ultimately ruining their credit), or open credit cards in children's names. Misuse of survivors' social security numbers is also common in the context of domestic violence. Abusers may fraudulently use survivors' social security numbers to stalk, harass, or threaten survivors. Read more to learn how to protect yourself if you are experiencing this type of abuse.

Survivors experiencing abuse should contact their local domestic violence program for immediate support. Check your local yellow pages or call the National Domestic Violence Hotline (operated by the Texas Council on Family Violence) at 800-799-SAFE to be connected to the program in your area.

Steps to Take to Protect Your Identity

Relocate: Moving across town, across the state, or across the country puts physical distance between you and the abuser. Be sure to obtain an unlisted phone number and be aware of the full faith and credit provisions in your restraining order, which make the order valid when you travel to another state or tribal jurisdiction.

Apply to the address confidentiality program in your state: These types of programs allow individuals who have experienced domestic violence, sexual assault, stalking, or other types of crime to receive mail at a confidential address, while keeping their actual address undisclosed. Rules and eligibility vary from state to state.

Open a post office box to receive mail: Abusers may be able to open fraudulent credit cards by responding to credit card offers received in the mail. A post office box may prevent this if only you have access to it. Be wary of the confidentiality policies of nongovernment post office box centers such as Mail Boxes, Etc. and the fact that it may not be possible to remain anonymous in rural towns while accessing the post office.

Protect your incoming and outgoing mail: Shred all credit card offers that come in the mail along with other documents that have your name, address, and/or social security number on them. Mail bills and other sensitive documents directly from the post office instead of from the mailbox on your porch or at the end of your driveway. Call 800-5OPT-OUT to stop receiving credit card offers in the mail.

Guard your social security number: Do not use your social security number as a general ID, personal identification number (PIN), or password. Request to have your social security number removed from documents you receive in the mail and ID cards for health insurance, driving, work, etc.

Check your credit report: The best way to determine if someone has committed fraud against you is to check your credit report with all three credit bureaus at least once per year. You can also make a request to have a fraud alert placed on your credit report.

Report suspected fraud: Contact local law enforcement if you know of or suspect fraud and ask to file a report. Check and/or close accounts you believe have been tampered. File a report with the Federal Trade Commission at 877-ID-THEFT and the Social Security Administration Fraud Hotline at 800-269-0271. File copies of police reports with credit bureaus.

Protect information you give out: Never give any identifying information over the phone or through e-mail or the internet unless you initiated the call or have verification that the website or e-mail communication is secure.

Section 45.2

Address Confidentiality Programs

Excerpted from "Address Confidentiality Programs," © 2007 National Coalition Against Domestic Violence. All rights reserved. Reprinted with permission. For additional information, visit www.ncadv.org. Reviewed by David A. Cooke, M.D., FACP, July 2012.

Why It Matters

Domestic violence is a pattern of behaviors involving physical, sexual, economic, and emotional abuse by an intimate partner for the purpose of establishing and maintaining power and control over the other partner.[1] Violence frequently escalates when batterers believe that they are losing control of their victims, thus exposing victims to the greatest risk of serious injury or death when victims attempt to flee violent relationships.[2] Because many states allow information from voter registration and drivers' licenses to be accessible by the public, batterers often search public records to obtain their victims' physical addresses in order to stalk them. State-operated Address Confidentiality Programs (ACPs) provide victims of domestic violence—and in some states, stalking and sexual assault—with a legal substitute address to prevent their perpetrators from using public records to track them down.

What Do ACPs Do?

ACPs provide victims with a substitute address, often the Secretary of State's address or a P.O. box on public records, thereby retaining confidentiality of their location.

The Secretary of State's office or other government agency serves as an agent that collects and forwards all first-class mail to victims.

There are narrowly statutorily specified circumstances in which the actual address may be disclosed:

- Law-enforcement officials

- Government officials, upon a showing of a bona fide statutory or administrative requirement for the physical address

- Other third parties pursuant to a court order.

Why Are ACPs Important?

- One in four women will experience domestic violence during her lifetime.[4]

- Eighty-one percent of women who are stalked by a current or former intimate partner are physically assaulted by that partner, and 31 percent are sexually assaulted.[5]

Registration Requirements

Many states require victims to apply for a confidential address through an enrolling agency, such as a domestic violence shelter/program, sexual assault crisis program, state or local agency, law enforcement office, certified advocate groups or victim assistance programs, or through an enrolling agent such as an application assistant or trained advocate.

While some states require victims to report the abuse to law enforcement or to have obtained an order of protection, others only require eligibility to apply for a restraining order. Most states require that they have left the abuser and live at an unknown address.

Although a few states require that the perpetrator be an intimate partner or family member, most states allow ACP registration for those who are victims of domestic violence, sexual assault, or stalking.

A few states require victims to register a post office box, as opposed to a government agency, as their substitute address.

Real ID Act of 2005

The passage of the Real ID Act in 2005 endangers victims of domestic violence, sexual assault, and stalking by jeopardizing their confidentiality:

- Section 206 (b)(6) of the act requires that all applicants for drivers' licenses or state identification cards must furnish their principal residence address to obtain a federally valid license or ID card.

Section 827 of the Violence Against Women Act of 2005 includes a requirement for the Department of Human Services (DHS) to give special consideration to victims of domestic abuse, sexual assault, stalking, or trafficking who are entitled to enroll in state ACPs when the agency is "developing regulations or guidance with regard to identification documents, including drivers licenses." These groups include domestic violence and sexual assault victims.[6]

The DHS draft regulations of March 2007 provided an exemption for those individuals enrolled in a state ACP (p. 18) and proposed an exemption for individuals who are entitled to enroll in state ACPs (p. 36).[7]

Sources

1. Pirro, Jeanine Ferris, Westchester County DA (1997). *Commission on Domestic Violence Fatalities Report to the Governor.* Retrieved June 27, 2007 from New York State Office for the Prevention of Domestic Violence Website: http://www.opdv.state.ny.us/publications/fatality/part3.html

2. Farr, K. A. (2002). "Battered Women Who Were 'Being Killed and Survived it': Straight Talk from Survivors," *Violence & Victims*, 17:267–81.

3. (2003) *Address Confidentiality Program for Victims Fleeing Violence.* Retrieved June 27, 2007 from Pennsylvania Coalition Against Domestic Violence Website: http://www.pcadv.org/publications/AddConf.faxable.pdf.

4. Thoennes, N., and Tjaden, P. (2000). "Extent, Nature and Consequences of Intimate Partner Violence," National Institute of Justice and Centers for Disease Control and Prevention, 5.

5. Thoennes, N., and Tjaden, P. (1998). "Stalking in America: Findings from the National Violence Against Women Survey," National Institute of Justice and Centers for Disease Control and Prevention, 2.

6. Title VII, Subtitle C, Sec. 827 (Pub. L 109–162, 119 Stat. 2960, 3066, Jan. 5, 2006).

7. "Minimum Standards for Driver's Licenses and Identification Cards Acceptable by Federal Agencies for Official Purposes; Notice of Proposed Rulemaking." 72 Federal Register 46 (9 March 2007), pp. 18, 36.

Section 45.3

Applying for a New Social Security Number

Excerpted from "New Numbers for Domestic Violence Victims,"
U.S. Social Security Administration, August 2011.

People in all walks of life can be victims of family violence or harassment, abuse, or life-endangering situations. If you are a victim of family violence, Social Security may be able to help you.

Public awareness campaigns stress how important it is for victims to develop safety plans that include gathering personal papers and choosing a safe place to go. Sometimes the best way to evade an abuser and reduce the risk of further violence may be to relocate and establish a new identity. Following these changes, it also may be helpful to get a new Social Security number.

Although Social Security does not routinely assign new numbers, we will do so when evidence shows you are being harassed or abused or your life is endangered.

How to Apply for a New Number

You must apply in person at any Social Security office. We will help you complete a statement explaining why you need a new number and an application for a new number.

You will need to present the following things:

- Evidence documenting the harassment or abuse

- Your current Social Security number

- Original documents establishing your:
  - U.S. citizenship or immigration status;
  - age;
  - identity; and
  - evidence of your legal name change if you have changed your name.

Also, we will need to see original documents showing you have custody of any children for whom you are requesting new numbers and documentation, proving their U.S. citizenship, ages, and identities.

Citizenship or Immigration Status

U.S. citizen: We can accept only certain documents as proof of U.S. citizenship. These include a U.S. birth certificate or a U.S. passport.

Noncitizen: To prove your U.S. immigration status, show us the current immigration document, I-94, Arrival/Departure Record, issued to you when you arrived in the United States. If you are an F-1 or M-1 student, you also must show us your I-20, Certificate of Eligibility for Nonimmigrant Student Status. If you are a J-1 or J-2 exchange visitor, show us your DS-2019, Certificate of Eligibility for Exchange Visitor Status.

Age

You must present your birth certificate.

Identity

We can accept only certain documents as proof of identity. An acceptable document must be current (not expired) and show your name, identifying information, and preferably a recent photograph.

U.S. citizen: Social Security will ask to see a U.S. driver's license, state-issued nondriver identification card, or U.S. passport as proof of identity. If you do not have the specific documents we ask for, we will ask to see other documents, including:

- employee ID card;
- school ID card;
- health insurance card (not a Medicare card);
- U.S. military ID card; or
- adoption degree.

Noncitizen: Social Security will ask to see your current U.S. immigration documents. Acceptable immigration documents include your:

- form I-551 (includes machine-readable immigrant visa and unexpired foreign passport);

- I-94 with your unexpired foreign passport; or

- I-766 (work permit from the Department of Homeland Security [DHS]).

How to Change Your Name on Your Card

If you legally change your name because of marriage, divorce, court order, or any other reason, you need to tell Social Security so that you can get a corrected card.

If you need to change your name on your Social Security card, you must show us a recently issued document as proof of your legal name change. Documents Social Security may accept to prove a legal name change include marriage document, divorce decree, certificate of naturalization showing a new name, or court order for a name change.

If the evidence of a legal name change does not give us enough information to identify you in our records or if your document was issued more than two years ago, you also must show us an identity document in your old name (as shown in our records).

Blocking Access to Your Record

You can choose to block electronic access to your Social Security record. When you do this, no one, including you, will be able to get or change your personal information on the internet or through our automated telephone service. If you block access to your record and then change your mind in the future, you can contact Social Security and ask us to unblock it.

Chapter 46

Life after Abuse: Looking after Yourself and Moving On

When the violence is finally over—you have arranged all the practical things like housing, money, schools for the children, and you feel reasonably sure that your abuser has stopped harassing you—you may be expecting to feel great. But that is unlikely to happen straight away. Recovering from abuse by someone who was close to you is a long process, and the damage may stay with you and your children for years.

Once you are away from the abuse, and it is safe to feel again, you may have a sense of anti-climax. You are likely to experience grief, pain, and a deep sense of loss: your trust will have been betrayed, your self-esteem and confidence are shattered. In many ways it is like being bereaved—and as with a bereavement, healing will take time.

Looking After Yourself

Treat yourself gently: don't rush the healing process, and don't expect to achieve everything you want straight away. Maybe you want to make huge changes—by changing your whole lifestyle, joining local organizations, returning to education, looking for a (different) job. This is all fine if that is how you are feeling, but if you don't want to change anything else at this point, that is fine too. It's good to have hopes and ambitions for the future, but try to set realistic goals and move at your own pace, rather than being concerned about what others might be thinking.

You may feel lonely and isolated: sometimes when you come home to an empty house or flat, it might seem that even an abusive partner was better than no one. Perhaps your partner cut you off from friends and family, so now you feel there is no one you can talk to or go out with. It may not be too late to reestablish contact with past friends—and in any case, you can think about making new friends and acquaintances.

Some of the things you might like to do:

- Take time and space for yourself each day.
- Reward yourself.
- Do something you enjoy and are good at.
- Take regular exercise (for example, try swimming, dancing, walking, or climbing).
- Learn a new skill (for example, yoga, meditation, self-defense).
- Be creative: try drawing, painting, writing.
- Practice relaxation exercises (for example, breathing exercises, tai chi, self-hypnosis, or massage).

It's also important to eat well and to get enough sleep, if you can.

Gaining Confidence

Living with someone who is always putting you down, criticizing you, controlling you, and being abusive or violent towards you will have sapped your self-confidence and your belief in yourself. You may find it hard (or impossible) to make decisions, even about small things—because your abuser did not allow you to make choices for yourself. You may find managing money very difficult: maybe your ex-partner controlled all the household finances; you are probably having to manage on a very limited income; and perhaps you had to leave behind many of your personal possessions.

You have already taken a huge step in leaving your abuser. Give yourself credit for that. Then think of all the other things you have achieved in your life, and build up a mental list that you can return to when you are feeling low.

You may find it helpful to talk about your experiences with other women who have also been in violent relationships. Look for a support group in your area.

Products focusing on building self-confidence (such as self-help books, CDs, and courses) are widely available. Some of these may be effective, at least in the short term, but none appear to have been fully evaluated (Emler, 2005).

Moving On

While you were with your abuser, you may not have been free to decide for yourself what kind of work you did, whether you took on paid employment or not, what leisure activities you engaged in, whether to study for more qualifications or to join an evening class just for pleasure. Now you have only yourself and your children to consider—but you may find it frightening suddenly to be responsible for making your own choices.

You might have had to give up your job because you had to go into a refuge, or move away to a different area to get away from your abuser. If you are claiming benefits, it may not be financially worthwhile to look for paid work at the moment—particularly if you have childcare to consider. Maybe you would like to re-train for a different kind of work, or go back into education, or do some voluntary work for a while. Or perhaps you don't feel ready to take any of these steps just yet.

You might find it helpful to look at some of the information and support available for single parents.

Helping Your Children

Your children, too, will probably take some time to adjust to the new situation. They will almost certainly have been affected by the abuse they witnessed or experienced directly. If you have moved to a different area, they will probably have to attend a new school and make new friends. They may be finding it really difficult to cope with all the changes in their lives—such as leaving their home and friends, and perhaps some of their possessions—and they will look to you to give them the answers they need.

You may find coping with your children's needs very difficult at a time when you are trying to deal with your own problems. On the other hand, you may find it a helpful distraction, or even see it as a reason for carrying on. Be as honest with your children as possible; let them know how you are feeling and tell them that you love them. Try to establish a "normal" routine as soon as you can, and show them that you can be relied upon even though their father or stepfather has let them down. Listen to your children's concerns, and help them to find other sources of support (for example, from grandparents or other relatives, from teachers or youth workers, or from workers and volunteers at a domestic violence outreach service).

Although your children will undoubtedly be relieved that the abuse has stopped, they may still miss their father or stepfather, and may blame you for taking them away from him. If they want to see him, that is fine if you feel it is safe for them to do so.

References

Emler, Nicholas (2001) "Self esteem: the costs and causes of low self worth." York: Joseph Rowntree Foundation); summary available at http://www.jrf.org.uk/knowledge/findings/socialpolicy/n71.asp.

NiCarthy, G. (1990) "Getting free: A handbook for women in abusive situations." Edited and adapted from the original American edition by Jane Hutt. London: Journeyman Press.

Part Six

Additional Help and Information

Chapter 47

Glossary of Terms Related to Domestic Abuse

There may be other definitions for these words but these are the meanings used in relation to domestic violence.

advocate: A person who works for an organization that provides help to domestic violence victims. The advocate must have received specialized training in counseling domestic violence victims. The advocate provides confidential, free help and will go to court with the domestic violence victim. A domestic violence advocate provides legal advocacy services for victims of abuse. Advocates help victims by notifying them of, and going with them to, court hearings; educating them about the court system and domestic violence; helping them fill out applications for restraining orders; helping them communicate with prosecutors, probation officers, and court personnel; and safety planning.

anger management class: An older term used to refer to what are now called batterer's intervention programs. The name has been changed to reflect current understanding that abuse is not only about anger but about control issues with many different causes.

batterer: Someone who abuses another person. Abuse can be physical, financial, or emotional.

child abuse: Maltreatment or neglect of a child, including nonaccidental physical injuries, sexual abuse/exploitation, severe or general neglect, unjustifiable mental suffering/emotional abuse, and willful cruelty or unjustifiable punishment of a child.

civil harassment restraining order: A restraining order that protects one person from another. Example: neighbor against neighbor, person against ex-spouse/girlfriend/ex-boyfriend's new partner.

civil standby: When a law enforcement agency comes to a location (normally the home shared by the protected person and restrained person) to keep the peace. This is usually so that one of the parties may pick up a few personal items or follow another court order.

criminal protective order: An order a judge makes to protect a witness or victim of a crime.

dating violence: Intimate partner violence (IPV) between people who are dating. The abusive behaviors between dating partners include verbal, physical, emotional, sexual, financial, and/or electronic harassment. The gender or sexual orientation of the parties doesn't matter.

defendant: The person accused of a crime in a criminal case. The person or company being sued in a civil case. In a civil case, the term used is "respondent."

dependent adult abuse: Physical abuse (including sexual), financial abuse, neglect, abandonment, isolation, abduction, treatment that causes physical harm, pain or mental suffering, and withholding of things or services by a care custodian of a dependent adult.

domestic violence agency: A nonprofit organization that provides free, confidential domestic violence services to victims. Services include: a twenty-four-hour crisis line, emergency and confidential shelter, legal advocacy, safety planning, peer counseling, therapy, and resource and referral. Domestic violence agencies have historically offered services including confidential emergency shelter, counseling and education, and legal advocacy. Legal advocacy could mean providing people who go to court hearings with the victim or the help of attorneys, when needed. Because some victims of domestic violence do not call domestic violence agencies, new types of agencies have started to help clients where they are: in drug rehabilitation, courtrooms, jails, or prisons. These victims are often referred to existing traditional domestic violence agencies for confidential shelter, counseling, or specialized programs.

elder abuse: Physical abuse (including sexual), financial abuse, neglect, abandonment, isolation, abduction, treatment that causes physical harm or pain or mental suffering, and withholding of things or services by a care custodian of an elderly person.

elder abuse/dependent adult abuse restraining order: These restraining orders are meant to prevent mistreatment of an elderly person or a dependent adult—an adult who has physical or developmental disabilities, or failing physical or mental abilities caused by age.

emergency protective order (EPRO): This is a restraining order requested by law enforcement on an emergency basis at a domestic violence scene. An EPRO can protect a victim from stalking, violence, threats of violence, or a pattern of harassing behavior; protect the victim, their immediate family, and people who live with them; and say who has custody as long as the EPRO is in effect. Employers can ask for EPRO's to protect their workplace from someone who is threatening their employee.

emergency protective restraining order: See emergency protective order.

EPO: See emergency protective order.

EPRO: Emergency protective restraining order; see emergency protective order.

ex parte order: An order that the judge makes after meeting with, or reading legal forms submitted by, only one party in a case (an ex parte request).

family violence: A general term which includes the categories of child abuse, elder abuse, dependent adult abuse, domestic violence, and animal cruelty.

intimate partner: Current or former spouses (husband/wife/domestic partner), boyfriends, and girlfriends of any sexual orientation.

intimate partner violence: Violence between intimate partners. "Violence" includes physical violence or a verbal threat of physical violence by one intimate partner against the other. It includes death and other crimes— rape, sexual assault, robbery, aggravated assault, and simple assault.

kick-out order: See move-out order.

move-out order: When a judge, through a valid court order, requires the restrained person to move out of the home the restrained person and protected person share for the safety of the protected person(s).

moving party: The party who files a motion in a case asking for a court order. It can be either the petitioner/plaintiff or respondent/defendant.

no-contact order: A type of restraining order. This order protects the person from any type of contact with the abuser (i.e., personal, phone, or email). Any contact in violation of this order can lead to criminal charges against the person who violates the order.

opposing party: The "other" person in a court case. For example, if you are opening a new domestic violence case, the opposing party is the person you want protection from.

PD: See public defender or police department.

peaceful contact order: A type of restraining order which is given to a person by the court which allows the restrained person (abuser) to contact the protected person (victim) as long as all contact is peaceful. The restrained person can live with the protected person; *but* the restrained person cannot hit, grab, throw things, damage property, or pull the phone cord out of the wall; knock over or break furniture; swear at, or about, the protected person; tear up important papers; stop the protected person from leaving the house; make threats to hit, harm, or kill the protected person; argue with the protected person or a family member; argue or shout so loud that the neighbors are disturbed; have friends come over and do any of the above; and not do anything that makes the protected person, or the family, frightened, hurt, injured, upset, or disturbed.

petitioner: A person who presents a petition to the court; a person who files legal forms to start a court case.

plaintiff: The person or company that files a lawsuit.

probation: When a defendant who has been found guilty of a crime is released into the community and must follow certain conditions, such as jail time, paying a fine, doing community service, or attending a drug treatment program. Violation of the conditions can result in incarceration.

protected party: A person who is protected by a court order(s) that restrains another person (the restrained person) from harassing, annoying, striking, etc. the protected party.

protective order: See criminal protective order.

public defender: A lawyer who works for a state or local agency representing clients accused of a crime who cannot afford to pay.

respondent: If you are the person that answers the original petition, you are the respondent. Even if you later file an action of your own in that case, you are still the respondent for as long as the case is open.

response: A respondent's first answer to the complaint or petition that started the case.

restitution: When a defendant/abuser/restrained person is ordered by the court to repay financial loss a victim suffered as a result of something the defendant/respondent did.

restrained party: The person who cannot contact the protected party when the court makes a restraining order.

restrained person: See restrained party.

restraining order: Common term used to refer to the existence of an emergency protective order, criminal protective order, or civil harassment restraining order.

safety plan: A plan created by a domestic violence victim (with the help of an advocate) that shows the victim ways she or he can prevent or protect her- or himself during a violent incident and reduce the risk they are hurt or killed. Safety plans should be prepared for different situations such as: during a violent incident, when the victim is getting ready to leave, after the victim leaves the abuser, and at their work. Each of these situations has different risks. Advocates can help victims weigh the risks to their safety and personal freedom in each of these situations, come up with options, and evaluate those options. Evaluating options includes anticipating the consequences of each action and determining which option best increases safety and personal freedom. Safety plans should be individualized and realistic.

serve: When the moving party has someone, not him or herself, give the filed court papers to the other party.

spousal abuse: A more narrow term describing abuse between husbands and wives. Currently it is more often called domestic violence or intimate partner violence.

stalking: Willfully, maliciously, and repeatedly following or willfully, maliciously, and repeatedly harassing another person and making a credible threat with the intent to place that person in fear for his or her own safety, or the safety of his or her immediate family.

teen dating violence: Intimate partner violence between teens who are dating. Of concern for young victims is a lack of experience responding to violence and/or sexually coercive behavior. This type of intimate partner violence is not limited to any particular sexual orientation or identity.

victim: A person who is harmed, physically, emotionally or financially, or killed by another; a person who suffers from a destructive or injurious action; the person against whom a crime has been committed.

Chapter 48

Directory of Domestic Violence Resources

Abuse of Power.info
Website:
http://www.abuseofpower.info

Abused Deaf Women's Advocacy Services
8623 Roosevelt Way NE
Seattle WA 98115
Phone: 206-922-7088
Phone: 206-518-9361
(Hotline—Videophone)
TTY: 206-726-0093
Fax: 206-726-0017
Website: http://www.adwas.org
E-mail: adwas@adwas.org

Alabama Coalition Against Domestic Violence
P.O. Box 4762
Montgomery, AL 36101
Toll-Free: 800-650-6522
(24-hour Hotline)
Phone: 334-832-4842
Fax: 334-832-4803
Website: http://www.acadv.org
E-mail:info@acadv.org

Asian & Pacific Islander Institute on Domestic Violence
450 Sutter Street, Suite 600
San Francisco, CA 94108
Phone: 415-568-3315
Fax: 415-954-9999
Website: http://www.apiidv.org
E-mail: info@apiidv.org

Resources in this chapter were compiled from several sources deemed reliable. All contact information was verified and updated in July 2012.

Aurora Center for Advocacy and Education
University of Minnesota
407 Boynton Health Services
410 Church Street
Minneapolis, MN 55455
Phone: 612-626-2929
Phone: 612-626-9111 (Help Line)
Fax: 612-626-9933
Website:
http://www.umn.edu/aurora
E-mail: aurora@umn.edu

Break the Cycle
5777 West Century Boulevard
Suite 1150
Los Angeles, CA 90045
Phone: 310-286-3383
Fax: 310-286-3386
Website:
http://www.breakthecycle.org
E-mail: info@breakthecycle.org

Centers for Disease Control and Prevention (CDC)
National Center for Injury
Prevention and Control (NCIPC)
4770 Buford
Highway NE, MS F-63
Atlanta, GA 30341-3717
Toll-Free: 800-CDC-INFO
(800-232-4636)
Toll-Free TTY: 888-232-6348
Website: http://www.cdc.gov
E-mail: cdcinfo@cdc.gov

Centre for Research and Education on Violence Against Women and Children
1137 Western Road, Room 1118
Faculty of Education Building
Western University
London, Ontario
CANADA N6G 1G7
Phone: 519-661-4040
Fax: 519-850-2464
Website: http://www.crvawc.ca

Child Witness to Violence Project
Website: http://www
.childwitnesstoviolence.org

Corporate Alliance to End Partner Violence
2416 East Washington Street
Suite E
Bloomington, IL 61704
Phone: 309-664-0667
Fax: 309-664-0747
Website: http://www.caepv.org
E-mail: caepv@caepv.org

FaithTrust Institute
2900 Eastlake Avenue East
Suite 200
Seattle, WA 98102
Phone: 206-634-1903
Fax: 206-634-0115
Website:
http://www.faithtrustinstitute.org

*Florida Council Against
Sexual Violence*
1820 East Park Avenue
Suite 100
Tallahassee, FL 32301
Toll-Free: 888-956-7273
Phone: 850-297-2000
Fax: 850-297-2002
Website: http://www.fcasv.org
E-mail: information@fcasv.org

Futures Without Violence
100 Montgomery Street
The Presidio
San Francisco, CA 94129
Toll-Free TTY: 800-595-4889
Phone: 415-678-5500
Fax: 415-529-2930
Website: http://
www.futureswithoutviolence.org

*Gay Men's Domestic
Violence Project*
955 Massachusetts Avenue
PMB 131
Cambridge, MA 02139
Toll-Free: 800-832-1901 (Hotline)
Phone: 617-354-6056
Fax: 617-354-6072
Website: http://gmdvp.org
E-mail: support@gmdvp.org

*Houston Area Women's
Center*
1010 Waugh Drive
Houston, TX 77019
Toll-Free: 800-256-0551
(Domestic Violence Hotline)
Toll-Free: 800-256-0661
(Sexual Assault Hotline)
Phone: 713-528-2121
(Domestic Violence Hotline)
Phone: 713-528-7273
(Sexual Assault Hotline)
TDD: 713-528-3625
(Domestic Violence Hotline)
TDD: 713-528-3691
(Sexual Assault Hotline)
Website: http://www.hawc.org

*Indiana Coalition Against
Sexual Assault (INCASA)*
26 North Arsenal Avenue
3rd Floor
Indianapolis, IN 46201
Toll Free 800-691-2272
Phone: 317-423-0233
Fax: 317-423-0237
Website: http://www.incasa.org
E-mail: incasa@incasa.org

*Institute on Domestic
Violence in the African
American Community*
University of Minnesota
School of Social Work
290 Peters Hall
1404 Gortner Avenue
St. Paul, MN 55108-6142
Toll-Free: 877-643-8222
Phone: 612-624-5357
Fax: 612-624-9201
Website: http://www.idvaac.org
E-mail: info@idvaac.org

Loveisrespect.org
Toll-Free: 866-331-9474
Toll-Free TTY: 866-331-8453
Website:
http://www.loveisrespect.org

Minnesota Coalition for Battered Women
60 East Plato Boulevard
Suite 130
St. Paul, MN 55107
Toll-Free: 800-289-6177
Phone: 651-646-6177
Fax: 651-646-1527
Website: http://www.mcbw.org

Muslim Advocacy Network Against Domestic Violence (MANADV)
Peaceful Families Project
P.O. Box 771
Great Falls, VA 22066
Phone: 703-474-6870
Website:
http://www.manadv.org
E-mail: info@manadv.org or
info@peacefulfamilies.org

National Center for Victims of Crime
2000 M Street NW, Suite 480
Washington, DC 20036
Phone: 202-467-8700
Fax: 202-467-8701
Website: http://www.ncvc.org

National Center on Domestic and Sexual Violence
4612 Shoal Creek Boulevard
Austin, Texas 78756
Toll-Free: 800-799-SAFE
(800-799-7233)
Toll-Free TTY: 800-787-3224
Phone/Fax: 512-407-9020
Phone: 206-787-3224 (Video
Phone Hotline)
Website: http://www.ncdsv.org or
http://www.thehotline.org

National Coalition Against Domestic Violence
One Broadway, Suite B210
Denver, CO 80203
Phone: 303-839-1852
TTY: 303-839-8459
Fax: 303-831-9251
Website: http://www.ncadv.org
E-mail: mainoffice@ncadv.org

National Council on Child Abuse & Family Violence
1025 Connecticut Avenue
Suite 1000
Washington, DC 20036
Phone: 202-429-6695
Fax: 202-521-3479
Website: http://www.nccafv.org
Email: info@nccafv.org

National Crime Prevention Council
2001 Jefferson Davis Highway
Suite 901
Arlington, VA 22202
Phone: 202-466-6272
Fax: 202-296-1356
Website: http://www.ncpc.org

National Latino Alliance for the Elimination of Domestic Violence (Alianza)
P.O. Box 2787
Española, NM 87532
Phone: 505-753-3334
Fax: 505-753-3347
Website:
http://www.dvalianza.org
E-mail: info@dvalianza.org

National Network to End Domestic Violence
2001 S Street NW, Suite 400
Washington, DC 20009
Phone: 202-543-5566
Fax: 202-543-5626
Website: http://nnedv.org

National Resource Center on Domestic Violence
Website: http://www.nrcdv.org

New York City Alliance Against Sexual Assault
32 Broadway, Suite 1101
New York, NY 10004
Phone: 212-229-0345
Fax: 212-229-0676 fax
Website:
http://www.svfreenyc.org
E-mail: contact-us@svfreenyc.org

New York State Coalition Against Domestic Violence
350 New Scotland Avenue
Albany, New York 12208
Toll-Free: 800-942-6906 (Hotline)
Toll-Free TTY: 800-942-6906 (Hotline)
Phone: 518-482-5465
Fax: 518-482-3807
Website: http://nyscadv.org
E-mail: nyscadv@nyscadv.org

New York State Office for the Prevention of Domestic Violence
Alfred E. Smith Building
80 South Swan Street
11th Floor
Room Number 1157
Albany, NY 12210
Phone: 518-457-5800
Fax: 518-457-5810
Website: www.opdv.ny.gov/

Peaceful Families Project
P.O. Box 771
Great Falls, VA 22066
Phone: 703-474-6870
Website:
http://www.peacefulfamilies.org
E-mail: info@
peacefulfamilies.org

Rape, Abuse & Incest National Network (RAINN)
2000 L Street NW, Suite 406
Washington, DC 20036
Toll-Free: 800-656-HOPE
(800-656-4673) (National Sexual
Assault Hotline)
Phone: 202-544-1034
Fax: 202-544-3556
Website: http://www.rainn.org
E-mail: info@rainn.org

Safe@Work Coalition
Website: http://
www.safeatworkcoalition.org

South Carolina Coalition Against Domestic Violence and Sexual Assault
P.O. Box 7776
Columbia, SC 29202
Phone: 803-256-2900
Website: http://
www.sccadvasa.org

Stop Abuse For Everyone
10030 Scenic View Terrace
Vienna, VA 22182
Phone: 503-853-8686
Website: http://www.safe4all.org
E-mail: safe@safe4all.org

U.S. Department of Health and Human Services Office on Women's Health
200 Independence Avenue SW
Washington, DC 20201
Phone: 202-690-7650
Fax: 202-205-2631
Website: http://
www.womenshealth.gov

Washington State Coalition Against Domestic Violence (WSCADV)
1402 Third Avenue
Suite 406
Seattle, WA 98101
Phone: 206-389-2515
TTY: 206-389-2900
Fax: 206-389-2520
Website: http://www.wscadv.org
E-mail: wscadv@wscadv.org

Women's Justice Center
P.O. Box 7510
Santa Rosa, CA 95407
Phone: 707-575-3150
Website:
http://www.justicewomen.com
E-mail: rdjustice@monitor.net

Child Abuse

Child Welfare Information Gateway
Children's Bureau/ACYF
1250 Maryland Avenue SW
Eighth Floor
Washington, DC 20024
Toll-Free: 800-394-3366
Website:
http://www.childwelfare.gov
E-mail: info@childwelfare.gov

Child Witness to Violence Project
Department of Pediatrics
Boston Medical Center
88 East Newton Street
Vose Hall
Boston, MA 02118
Phone: 617-414-4244
Website:
http://www.childwitnessto
violence.org/contact-us.html

National Children's Advocacy Center
210 Pratt Avenue
Huntsville, AL 35801
Phone: 256-533-KIDS
(256-533-5437)
Fax: 256-534-6883
Website:
http://www.nationalcac.org
E-mail: prevention
@nationalcac.org (Prevention)
E-mail: intervention
@nationalcac.org (Intervention)

Elder Abuse

Clearinghouse on Abuse and Neglect of the Elderly (CANE)
University of Delaware
Department of Consumer Studies
Alison Hall West, Room 211
Newark, DE 19716
Website:
http://www.cane.udel.edu
E-mail: CANE-UD@udel.edu

National Center on Elder Abuse
National Association of State
Units on Aging
University of California—Irvine
Program in Geriatric Medicine
101 The City Drive South
200 Building
Orange, CA 92868
Toll-Free: 855-500-ELDR
(855-500-3537)
Fax: 714-456-7933
Website: http://www.ncea.aoa.gov
E-mail: ncea-info@aoa.hhs.gov

National Clearinghouse on Abuse in Later Life
307 South Paterson Street
Suite 1
Madison, WI 53703-3517
Phone: 608-255-0539
TTY/Fax: 608-255-3560
Website: http://www.ncall.us
E-mail: ncall@wcadv.org

**National Committee for the
Prevention of Elder Abuse
(NCPEA)**
151 First Avenue, #93
New York, NY 10003
Phone: 646-462-3603
Fax: 212 420-6026
Website:
http://www.preventelderabuse.org
Email:
info@preventelderabuse.org

Chapter 49

Domestic Violence Hotlines

National Domestic Abuse Hotlines

National Domestic Violence Hotline
Toll-Free: 800-799-SAFE (800-799-7233)
TTY: 800-787-3224

Rape, Abuse, and Incest National Network (RAINN)
National Hotline
Toll-Free: 800-656-HOPE (800-656-4673)

Safe Horizon Domestic Violence Hotline
Toll-Free: 800-621-HOPE (800-621-4673)
TDD: 866-604-5350

Domestic Violence Hotlines by State

If your state is not listed below, call the National Domestic Violence Hotline (listed above).

Alabama Coalition Against Domestic Violence
Toll-Free: 800-650-6522

Information in this chapter was compiled from sources deemed accurate. All contact information was verified and updated in July 2012.

Alaska Network on Domestic Violence and Sexual Assault
Phone: 907-586-3650

Arizona Coalition Against Domestic Violence
Toll-Free: 800-782-6400
TTY: 602-279-7270

Arkansas Coalition Against Domestic Violence
Toll-Free: 800-269-4668

California—Support Network for Battered Women
Toll-Free: 800-572-2782

Florida Coalition Against Domestic Violence
Toll-Free: 800-500-1119 (Florida callers only)
TTY: 800-621-4202

Hawaii State Coalition Against Domestic Violence
Hilo: 808-959-8864
Kauai: 808-245-6362
Kona: 808-322-SAFE (7233)
Maui/Lanai: 808-579-9581
Molokai: 808-567-6888
Oahu: 808-841-0822 (Town/Leeward) 808-526-2200 (Windward)

Iowa Coalition Against Domestic Violence
Toll-Free: 800-942-0333

Idaho Coalition Against Sexual and Domestic Violence
Toll-Free: 800-669-3176

Kansas
Toll-Free: 888-END-ABUSE (888-363-2287) (Kansas callers only)

Maine Coalition to End Domestic Violence
Toll-Free: 866-834-HELP (866-834-4357) (Maine callers only)

Massachusetts
Toll-Free: 877-785-2020

Minnesota Day One Domestic Violence Crisis Line
Toll-Free: 866-223-1111

Mississippi State Coalition Against Domestic Violence
Toll-Free: 800-898-3234 (Mon-Fri 8 a.m.–5 p.m.) (Mississippi callers only)

New Hampshire Coalition Against Domestic and Sexual Violence
Toll-Free: 866-644-3574
Toll-Free: 800-277-5570 (Sexual Assault)

New York State Coalition Against Domestic Violence
Toll-Free (English): 800-942-6906
TTY (English): 800-818-0656
Toll-Free (Spanish): 800-942-6908
TTY (Spanish): 800-780-7660

North Dakota Council on Abused Women's Services
Toll-Free: 800-472-2911 (North Dakota callers only)

Ohio Domestic Violence Network
Toll-Free: 800-934-9840

Oregon Coalition Against Domestic Violence and Sexual Assault
Toll-Free: 888-235-5333 (Statewide Crisis Center)

Rhode Island Coalition Against Domestic Violence
Toll-Free: 800-494-8100

South Dakota Coalition Against Domestic Violence and Sexual Assault
Toll-Free: 800-572-9196

Utah LINK Line
Toll-Free: 800-897-LINK (800-897-5465)

Vermont Network Against Domestic and Sexual Violence
Toll-Free: 800-228-7395 (Domestic Violence)
Toll-Free: 800-489-7273 (Sexual Violence)

Virginia Family Violence and Sexual Assault Hotline
Toll-Free: 800-838-VADV (800-838-8238) (Voice/TTY)

Washington State Domestic Violence Hotline
Toll-Free: 800-562-6025

Elder Abuse Resources

Eldercare Locator
Toll-Free: 800-677-1116
TTY: 800-677-1116
Website: http://www.eldercare.gov/ELDERCARE.NET/Public/About/
Services.aspx
E-mail: eldercarelocator@n4a.org

Elder Abuse Resources by State
For state reporting numbers, government agencies, state laws, state-specific data and statistics, and other resources, visit http://www.ncea
.aoa.gov/ncearoot/main_site/Find_Help/State_Resources.aspx.

Chapter 50

State Child Abuse Reporting Numbers

State contact numbers for specific agencies designated to receive and investigate reports of suspected child abuse and neglect.

Alabama
Phone: 334-242-9500
Website: http://dhr.alabama.gov/ services/Child_Protective_Services /Abuse_Neglect_Reporting.aspx

Visit the website above for information on reporting or call Childhelp® (800-422-4453) for assistance.

Alaska
Toll-Free: 800-478-4444
Website: http://www.hss.state.ak .us/ocs/default.htm

Arizona
Toll-Free: 888-SOS-CHILD (888-767-2445)
Website: https://www.azdes.gov/ dcyf/cps/reporting.asp

Arkansas
Toll-Free: 800-482-5964
Website: http://www.arkansas.gov/ reportARchildabuse

California
Website: http://www.dss.cah-wnet.gov/cdssweb/PG20.htm

Visit the website above for information on reporting or call Childhelp® (800-422-4453) for assistance.

Reprinted from "State Child Abuse Reporting Numbers," U.S. Department of Health and Human Services, January 5, 2012. All contact information was verified and updated in July 2012.

Colorado

Phone: 303-866-5932

Website: http://www.cdhs.state
.co.us/childwelfare/FAQ.htm

Visit the website above for information on reporting or call Childhelp® (800-422-4453) for assistance.

Connecticut

Toll-Free: 800-842-2288

Toll-Free TDD: 800-624-5518

Website: http://www.state.ct.us/
dcf/HOTLINE.htm

Delaware

Toll-Free: 800-292-9582

Website: http://kids.delaware.gov/
services/crisis.shtml

District of Columbia

Phone: 202-671-SAFE
(202-671-7233)

Website: http://cfsa.dc.gov/DC/
CFSA/Support+the+Safety+Net/
Report+Child+Abuse+and
+Neglect

Florida

Toll-Free: 800-96-ABUSE
(800-962-2873)

Website: http://www.dcf.state.
fl.us/abuse

Georgia

Website: http://dfcs.dhs.georgia
.gov

Visit the website above for information on reporting or call Childhelp® (800-422-4453) for assistance.

Hawaii

Phone: 808-832-5300

Website: http://www.hawaii.gov/
dhs/protection/social_services/
child_welfare

Idaho

Toll-Free: 800-926-2588

TDD: 208-332-7205

Website: http://healthandwelfare
.idaho.gov/Children/AbuseNeglect/
ChildProtectionContactPhone
Numbers/tabid/475/Default.aspx

Illinois

Toll-Free: 800-25-ABUSE
(800-252-2873)

Phone: 217-785-4020

Website: http://www.state.il.us/
dcfs/child/index.shtml

Indiana

Toll-Free: 800-800-5556

Website: http://www.in.gov/dcs/
protection/dfcchi.html

Iowa

Toll-Free: 800-362-2178

Website: http://www.dhs.state
.ia.us/dhs2005/dhs_homepage/
children_family/abuse_reporting/
child_abuse.html

Kansas

Toll-Free: 800-922-5330

Website: http://www.dcf.ks.gov/
Pages/Default.aspx

Kentucky
Toll-Free: 1-877-KYSAFE1
(877-597-2331)
Website: http://chfs.ky.gov/dcbs/
dpp/childsafety.htm

Louisiana
Toll-Free: 855-4LA-KIDS
(855-452-5437)
Website: http://dss.louisiana.gov/
index.cfm?md=pagebuilder
&tmp=home&pid=109

Maine
Toll-Free: 800-452-1999
Toll-Free TTY: 800-963-9490
Website: http://www.maine.gov/
dhhs/ocfs/hotlines.htm

Maryland
Website: http://www.dhr.state.md
.us/cps/report.htm

Visit the website above for information on reporting or call Childhelp® (800-422-4453) for assistance.

Massachusetts
Toll-Free: 800-792-5200
Website: http://www.mass.gov/
eohhs/consumer/family-services/
child-abuse-neglect

Michigan
Toll-Free: 855-444-3911
Website: http://www.michigan
.gov/dhs/0,1607,7-124-5452_
7119---,00.html

Minnesota
Website: http://www.dhs.state
.mn.us/main/idcplg?IdcService=
GET_DYNAMIC_CONVERSI
ON&RevisionSelectionMethod
=LatestReleased&dDocName=
id_000152

Visit the website above for information on reporting or call Childhelp® (800-422-4453) for assistance.

Mississippi
Toll-Free: 800-222-8000
Phone: 601-432-4570
Website: http://www.mdhs.state
.ms.us/fcs_prot.html

Missouri
Toll-Free: 800-392-3738
Phone: 573-751-3448
Website: http://www.dss.mo.gov/
cd/rptcan.htm

Montana
Toll-Free: 866-820-5437
Website: http://www.dphhs.mt
.gov/cfsd/index.shtml

Nebraska
Toll-Free: 800-652-1999
Website: http://dhhs.ne.gov/chil
dren_family_services/Pages/
children_family_services.aspx

Nevada
Toll-Free: 800-992-5757
Phone: 702-399-0081
Website: http://dcfs.state.nv.us/
DCFS_ReportSuspectedChild
Abuse.htm

New Hampshire
Toll-Free: 800-894-5533
Toll-Free TDD: 800-735-2964
Phone: 603-271-6556
Fax: 603-271-6565 (Report Child Abuse Fax)
Website: http://www.dhhs.state
.nh.us/dcyf/cps/contact.htm

New Jersey
Toll-Free: 877-NJ ABUSE
(877-652-2873)
Toll-Free TDD/TTY:
800-835-5510
Website: http://www.state.nj.us/
dcf/abuse/how

New Mexico
Toll-Free: 855-333-SAFE
(855-333-7233)
Website: http://www.cyfd.org/
content/reporting-abuse-or
-neglect

New York
Toll-Free: 800-342-3720
Toll-Free TDD/TTY:
800-638-5163
Phone: 518-473-7793
Website: http://www.ocfs.state.ny
.us/main/cps

North Carolina
Website: http://www.dhhs.state
.nc.us/dss/cps/index.htm

Visit the website above for information on reporting or call Childhelp® (800-422-4453) for assistance.

North Dakota
Website: http://www.nd.gov/
dhs/services/childfamily/
cps/#reporting

Visit the website above for information on reporting or call Childhelp® (800-422-4453) for assistance.

Ohio
Website: http://jfs.ohio.gov/County/
County_Directory.pdf

Contact the county Public Children Services Agency or call Childhelp® (800-422-4453) for assistance.

Oklahoma
Toll-Free: 800-522-3511
Website: http://www.okdhs
.org/programsandservices/cps/
default.htm

Oregon
Website: http://www.oregon.gov/
DHS/children/abuse/cps/report
.shtml

Visit the website above for information on reporting or call Childhelp® (800-422-4453) for assistance.

Pennsylvania
Toll-Free: 800-932-0313
Toll-Free TDD: 866-872-1677
Website: http://www.dpw.state.pa
.us/forchildren/childwelfareser
vices/calltoreportchildabuse!/
index.htm

Puerto Rico
Toll-Free: 800-981-8333
Phone: 787-749-1333
Website (Spanish):
http://www.gobierno.pr/GPRPortal/
StandAlone/AgencyInformation
.aspx?Filter=177

Rhode Island
Toll-Free: 800-RI-CHILD
(800-742-4453)
Website: http://www.dcyf.ri.gov/
child_welfare/index.php

South Carolina
Phone: 803-898-7318
Website: http://dss.sc.gov/content/
customers/protection/cps/index
.aspx

Visit the website above for information on reporting or call Childhelp® (800-422-4453) for assistance.

South Dakota
Website: http://dss.sd.gov/cps/
protective/reporting.asp

Visit the website above for information on reporting or call Childhelp® (800-422-4453) for assistance.

Tennessee
Toll-Free: 877-237-0004 or
877-54ABUSE (877-542-2873)
Website: https://reportabuse
.state.tn.us

Texas
Department of Family and Protective Services
Toll-Free: 800-252-5400
Toll-Free TTY: 800-735-2989
Website: https://www.dfps.state
.tx.us/Child_Protection/
About_Child_Protective_Services/
reportChildAbuse.asp
Spanish: http://www.dfps.state
.tx.us/default-sp.asp

Utah
Toll-Free: 855-323-3237
Website: http://www.hsdcfs.utah
.gov

Vermont
After hours: 800-649-5285
Website: http://www.dcf.state
.vt.us/fsd/reporting_child_abuse

Virginia
Toll-Free: 800-552-7096
Phone: 804-786-8536
Website: http://www.dss.virginia
.gov/family/cps/index.html

Washington
Toll-Free: 800-562-5624 or
866-END-HARM (866-363-4276)
Toll-Free TTY: 800-624-6186
Website: http://www1.dshs.wa
.gov/ca/safety/abuseReport.asp?2

West Virginia
Toll-Free: 800-352-6513
Website: http://www.wvdhhr.org/
bcf/children_adult/cps/report.asp

Wisconsin

Website: http://dcf.wisconsin.gov/
children/CPS/cpswimap.HTM

Visit the website above for information on reporting or call Childhelp® (800-422-4453) for assistance.

Wyoming

Website: http://dfsweb.state.
wy.us/protective-services/cps/
index.html

Visit the website above for information on reporting or call Childhelp® (800-422-4453) for assistance.

Chapter 51

Programs Providing Shelter for Pets of Domestic Violence Victims

If you are concerned about your pet's safety, check our list for a shelter near you that allows pets.

If you don't see a program listed in your area, contact your local domestic violence shelter, animal shelter, veterinarian, or boarding kennel to see if they have a Safe Haven for Animals program or can provide temporary care for your pet.

Alabama

Tuscaloosa
Organization: Tuscaloosa Metro Animal Shelter
3140 35th Street
Tuscaloosa, AL 35401
Phone: 205-752-9101
Website: http://www.metroanimalshelter.org/index.html
E-mail: mas@dbtech.net

Alaska

Dillingham
Program: Safe and Fear Free Environment, Inc.
P.O. Box 94
Dillingham, AK 99576
Toll-Free: 800-478-2316
(24-hour Crisis Line)
Phone: 907-842-2320
Fax: 907-842-2198
Website: http://www.safebristolbay.org

Arizona

Casa Grande

Organization: Valley Humane
Society, Inc.*
15699 West Aniceto Road
Casa Grande, AZ 85193
Phone: 520-836-0904
Fax: 520-836-7261
Website: http://www.petfinder
.com/shelters/vhs.html
E-mail: vhsanimals@yahoo.com
*Animals are welcome on a
space-available basis.

Page

Organization: Page Regional
Domestic Violence Services
P.O. Box 3686
Page, AZ 86040
Phone: 928-645-5300 (24-hour
Hotline)
Fax: 928-645-3414
Website: http://pageregional
domesticviolenceservices.org
E-mail: info@pageregional
domesticviolenceservices.org or
AnotherWay@cableone.net

Phoenix

Program: Project Safe House
Organization: Arizona Humane
Society
9226 North 13th Avenue
Phoenix, AZ 85021
Phone: 602-997-7586 ext. 2058
(Manager of Alternative Place-
ment and Animal Care)
Fax: 602-870-1999
Website: http://www.azhumane
.org/artman2/publish/programs/
alternative-placement.shtml

Program: MSCO Animal Safe
Haven (MASH)
Organization: Maricopa County
Sheriff's Office
First Avenue and Madison
Street
Phoenix, AZ 85003
Phone: 602-876-1212
Website: http://www.mcso.org/
Mash/default.aspx
E-mail:
MASH@mcso.maricopa.gov

Tucson

Program: Safe Haven Animal
Foster Care Program
Organization: Humane Society
of Southern Arizona
Contact: Safe Haven Coordinator
3450 North Kelvin Boulevard
Tucson, AZ 85716-1326
Phone: 520-327-6088 ext. 100
Fax: 520-325-7190
Website: http://www.hssaz.org/
sitePageServer?pagename
=hssaz_homepage

California

Encinitas

Program: Animal Safehouse
Program (ASP)
Organization: Rancho Coastal
Humane Society
389 Requeza Street
Encinitas, CA 92023
Phone: 760-753-6476
Fax: 760-753-6664
Website: http://www.rancho
coastalasp.org
E-mail: safehouse@
rchumanesociety.org

Novato
Program: Companions in Crisis
Organization: Marin Humane Society
71 Bel Marin Keys Boulevard
Novato, CA 94949
Phone: 415-883-4621
(24-hour Hotline)
Website: http://www.marinhuma
nesociety.org/site/c.aiIOI3NLK
gKYF/b.7727631/.66AF/Compan
ions_in_Crisis.htm

Placerville
Program: Safe Pet Program
Organization: Center for Violence-Free Relationships
344 Placerville Drive, Suite 11
Placerville, CA 95667
Phone: 530-626-1131 or
916-939-6616 (24-hour Help Lines)
Fax: 530-626-6895
Website: http://thecenternow
.org/what-we-do/services/safe
-pet-program/

Redding
Organization: Haven Humane Society
7449 Eastside Road
Anderson, CA 96007
Phone: 530-241-1653
Website:
http://www.havenhumane.net
E-mail:
rescue@havenhumane.org

San Diego
Program: PATH (Protecting Animals through Temporary Housing)
2317 Shamrock Street
San Diego, CA 92105
Phone: 717-650-7715

San Francisco
Program: Safe Pets Program
Organization: San Francisco Department of Animal Care and Control
Contact: Shelter Office Supervisor
1200 15th Street
San Francisco, CA 94103
Phone: 415-554-9401
(Shelter Office Supervisor) or
415-554-6364 (General)
Fax: 415-864-2863 or
415-557-9950
Website: http://www.sfgov2.org/
index.aspx?page=942

San Mateo
Program: Safe Pets Program
Organization: Peninsula Humane Society and SPCA
12 Airport Boulevard
San Mateo, CA 94401-1006
Phone: 650-340-7022 ext. 378
Fax: 650-685-0102
Website: http://www
.peninsulahumanesociety.org

Sonora
Organization: Victim/Witness Assistance Center at Tuolumne County District Attorney's Office*
423 North Washington Street
Sonora, CA 95370-5525
Phone: 209-588-5440
Fax: 209-588-5455
*Helps pay for people and pets to stay at a local hotel for two nights.

Colorado

Boulder
Program: Safehouse Progressive
Alliance for Nonviolence
Organization: Humane Society
of Boulder Valley
Contact: HSBV Behavior and
Health Department
2323 55th Street
Boulder, CO 80301-2806
Phone: 303-442-4030 ext. 657
Fax: 303-565-5151
Website:
http://www.boulderhumane.org
E-mail: health.behavior
@boulderhumane.org

Colorado Springs
Program: Safe Pets Program
through the TESSA Safe House
Organization: Humane Society
of the Pikes Peak Region
610 Abbott Lane
Colorado Springs, CO 80905
Phone: 719-473-1741 ext. 8750
(Humane Society) or
719-633-3819 (TESSA 24-hour
Crisis Line)
Fax: 719-444-0179 (Humane
Society)
Websites: http://www.tessacs.org
and http://www.hsppr.org

Denver
Program: Pet Assistance Pro-
gram
Organization: Dumb Friends
League
2080 South Quebec Street
Denver, CO 80231
Phone: 303-696-4941 ext. 7291

Phone: 303-751-5775 ext. 7300
(Animal Care Manager) or 303-
751-5772 (Foster Department)
Fax: 303-696-0063
Website: http://www.ddfl.org

Fort Collins
Program: Crosstrails
Organization: Crossroads
Safehouse, Inc.
P.O. Box 993
Fort Collins, CO 80522-0993
Toll-Free: 888-541-7233
(24-hour Hotline)
Phone: 970-482-3502
(24-hour Hotline)
Fax: 970-482-3028
Website: http://www.crossroads
safehouse.org

Longmont
Program: Safekeep Program
Organization: Longmont
Humane Society
9595 Nelson Road
Longmont, CO 80501
Phone: 303-772-1232 ext. 26
Fax: 303-772-2219
Website: http://www.longmont
humane.org

Rangely
Program: Rangely Animal Shelter
Organization: Rangely Victim
Services
P.O. Box 194
Rangely, CO 81648
Phone: 970-675-8476
Website: http://www.rangely.com/
animal-shelter.htm
E-mail: rangelyinfo@
rangelygovt.com

District of Columbia

Program: Safety Network For Abused Animals And People (SNAAP)
Organization: Washington Humane Society
Contact: Director of Safe Haven Program
7319 Georgia Avenue NW
Washington, DC 20012-1719
Phone: 202-BE-HUMANE (24-hour Animal Cruelty Hotline) or 202-234-8626 ext. 230 (Director of Safe Haven Program)*
Fax: 202-723-5409
Website: http://www .safeanimalssafepeople.org
* To enroll in the Safe Haven Program, have your domestic violence advocate contact the Washington Humane Society at (202) 234-8626.

Florida

Brevard

Organization: Animal Safehouse of Brevard
Phone: 407-620-6865
Website: http://www.animalsafe housebrevard.org
E-mail: animalsafehouse@ gmail.com

Fort Lauderdale

Program: Companion Animal Rescue Efforts (CARE)
Organization: Humane Society of Broward County
2070 Griffin Road
Fort Lauderdale, FL 33312
Phone: 954-237-0223
(Senior Director of Operations) or 954-989-3977 (General Number)
Fax: 954-989-3991
Website: http://www.humanebroward.com
E-mail: info@humanebroward.com

Fort Walton Beach

Program: Safe People, Safe Pets
Organization: PAWS— Panhandle Animal Welfare Society
752 Lovejoy Road
Fort Walton Beach, FL 32548
Phone: 850-243-1525
(Executive Director of Animal Services, ext. 20 or Director of the Humane Society & Adoption Center, ext. 12)
Fax: 850-664-0445
Website: http://www.paws -shelter.com
E-mail: acoatpaws@ embarqmail.com

Partner Organization: Shelter House, Inc.
P.O. Box 220
Fort Walton Beach, FL 32549
Toll-Free: 800-442-2873 (24-Hour Crisis Hotline)
Phone: 850-863-4777 (24-Hour Crisis Hotline)
Fax: 850-243-6756
Website: http://www.shelterhousenwfl .org
E-mail: info@ shelterhousenwfl.org

Largo

Organization: SPCA
of Tampa Bay
9099 130th Avenue N
Largo, FL 33773
Phone: 727-586-3591 ext. 161
(Director of Animal Care and
Facilities)
Fax: 727-499-0368
Website: http://
www.spcatampabay.org

Miami

Program: Project Safe Families,
Safe Pets
Organization:
Humane Society of
Greater Miami
16101 West Dixie Highway
North Miami, FL 33160
Phone: 305-749-1818
(Senior Shelter Manager)
Website: http://
www.humanesocietymiami.org

Naples

Program: On-Site Kennel for
Pets of Shelter Residents
Organization: Shelter for Abused
Women and Children
P.O. Box 10102
Naples, FL 34101-0102
Phone: 239-280-1350
(Director of Operations) or
239-775-1101
(24-hour Crisis Line)
TTY: 239-775-4265 (24-hour
Crisis Line)
Fax: 239-775-3061
Website:
http://www.naplesshelter.org
E-mail: info@naplesshelter.org

Newberry

Organization: West End Animal
Hospital
15318 West Newberry Road
Newberry, FL 32669
Phone: 352-472-7626
Fax: 352-472-5471
Website: http://
www.westendanimal.com
E-mail: weahinfo@gmail.com

St. Augustine

Organization: St. Johns County
Animal Control/Pet Center
130 North Stratton Road
St. Augustine, FL 32095
Phone: 904-209-0746 (Animal
Control) or 904-209-6190
(Pet Center)
Website: http://www.co.st-johns
.fl.us/AnimalControl/index.aspx
E-mail: info@sjcfl.us

St. Petersburg

Organization: CASA,
Department of Children and
Family Services
P.O. Box 414
St. Petersburg, FL 33731
Phone: 727-895-4912 ext. 111
Fax: 727-821-7101
Website: http://www.casa
-stpete.org
E-mail: info@casa-stpete.org

Vero Beach

Program: Foster Pet Program
Organization: Humane Society
of Vero Beach and Indian River
County
6230 77th Street
Vero Beach, FL 32967

Phone: 772-388-3331
(Director of Animal Protective
Services, ext. 28 or Director of
Animal Care, ext. 31)
Fax: 772-388-3981
Website: http://hsvb.org/
default3.htm

Georgia

Atlanta
Organization: Ahimsa House,
Inc.
P.O. Box 8181
Atlanta, GA 31106
Phone: 404-496-4038
(Administrative Line) or
404-452-6248 (24-hour Hotline)
Fax: 404-671-8599
Website: http://
www.ahimsahouse.org
E-mail: info@ahimsahouse.org

Blairsville
Organization: Support in
Abusive Family Emergencies,
Inc. (SAFE)
P.O. Box 11
Blairsville, GA 30514
Phone: 706-379-3000 (24-hour
Hotline) or 706-379-1901
(Administrative)
Fax: 706-379-1910
Website:
http://www.gnesa.org/safe
E-mail: info@safeservices.org

Hawaii

Honolulu
Program: Emergency Foster
Care

Organization: Hawaiian
Humane Society
2700 Waialae Avenue
Honolulu, HI 96826
Phone: 808-356-2229 (Foster
Care) or 808-946-2187 (Humane
Society)
Fax: 808-955-6034
Website: http://
www.hawaiianhumane.org/
Foster-Care.html
E-mail:
hhs@hawaiianhumane.org

Idaho

Rexburg
Organization:
Family Crisis Center
16 East Main Street
Rexburg, ID 83440
Phone: 208-356-0065
E-mail:
familycrisiscenterrexburg@
gmail.com

Illinois

Decatur
Organization: Dove, Inc.
788 East Clay Street
Decatur, IL 62521
Phone: 217-428-6616
Fax: 217-428-7256
Website: http://www.doveinc.org
E-mail: dove@doveinc.org

DeKalb
Program: Safe Pets Program
Organization: Tails Humane
Society (in partnership with the
Safe Passage Domestic Violence
Center)

2250 Barber Greene Road
DeKalb, IL 60115
Phone: 815-758-2457
Fax: 815-787-4888
or 815-487-4944
Website: http://
www.tailshumanesociety.org
E-mail: info@
tailshumanesociety.org

Naperville
Program: Safe Pets Program
Organization: Naperville Area
Humane Society
1620 West Diehl Road
Naperville, IL 60563
Phone: 630-420-8989
Fax: 630-420-9380
Website: http://www.naperville
humanesociety.org
E-mail: info@
napervilleareahumanesociety.org

Princeton
Program: Safe Animal Fostering
Environment (SAFE)
Organization: Friends of Strays,
Inc.
2845 North Main Street
Princeton, IL 61356
Phone: 815-872-7387
Website: http://www.friendsof
straysshelter.org
E-mail: fos3@frontier.com

Indiana

Evansville
Program: Safe Pets
Organization: Vanderburgh
Humane Society
400 Millner Industrial Drive

Evansville, IN 47710
Phone: 812-426-2563 ext. 203
(Operations Manager)
Website: http://www.vhslifesaver
.org/help/volunteer_programs
.html
E-mail: info@vhslifesaver.org

Fort Wayne
Program: Safe Haven
for Domestic Violence
Organization: City of Fort Wayne
Animal Care and Control
3020 Hillegas Road
Fort Wayne, IN 46808
Phone: 260-427-1244
Fax: 260-427-5514
Website: http://
www.cityoffortwayne.org/animal
-care-and-control.html

West Lafayette
Program: Animals in Crisis
(PetSafe)
Organization: Center for the
Human-Animal Bond
Purdue University School of
Veterinary Medicine
625 Harrison Street
West Lafayette, IN 47907
Phone: 765-494-1107
(Purdue Small Animal Hospital)
Website: http://www.vet.purdue
.edu/chab/petsafe.htm

Kansas

Newton
Organization: Caring Hands
Humane Society
1400 SE Third Street
Newton, KS 67114

Phone: 316-283-0839
Fax: 316-283-4050
Website: http://
www.caringhandshs.org

Kentucky

Covington
Program: Pet Protection
Program
Organization: Women's Crisis
Center, Inc.
835 Madison Avenue
Covington, KY 41011
Toll-Free: 800-928-3335
(24-hour Crisis Line)
Phone: 859-491-3335 (24-hour
Crisis Line)
TDD: 859-655-2657
(24-hour Crisis Line)
Fax: 859-655-2655
Website: http://www.wccky.org

Louisville
Program: Kentucky Humane
Society in Partnership with the
Safe Haven for Pets
Organization: The Center for
Women and Families
P.O. Box 2048
927 South 2nd Street
Louisville, KY 40201
Toll-Free: 877-803-7577
(24-hour Crisis Line)
Phone: 502-581-7200 (Business)
or 502-581-7222 (24-hour)
Websites: http://www.thecenter
online.org/get-help (Center for
Women and Families) and
http://www.kyhumane.org (Hu-
mane Society)
E-mail: info@cwfempower.org

Louisiana

Lake Charles
Organization: OASIS—A Safe
Haven for Survivors of Domestic
and Sexual Violence
(formerly known as Calcasieu
Women's Shelter)
P.O. Box 276
Lake Charles, LA 70602
Toll-Free: 800-223-8066
(24-hour Crisis Hotline)
Phone: 337-436-4552 (24-hour
Crisis Hotline)
Fax: 337-436-8327
Website: http://
www.cwshelter.org
E-mail: cws@cwshelter.org

Maine

Brunswick
Program: Crisis Care
Organization: Coastal Humane
Society
30 Range Road
Brunswick, ME 04011
Phone: 207-725-5051
Fax: 207-725-4111
Website: http://
www.coastalhumanesociety.org
E-mail: info@
coastalhumanesociety.org

Lewiston
Organization: Greater
Androscoggin Humane Society
55 Strawberry Avenue
Lewiston, ME 04240
Phone: 207-786-4713
(Shelter Director) or
207-783-2311 (Main Number)

Fax: 207-782-5521
Website: http://
www.gahumane.org
E-mail: info@gahumane.org

Portland/Westbrook
Program: PAST Foster Care
Program
Organizations: Animal Refuge
League of Greater Portland and
Family Crisis Services (Contact
a counselor with Family Crisis
Services to arrange shelter with
the Animal Refuge League.)
449 Stroudwater Street
Westbrook, Maine 04092
Toll-Free: 866-834-4357 (24-hour
Hotline—TTY Accessible Family
Crisis Services)
Phone: 207-767-4952
(Family Crisis Administrative) or
207-874-1973 (24-hour Hotline)
or 207-854-9771 (Animal Refuge
League)
Fax: 207-767-8109
Websites: http://www.familycrisis
.org and http://www.arlgp.org
E-mail: familycrisis@
familycrisis.org

Rockland
Organization: New Hope for
Women
P.O. Box A
5 Beech Street
Rockland, ME 04841
Toll-Free: 800-522-3304
(24-hour Hotline)
Phone: 207-594-2128
Fax: 207-594-0811
Website: http://www.new
hopeforwomen.org/services.php

Waterville
Program: PAC—People
and Animals in Crisis
Organization: Humane Society
Waterville Area
100 Webb Road
Waterville, ME 04901
Phone: 207-873-2430
Fax: 207-873-1266
Website: http://www.hswa.org

West Kennebunk
Program: Pets and Women to
Safety (PAWS)
Organization: Animal Welfare
Society
P.O. Box 43
West Kennebunk, ME 04094
Phone/Fax: 207-985-3244
Website: http://www
.animalwelfaresociety.org

Maryland

Baltimore
Program: Safe House Program
Organization: House of Ruth
Maryland
2201 Argonne Drive
Baltimore, MD 21218
Phone: 410-889-0840
(Administrative Line) or
410-889-7884 (24-hour Hotline)
Fax: 410-889-9347
Website: http://www.hruth.org
E-mail: info@hruthmd.org

Chesapeake City/Elkton
Program: Domestic
Abuse Assistance
Organization: Cecil County
SPCA, Inc.

Contact: Have a social worker contact the SPCA to make arrangements
3280 Augustine Herman Highway
Chesapeake City, MD 21915
Phone: 410-398-9555 or 410-885-2342
Fax: 410-885-2910
Website: http://www.cecilcountyspca.org/services.html
E-mail: cecilcospca@verizon.net

Partnering organization:
Cecil County Domestic Violence/ Rape Crisis Center
P.O. Box 2137
Elkton, MD 21922
Phone: 410-996-0333
(24-hour Hotline)
Fax: 410-885-2910

Columbia
Program: Pet Safe Project
Organization: Domestic Violence Center of Howard County
5457 Twin Knolls Road
Suite 310
Columbia, MD 21045
Toll-Free: 800-752-0191
(24-hour Hotline)
Phone: 410-997-0304
(Administrative Line) or
410-997-2272 (24-hour Hotline)
Fax: 410-997-1397
Website: http://www.dvcenter.org
E-mail: dvc@dvcenter.org

Denton
Program: Safe Pet Sheltering Program
Organization: Mid-Shore Council on Family Violence

P.O. Box 5
Denton, MD 21629
Toll-Free: 800-927-4673
(24-hour Hotline)
Phone: 410-479-1149
(Administrative Line)
Fax: 410-479-2064
Website: http://www.mscfv.org/joomla

Hartford County
Program: Safe Haven for Pets
Organization: SARC-Sexual Assault/Spouse Abuse Resource Center
Contact: Safe House Supervisor
P.O. Box 1207
Bel Air, MD 21014
Phone: 410-836-8430
(24-hour Hotline)
Fax: 410-838-9484
Website: http://www.sarc-maryland.org
E-mail: information@sarc-maryland.org

Towson
Organization: TurnAround, Inc.
401 Washington Avenue
Suite 300
Towson, MD 21204
Phone: 410-377-8111
(Administrative) or
410-828-6390 (24-hour Hotline)
Fax: 410-377-6806
Website: http://www.turnaroundinc.org
E-mail: info@turnaroundinc.org

Massachusetts

Pittsfield
Program: PetSafe

Organization: Berkshire
Humane Society
214 Barker Road
Pittsfield, MA 01201
Phone: 413-447-7878
Fax: 413-443-3347
Website: http://
berkshirehumane.org

Michigan

Ann Arbor

Organization: Domestic Violence
Project, Inc.
SafeHouse Center
4100 Clark Road
Ann Arbor, MI 48105
Phone: 734-973-0242 or
734-995-5444
(24-hour HelpLine)
TTY: 734-973-2227
(24-hour HelpLine)
Fax: 734-973-7817
Website: http://www.dvpsh.org

Battle Creek

Program: SAFE Place Shelter
(Individuals must go through
SAFE Place first.)
Organization: Humane Society
of South Central Michigan
2500 Watkins Road
Battle Creek, MI 49015
Phone: 269-965-6093 (SAFE
Place) or 269-963-1796 ext. 13
(Executive Director,
Humane Society)
Fax: 269-963-3365
(Humane Society)
Websites: http://www.safeplace
shelter.org
and http://www.hs-scm.org/

Howell

Program: Safe Pet Place
Organization: LACASA
2895 West Grand River Avenue
Howell, MI 48843
Toll-Free: 866-522-2725
(24-hour Crisis Line)
Phone: 517-548-1350
(Administrative Line)
TTY: 517-548-0781
Fax: 517-548-3034
Website: http://www.lacasa
center.org/safe-pet-place
E-mail: info@lacasacenter.org

Cadillac

Program: Wonderland Pet Haven
Organization: Wonderland
Humane Society (in cooperation
with OASIS/Family Resource
Center)
Wonderland Humane Society
P.O. Box 935
Cadillac, MI 49601
Toll-Free: 800-775-4646
(OASIS 24-hour Crisis Line)
Phone: 231-920-6405(Humane
Society) or
231-775-SAFE (231-775-7233)
(OASIS 24-hour Crisis Line)
Fax: 231-920-6405
Website: http://www.cadillac
oasis-frc.org/dv_services.asp

Kalamazoo

Program: Domestic Violence
Emergency Pet Sheltering
Program
Organization: Kalamazoo
Humane Society (in collabora-
tion with the YWCA of Kalama-
zoo Domestic Assault Program)

Kalamazoo Humane Society
4239 South Westnedge Avenue
Kalamazoo, MI 49008
Phone: 269-385-2869 (YWCA
Domestic Assault Program*) or
269-385-3587 (YWCA 24-hour
Crisis Line)
Fax: 269-345-8230
Websites: http://www.kazoo
humane.org/Services/
TemporarySheltering.aspx
and http://www.ywca.org/site/
pp.asp?c=bpLJJTOvHmE
&b=420791
E-mail: info@ywcakalamazoo.org
*If you feel you may qualify for
the Emergency Pet Sheltering
Program, please contact a staff
member of the YWCA Domestic
Assault Program.

Petoskey
Program: PetSafe
Organization: Women's Resource
Center of Northern Michigan
423 Porter Street
Petoskey, MI 49770-2844
Toll-Free: 800-275-1995
(Crisis Line)
Phone: 231-347-0082
(Safe Home Coordinator;
24-hour Crisis Line)
Fax: 231-347-5805
Website: http://www.wrcnm.org
E-mail: safe@wrcnm.org

Minnesota

Bloomington
Organization: Cornerstone
1000 East 80th Street
Bloomington, MN 55420

Phone: 952-884-0376 or
952-884-0330 (24-hour Helpline)
Fax: 952-884-2135
Website: http://
www.cornerstonemn.org
E-mail: info@cornerstonemn.org

Mississippi

Tupelo
Organization: S.A.F.E., Inc.
P.O. Box 985
Tupelo, MS 38802
Toll-Free: 800-527-7233
(24-hour Crisis Line)
Phone: 662-841-9138
Fax: 662-680-5785
Website: http://safeshelter.net

Tylertown
Program: Animal Safehouse
Program (ASP)
Organization: Saint Francis
Animal Sanctuary (SFAS)
97 Obed Magee Road
Tylertown, MS 39667
Phone: 601-222-1927
Website: http://www.sfas.org
E-mail: safehouse@sfas.org

Missouri

Cape Girardeau
Program: The P.A.W.S. Program
Organization: Safe House for
Women, Inc.
230 North Spring Street
Cape Girardeau, MO 63702
Toll-Free: 800-341-1830
(24-hour hotline)
Phone: 573-651-1614
(24-hour Hotline)

Fax: 573-335-6435
Website: http://www.semosafe
house.org/Shelter%20for%20
Your%20Pets.aspx

Kansas City

Organization: Rose Brooks
Center
P.O. Box 320599
Kansas City, MO 64132
Phone: 816-523-5550 (Offices) or
816-861-6100 (Crisis Line)
Website: https://www.rosebrooks
.org/index.html

Lebanon

Organization: COPE, Inc.
P.O. Box 1281
Lebanon, MO 65536
Toll-Free: 877-275-0930
(24-hour Hotline)
Phone: 417-532-2885
Website: http://
www.copeoflebanon.com/

St. Louis

Program: Domestic Violence Pet
Assistance Program
Organization: Animal Protective
Association of Missouri
1705 South Hanley Road
St. Louis, MO 63144
Phone: 314-645-4610
Fax: 314-645-3292
Website: http://www.apamo.org/
CommunityPrograms.aspx
E-mail: education@apamo.org

Montana

Glasgow

Organization: Women's Resource
Center
114 5th Street South
Glasgow, MT 59230
Toll-Free: 877- 972-3232
(Crisis Line)
Phone: 406-228-8401 (Business)
or 446-228-8400 (Crisis Line)
Fax: 406-228-8407
Website: http://www.thewrc.org/
safe_home.htm
E-mail: women@nemontel.net

Missoula

Program: YWCA Pathways of
Missoula
Organization: YWCA of Missoula
Contact: Shelter Manager or Pet
Advocate Program Coordinator
1130 West Broadway Street
Missoula, MT 59802
Phone: 406-543-6691
Fax: 406-543-6777
Website: http://
www.ywcaofmissoula.org

Nebraska

Columbus

Organization: Center for Sexual
Assault and Domestic Violence
Survivors
P.O. Box 42
Columbus, NE 68602
Toll-Free: 800-658-4482
Phone: 402-564-2155
Fax: 402-563-1719
Website: http://
centerforsurvivors.net/site/
E-mail: centerforsurvivors@
citlink.net

Gering

Organization: DOVES

2035 10th Street
Gering, NE 69341-2417
Phone: 308-436-2787
Fax: 308-436-2817
Website: http://
www.dovesprogram.com/

Lincoln

Program: Safe Way Out
Organization: Capital
Humane Society
2320 Park Boulevard
Lincoln, NE 68502
Phone: 402-441-4488
Fax: 402-438-6182
Website: http://
www.capitalhumanesociety.org
E-mail: edvol@
capitalhumanesociety.org

Omaha

Program: Project Pet Safe
Organization: Nebraska
Humane Society
8929 Fort Street
Omaha, NE 68134
Phone: 402-444-7800
Fax: 402-546-1476
Website: http://nhs.convio.net/site/
PageServer?pagename=
programs_Project_Pet_Safe
E-mail: nhs@nehumanesociety
.org

Nevada

Las Vegas

Program: Noah's Animal House
Organization: The Shade Tree
Women and Children's Shelter
1 West Ownes Avenue
North Las Vegas, NV 89030

Phone: 702-385-0072
Fax: 702-385-2337
Website: http://noahs.the
shadetree.org
and http://www.theshadetree.org
E-mail: noahs@theshadetree.org
or fd@theshadetree.org

New Hampshire

Bedford

Organization: Animal Rescue
League of New Hampshire
545 Route 101
Bedford, NH 03110
Phone: 603-471-0888
Website: http://
www.rescueleague.org

Conway

Organization: Animal Rescue
League of New
Hampshire - North
P.O. Box 260
Conway, NH 03818
Phone: 603-447-5955
Website: http://
www.conwayshelter.org

Enfield

Program: Wise
Organization: Upper Valley
Humane Society
Contact: Animal Services
Manager
300 Old Route 10
Enfield, NH 03748
Phone: 603-448-6888
Fax: 603-448-0180
Website: http://www.uvhs.org/
home.php
E-mail: info@uvhs.org

Penacook

Organization: Concord-
Merrimack County SPCA
130 Washington Street
Penacook, NH 03303
Phone: 603-753-6751
Website: http://
www.concordspca.org

Salem

Program: Safe Home, Safe Pets
Organization: Salem Animal
Rescue League
4 Sarl Drive
Salem, NH 03079
Phone: 603-893-3210
Fax: 603-890-8717
Website: http://sarl-nh.org/about
-us/community-programs/safe
-home-safe-pet-program.html

Stratham

Program: A Safe Pet
Organization: New Hampshire
SPCA
Contact: Manager of Animal
Care
P.O. Box 196
Stratham, NH 03885-0196
Phone: 603-772-2921
Fax: 603-772-5920
Website: http://www.nhspca.org

Swanzey

Program: Project Safe
Organization: Monadnock Hu-
mane Society
101 West Swanzey Road
Swanzey, NH 03446
Phone: 603-352-9011
Website: http://www.monadpets
.org/index.html

E-mail: monadpets@
humanecommunity.org

New Jersey

East Hanover

Program: SASHA—Safe and
Sound Housing for Animals
Organization: Mt. Pleasant
Animal Shelter
Contact: Shelter Director
194 Route 10 West
East Hanover, NJ 07936
Phone: 973-386-0590
Fax: 973-503-9697
Website: http://njshelter.arceye
.net/programs/community
-outreach/
E-mail: info@njshelter.org

New Mexico

Albuquerque (and statewide)

Program: Companion Animal
Rescue Effort (CARE)
Organization: Animal Protection
of New Mexico (APNM)
P.O. Box 11395
Albuquerque, NM 87192
Phone: 505-307-2314
Fax: 505-265-2488
Website: http://www.apnm.org/
programs/care

Santa Fe

Program: Safe Pets
Organization: Santa Fe Animal
Shelter and Humane Society
Contact: Director of Licensing
and Receiving
100 Caja del Rio Road

Santa Fe, NM 87505
Phone: 505-983-4309 ext. 200
Fax: 505-820-6901
Website: http://
www.sfhumanesociety.org

New York

A comprehensive list of additional Safe Havens for the pets of domestic violence victims in New York has been compiled by the SUNY Buffalo Law School (Website: http://law.buffalo.edu/familyviolence/animalShelterDB.asp).

Albany and Rensselaer Counties
Organization: Mohawk and Hudson River Humane Society
3 Oakland Avenue
Menands, NY 12204
Phone: 518-434-8128
Website: http://
www.mohawkhumane.org

Fairport
Program: Mary Ellen Program
Organization: Lollypop Farm, Humane Society of Greater Rochester
Contact: Shelter Manager
99 Victor Road
Fairport, NY 14450
Phone: 585-223-1330
or 585-223-6500 (24-hour Animal Cruelty Hotline)
Fax: 585-425-4183
Website: http://www.lollypop
.org/site/c.clKUI9OQIoJcH/
b.6179485/k.BEF3/Home.htm

Lowville
Program: Safe Pet Program
Organization: Lewis County Opportunities, Inc.
8265 State Route 812
Lowville, NY 13367
Phone: 315-376-8202 or
315-376-4357 (24-hour Hotline; Collect calls accepted)
Fax: 315-376-8421
Website: http://www
.lewiscountyopportunities.com
E-mail: dpo@lcopps.org

Owego
Program: Companion Animal Program
Organization: A New Hope Center
20 Church Street
Owego, NY 13827
Toll-Free: 800-696-7600
(24-hour Hotline)
Phone: 607-687-6887 (Business Line) or 607-687-6866 (24-hour Hotline)
Fax: 607-687-6119
Website: http://www
.anewhopecenter.org/canimal
program.php
E-mail: info@
anewhopecenter.org

Saratoga Springs
Program: Safe Pet Partnership
Organization: Domestic Violence and Rape Crisis Services of Saratoga County
480 Broadway LL 20
Saratoga Springs, NY 12866
Phone: 518-583-0280 (Business Line) or 518-584-8188 (24-hour

Hotline)
Fax: 518-583-2215
Website:
http://www.dvrcsaratoga.org/
services_dv.html
E-mail: dvrc@crisny.org

Scotia
Program: Pet Guardian Program
Organization: Animal Protective
Foundation in partnership with
the YWCA of Schenectady
53 Maple Avenue
Scotia, NY 12302
Phone 518-374-3944
(Animal Protective Foundation)
or 518-374-3386 (YWCA)
Fax: 518-346-2120
Website: http://www
.animalprotective.org/index.php/
programs/pet-guardian
E-mail: info@
animalprotective.org

Tonawanda
Program: SAFE Haven—Safely
Assisting Friends in Emergencies
Organization: SPCA Serving
Erie County
205 Ensminger Road
Tonawanda, NY 14150
Phone: 716-875-7360 (SPCA) or
716-629-3535 (Admissions/Ani-
mal Rescue Supervisor)
Fax: 716-875-8100
Website: http://www.yourspca.org

North Carolina

Asheville
Program: Safe Pets Program
a/k/a Anna Marie Goodman

Foundation (for Buncombe
County residents only)
Organization: Asheville Humane
Society
Asheville Humane Society
14 Forever Friend Lane
Asheville, NC 28806
Phone: 828-761-2001 (Humane
Society) or 828-250-6430 (Anna
Marie Goodman Foundation)
Fax: 828-761-2009 (Humane
Society) or 828-253-6383 (Anna
Marie Goodman Foundation)
Website:
http://www.ashevillehumane.org

Charlotte
Program: Domestic Violence Safe
Haven for Animal Sheltering
Organization: Charlotte-
Mecklenburg Police Animal Care
and Control Division
8315 Byrum Drive
Charlotte, NC 28217
Phone: 704-336-6698
(General Line)
Fax: 704-336-5709
Website: http://charmeck.org/
city/charlotte/CMPD/
organization/Support/
AnimalControl/newsevents/
Pages/EventsPage.aspx

Monroe
Program: Pet Safe
Organization: Turning Point of
Union County
P.O. Box 952
Monroe, NC 28111-0952
Phone: 704-283-9150 (Business
Line) or 704-283-7233 (24-hour
Crisis Hotline)

Fax: 704-225-8857
Website: http://www
.unioncountyturningpoint.org
E-mail: info@turntoday.net

Winston-Salem

Program: Safe Haven Family
Services, Inc.
Organization: Forsyth County
Animal Control
5570 Sturmer Park Circle
Winston-Salem, NC 27105
Phone: 336-763-8125 (Temporary
Shelter Arrangement) or
336-723-8125 (24-hour Hotline)
Fax: 336-661-6414
Website: http://www.co.forsyth
.nc.us/animalcontrol/safe_haven
.aspx

North Dakota

Ellendale

Organization: Kedish House
Domestic Violence Program
P.O. Box 322
Ellendale, ND 58436
Toll-Free: 877-349-4729
Phone: 701-349-4729 (Business
Line) or 701-349-4118
(24-hour Crisis Line)
Fax: 701-349-3562
Website: http://www
.ellendalend.com/index
.asp?Type=NONE&SEC=
{700D2671-BD9B-476C
-BB6B-4633EC775135}

Ohio

Bowling Green

Program: Safe Pets

Organization: Wood County Humane Society
801 Van Camp Road
Bowling Green, OH 43402
Phone: 419-352-7339
Fax: 419-352-2359
Website: http://www
.woodcountyhumanesociety.org
E-mail: woodcountyhumane
society@gmail.com

Chardon

Program: Pet Safe
Organization: Women Safe, Inc.
12041 Ravenna Road
Chardon, OH 44024
Toll-Free: 888-285-5665
(COPEline 24-hour Support
and Crisis Management)
Phone: 440-286-7154
Fax: 440-286-1037
Website: http://
www.womensafe.org

Dayton

Program: Safe Pets Program
Organization: Animal Resource
Center of Montgomery County
6790 Webster Street
Dayton, OH 45414
Phone: 937-898-4457
Fax: 937-454-8139
Website: http://www.mcohio.org/
animalshelter
E-mail: AnimalShelter@
mcohio.org

Cleveland

Organization: Safety for Animals
and Families in Emergencies
(SAFE)
P.O. Box 29295

Cleveland, OH 44129
Phone: 216-970-3035 (Hotline)
Website: http://www.safe
.cuyahogacounty.us
E-mail: info@safeoh.org

Hilliard

Program: Safe Haven for Pets
Organization: Capital Area
Humane Society
3015 Scioto-Darby Executive
Court
Hilliard, OH 43026
Phone: 614-315-0102
Website: http://www.cahs-pets
.org/programs/Safe_Haven.htm
E-mail: safehaven@cahs-pets.org

Marion

Organization: Turning Point
P.O. Box 875
Marion, OH 43302
Toll-Free: 800-232-6505
(24-hour Hotline)
Phone: 740-382-8988
Fax: 740-382-6554
Website: http://www.turning
point6.com

Oklahoma

Ardmore

Organization: Ardmore Animal
Care, Inc. Animal Shelter
321 Carol Brown Boulevard
Ardmore, OK 73401
Phone: 580-223-7070
Fax: 580-226-7737
Website: http://www.ardmore
animalshelter.org
E-mail: animalshelter
@cableone.net

Tulsa

Program: Domestic Violence
Intervention Services
Organization: Tulsa SPCA
Tulsa SPCA
2910 Mohawk Boulevard
Tulsa, OK 74110
Phone: 918-428-7722 (SPCA) or
918-743-5763 (24-hour Domestic
Violence Intervention Services
Hotline)
Fax: 918-428-2525
Websites: http://www.dvis.org/
dvis/default.asp
and http://tulsaspca.org
E-mail: info@tulsaspca.org

Oregon

Eugene

Program: Women Space
Domestic Violence Services
Organization: Greenhill Humane
Society and SPCA
88530 Greenhill Road
Eugene, OR 97402
Phone: 541-689-1503 ext. 117
(Greenhill Humane Society) or
541-485-6513 (Women Space
24-hour Crisis Line)
Website: http://www.green-hill
.org/emergency.html (Greenhill
Humane Society) or
http://www.enddomesticviolence
.com (Women Space)
E-mail: receiving@green-hill.org

Portland

Program: Red Cross Program
Organization: Oregon Humane
Society
1067 NE Columbia Boulevard

Portland, OR 97211-1411
Phone: 503-285-7722 (Dogs,
Birds, and Small Animals, ext.
293 or Cats, ext. 402)
Website: http://rosecityresource
.org/resources/pet-care/1438

Program: Yolanda House
Organization: YWCA of Greater
Portland
P.O. Box 19178
Portland, OR 97280
Phone: 503-535-3269 (24-hour
Crisis Line) or 503-294-7400
(Business Line)
Fax: 503-977-7828
Website: http://ywcapdx.org/
domestic_violence.html

Pennsylvania

Hanover
Program: SafePet Program
Organization: Safe Home
P.O. Box 824
Havover, PA 17331
Phone: 717-632-0007
Fax: 717-633-1016
E-mail: safehome@ywcahanover.org

Lahaska
Organization: Bucks County
SPCA
P.O. Box 277
Lahaska, PA 18931
Phone: 215-794-7425
Fax: 215-794-2750
Website: http://www.bcspca.org
E-mail: info@bcspca.org

Lancaster
Program: Safe Spaces/Foster
Care

Organization: Humane League
of Lancaster County
2195 Lincoln Highway East
Lancaster, PA 17602
Phone: 717-393-6551
Fax: 717-481-9976
Website: http://humaneleague.com
E-mail: info@humaneleague.com

Partner Organization: Domestic
Violence Services of Lancaster
County
P.O. Box 359
Lancaster, PA 17608
Phone: 717-299-9677
(Domestic Violence Advocate)
Fax: 717-290-6855

Pittsburgh
Organization: Women's
Center and Shelter of Greater
Pittsburgh
P.O. Box 9024
Pittsburgh, PA 15224
Phone: 412-687-8005
Fax: 412-687-3315
Website: http://
www.wcspittsburgh.org
E-mail: info@wcspittsburgh.org

Reading
Program: PetNet
Organization: The Humane
Society of Berks County, Inc.
1801 North Eleventh Street
Reading, PA 19604
Phone: 610-921-2348
Fax: 610-921-5833
Website: http://www
.berkshumane.net/cms/index
.php?option=com_content&view
=article&id=67&Itemid=131

York

Organization: ACCESS-York, Inc.
P.O. Box 743
York, PA 17405-0743
Toll-Free: 800-262-8444
(24-hour Hotline)
Phone: 717-846-5400
Website: http://www.ywcayork
.org/victim-services
E-mail: info@access-york.org

Rhode Island

Newport

Program: Pet Safe Program
Organization: Potter League for Animals
P.O. Box 412
Newport, RI 02840
Phone: 401-846-0592 ext. 115
(Executive Director)
Fax: 401-780-0940
Website: http://www.potter
league.org
E-mail: info@potterleague.org

Providence

Program: Safe Haven
Organization: Rhode Island Veterinary Medical Association
302 Pearl Street #108
Providence, RI 02907
Phone: 401-751-0944
Fax: 401-780-0940
Website: http://www.rivma.org
E-mail: rivma@rivma.org

South Carolina

Columbia

Organization: Sistercare, Inc.
P.O. Box 1029

Columbia, SC 29202
Phone: 803-765-9428
(Crisis Line)
Fax: 803-794-0948
Website: http://www.sistercare
.com

Texas

Houston

Program: Burnie's Buddies
Organization: Houston Humane Society
14700 Almeda Road
Houston, TX 77053
Phone: 713-433-6421
Website: http://www.houston
humane.org/burnies-buddies

Program: PetSafe
Organization: Houston SPCA
900 Portway Drive
Houston, TX 77024
Phone: 713-869-7722, ext. 122
(PetSafe Program Coordinator)
Website: http://www.houston
spca.org/site/PageNavigator/
animal_resources_petsafe

New Braunfels

Organization: Crisis Center of Comal County
P.O. Box 310344
New Braunfels, TX 78131-0344
Toll-Free: 800-434-8013
(24-hour Hotline)
Phone: 830-620-4357
(24-hour Hotline) or
830-620-7520 (General Questions)
Fax: 830-625-2984
Website:
http://www.ccccnbtx.org
E-mail: contact@ccccnbtx.org

Temple

Program: Temple Animal
Services Division
Organization: City of Temple
Texas
620 Mama Dog Circle
Temple, Texas 76501
Phone: 254-298-5732
Fax: 254-298-5741
Website: http://www.ci.temple
.tx.us/index.aspx?NID=91
E-mail: animalshelter
@ci.temple.tx.us

Victoria

Program: Family Violence
Program
Organization: Mid-Coast Family
Services
120 S. Main Street, Suite 310
Victoria, TX 77901
Toll-Free: 800-870-0368
(Hotline)
Phone: 361-575-7842 (Hotline)
Fax: 361-575-8218
Website: http://
www.midcoastfamily.org
E-mail: info@midcoastfamily.org

Utah

Brigham City

Program: Your Community in
Unity
Organization: New Hope Crisis
Center
435 East 700 South
Brigham City, UT 84302
Phone: 435-723-5600
Website: http://
www.newhopecrisis.org
E-mail: info@newhopecrisis.org

Vermont

South Burlington

Program: Good Neighbor
Program
Organization: Humane Society
of Chittenden County
142 Kindness Court
South Burlington, VT 05403
Phone: 802-862-0135 ext. 11
Fax: 802-860-5868
Website: http://
www.chittendenhumane.org/
programs-services/good
-neighbor-program
E-mail: bestfriends@
chittendenhumane.org

Virginia

Alexandria

Program: Safekeeping Program
Organization: Animal Welfare
League of Alexandria
Vola Lawson Animal Shelter
4101 Eisenhower Avenue
Alexandria, VA 22304
Phone: 703-746-4774
Fax: 703-746-4775
Website:
http://awla.convio.net
E-mail: staff@alexandria
animals.org

Partnering Organization:
Alexandria Domestic Violence
Program
421 King Street, Suite 400
Alexandria, VA 22314
Phone: 703-746-4911
(24-hour Hotline)
Website:
http://alexandriava.gov/Women

Arlington

Program: Safe Keeping Program
Organization: Animal Welfare
League of Arlington
2650 South Arlington Mill Drive
Arlington, VA 22206
Phone: 703-931-9241
Fax: 703-931-2568
Website: http://www.awla.org

Charlottesville

Program: Pet Safe
Organization: Shelter for Help in
Emergency
P.O. Box 1013
Charlottesville, VA 22902
Phone: 434-963-4676 or
434-293-8509 (24-hour Hotline;
Voice/TTY; Collect calls accepted)
Fax: 434-293-6624
Website: http://www.shelter
forhelpinemergency.org/page20
.html
E-mail: info@
shelterforhelpinemergency.org

Gate City

Program: Alice's Pet Haven
Organization: Hope House of
Scott County, Inc.
P.O. Box 1992
Gate City, VA 24251
Phone: 276-386-3334
Fax: 276-386-1252

Gloucester

Organization: Gloucester-
Mathews Humane Society
6620 Jackson Lane
Gloucester, VA 23061
Phone: 804-693-5520
Fax: 804-693-2009

Website: http://www.gloucester
mathewshumanesociety.org
E-mail: information
@gmhumanesociety.org

Loudoun County

Program: Emergency
Shelter for Pets
Organization: LAWS—
Loudoun Abused Women's
Shelter (working with Loudoun
County Department of Animal
Care and Control)
105 East Market Street
Leesburg, VA 20176
Phone: 703-777-6552
(24-hour Crisis Hotline;
Voice/TTY)
Fax: 703-771-7865
Website: http://lcsj.org/services/
domestic-violence
E-mail: laws@lcsj.org

Martinsville

Organization: Citizens Against
Family Violence (working with
the SPCA of Martinsville/
Houston County)*
P.O. Box 352
Martinsville, VA 24114
Phone: 276-632-8701
(24-hour Hotline)
Fax: 276-632-0529
Websites: http://www.cafv.info
(Citizens Against Family Vio-
lence) and
http://www.spcamhc.org (SPCA
of Martinsville/Houston County)
*Sheltering service includes
free spay/neuter and vaccinations
for pets of domestic violence
victims

Norton

Organization: Family Crisis
Support Services, Inc.
701 Kentucky Avenue SE
Norton, VA 24273
Toll-Free: 800-572-2278
(24-hour Hotline)
Phone: 276-679-7240
Fax: 276-679-1820
Website:
http://www.family-crisis.com/

Richmond

Program:
Sheltering Animals of
Abused Families (SAAF), a
project of the Richmond SPCA
Robins-Starr Humane Center
2519 Hermitage Road
Richmond, VA 23220
Phone: 804-643-6785
Website: http://
www.richmondspca.org/SAAF

Partnering Organizations:
Toll-Free: 800-838-8238
(Hanover Safe Place)
Phone: 804-643-0888 (YWCA
Richmond; 24-hour Hotline)
or 804-287-7877 (Safe Harbor;
24-hour Hotline)

Virginia Beach

Organization: Virginia Beach
SPCA
3040 Holland Road
Virginia Beach, VA 23453-2610
Phone: 757-427-6387
Fax: 757-427-5939
Website: http://vbspca.com/
modules/vbspcainfo/category
.php?categoryid=1

Washington

Coupeville

Organization: WAIF:
Whidbey Animals' Improvement
Foundation
P.O. Box 1108
Coupeville, WA 98239-1108
Phone: 360-678-1399
Website: http://
www.waifanimals.org
E-mail: shelter@waifanimals.org

Kelso

Organization: Emergency
Support Shelter
P.O. Box 877
Kelso, WA 98626
Phone: 360-425-1176
(24-hour Hotline)
Fax: 360-425-3970

Seattle

Program: Domestic Violence
Program
Organization: Seattle Animal
Shelter
2061 15th Avenue West
Seattle, WA 98119
Phone: 206-386-7387
Fax: 206-386-4285
Website: http://www.seattle.gov/
animalshelter/

Spokane

Organization: SpokAnimal
C.A.R.E.
714 North Napa Street
Spokane, WA 99202
Phone: 509-534-8133
Website: http://
www.spokanimal.org

E-mail: mailbox
@spokanimal.org
(Clients must have their local
caseworker contact SpokAnimal
to make arrangements.)

Tacoma

Program: Pet Housing Program
Organization: Family Renewal
Shelter
6832 Pacific Avenue
Tacoma, WA 98408-7206
Phone: 253-475-9010
(24-hour Crisis Line)
Fax: 253-475-0848
Website: http://
www.domesticviolencehelp.org
E-mail: staff@dvhelp.org

Organization: Tacoma-Pierce
County Humane Society
2608 Center Street
Tacoma, WA 98409
Phone: 253-284-5850
(Executive Director) or
253-383-2733 (General Informa-
tion)
Fax: 253-620-1564
Website: http://
www.thehumanesociety.org

Program: Domestic Violence
Emergency Women and
Children's Center
Organization: Korean Women's
Association
123 East 96th Street
Tacoma, WA 98445
Toll-Free: 888-508-2780
Phone: 253-535-4202 or
253-535-2731
TTY: 253-460-5045

Website: http://www.kwacares
.org/services/domestic-violence
-assistance

West Virginia

Charleston

Organization: Kanawha/
Charleston Humane Association
1248 Greenbrier Street
Charleston, WV 25311
Phone: 304-342-1576
or 304-347-0800 (After Hours
Emergency)
Fax: 304-342-3395
Website: http://
www.wvanimalshelter.com
E-mail:
wvanimalshelter@
suddenlinkmail.com

Wisconsin

Madison

Program: Sheltering Animals of
Abuse Victims (SAAV)
Organization: Sheltering
Animals of Abuse Victims
SAAV Program, Inc.
P.O. Box 5152
Madison, WI 53705
Toll-Free: 800-747-4045
(24-hour Helpline)*
Phone: 608-251-4445 (24-hour
Helpline)*
Website: http://
www.saavprogram.org
E-mail: info@saavprogram.org
*Victims interested in using The
SAAV Program should contact
this 24-hour helpline for Domes-
tic Abuse Intervention Services.

Menomonie

Organization:
The Bridge to Hope
1901 South Broadway
Menomonie, WI 54751
Toll-Free: 800-924-9918
(24-hour Hotline)
Phone: 715-235-9074
Fax: 715-235-9073
Website: http://
www.thebridgetohope.com
E-mail: manager@
thebridgetohope.org

Milwaukee

Program: Safe Haven Program
Organization: Wisconsin
Humane Society partnering with
the Sojourner Family Peace
Center
4500 West Wisconsin Avenue
Milwaukee, WI 53208-3156

Phone: 414-264-6257 (Wisconsin
Humane Society) or
414-933-2722 (Sojourner Family
Peace Center)
Website: http://
www.wihumane.org/volunteer/
SafeHavenProgram.aspx
E-mail: info@wihumane.org

Wyoming

Casper

Program: Pet Safe Harbor
Organization: Self Help
Center, Inc.
918 East 2nd Street
Suite 300
Casper, WY 82604
Phone: 307-235-2814
Fax: 307-472-4307
E-mail: selfhelp.center@
yahoo.com

Index

Index

Page numbers followed by 'n' indicate a footnote. Page numbers in *italics* indicate a table or illustration.

A

623

Health Reference Series